PHARMACEUTICAL PRODUCT LICENSING
Requirements for Europe

ELLIS HORWOOD SERIES IN PHARMACEUTICAL TECHNOLOGY

Editor: Professor M. H. RUBINSTEIN, School of Health Sciences, Liverpool Polytechnic

UNDERSTANDING EXPERIMENTAL DESIGN AND INTERPRETATION IN PHARMACEUTICS
N. A. Armstrong & K. C. James
MICROBIAL QUALITY ASSURANCE IN PHARMACEUTICALS, COSMETICS AND TOILETRIES
Edited by S. Bloomfield *et al.*
PHARMACEUTICAL PRODUCT LICENSING: Requirements for Europe
Edited by A. C. Cartwright & B. R. Matthews
DRUG DISCOVERY TECHNOLOGIES
C. Clark & W. H. Moos
PHARMACEUTICAL PRODUCTION FACILITIES: Design and Applications
G. Cole
PHARMACEUTICAL TABLET AND PELLET COATING
G. Cole
THE PHARMACY AND PHARMACOTHERAPY OF ASTHMA
Edited by P. F. D'Arcy & J. C. McElnay
GUIDE TO MICROBIOLOGICAL CONTROL IN PHARMACEUTICALS
Edited by S. P. Denyer & R. M. Baird
PHARMACEUTICAL THERMAL ANALYSIS: Techniques and Applications
J. L. Ford and P. Timmins
PHYSICO-CHEMICAL PROPERTIES OF DRUGS: A Handbook for Pharmaceutical Scientists
P. Gould
DRUG DELIVERY TO THE GASTROINTESTINAL TRACT
Edited by J. G. Hardy, S. S. Davis and C. G. Wilson
POLYPEPTIDE AND PROTEIN DRUGS: Production, Characterization and Formulation
Edited by R. C. Hider and D. Barlow
HANDBOOK OF PHARMACOKINETICS: Toxicity Assessment of Chemicals
J. P. Labaune
TABLET MACHINE INSTRUMENTATION IN PHARMACEUTICS: Principles and Practice
P. Ridgway Watt
PHARMACEUTICAL CHEMISTRY, Volume 1 Drug Synthesis
H. J. Roth *et al.*
PHARMACEUTICAL CHEMISTRY, Volume 2 Drug Analysis
H. J. Roth *et al.*
PHARMACEUTICAL TECHNOLOGY: Controlled Drug Release, Volume 1
Edited by M. H. Rubinstein
PHARMACEUTICAL TECHNOLOGY: Controlled Drug Release, Volume 2*
Edited by M. H. Rubinstein
PHARMACEUTICAL TECHNOLOGY: Tableting Technology, Volume 1
Edited by M. H. Rubinstein
PHARMACEUTICAL TECHNOLOGY: Tableting Technology, Volume 2*
Edited by M. H. Rubinstein
PHARMACEUTICAL TECHNOLOGY: Drug Stability
Edited by M. H. Rubinstein
PHARMACEUTICAL TECHNOLOGY: Drug Targeting*
Edited by M. H. Rubinstein
UNDERSTANDING ANTIBACTERIAL ACTION AND RESISTANCE
A. D. Russell and I. Chopra
RADIOPHARMACEUTICALS USING RADIOACTIVE COMPOUNDS IN PHARMACEUTICS AND MEDICINE
Edited by A. Theobald
PHARMACEUTICAL PREFORMULATION: The Physicochemical Properties of Drug Substances
J. I. Wells
PHYSIOLOGICAL PHARMACEUTICS: Biological Barriers to Drug Absorption
C. G. Wilson & N. Washington
PHARMACOKINETIC MODELLING USING STELLA ON THE APPLE™ MACINTOSH™
C. Washington, N. Washington & C. Wilson

* *In preparation*

3 0116 00371 1155

This book is due for return not later than the last date stamped below, unless recalled sooner.

2 8 MAY 1992 LONG LOAN	2 4 NOV 2003 MEDIUM LOAN	
2 7 MAY 2000 LONG LOAN	1 0 FEB 2004 LONG LOAN	
1 3 NOV 2000 LONG LOAN		

ASTON UNIVERSITY
LIBRARY SERVICES

WITHDRAWN
FROM STOCK

PHARMACEUTICAL PRODUCT LICENSING
Requirements for Europe

Editors
A. C. CARTWRIGHT and BRIAN R. MATTHEWS
both of the Medicines Control Agency
Department of Health, London

ELLIS HORWOOD
NEW YORK LONDON TORONTO SYDNEY TOKYO SINGAPORE

First published in 1991 by
ELLIS HORWOOD LIMITED
Market Cross House, Cooper Street,
Chichester, West Sussex, PO19 1EB, England

A division of
Simon & Schuster International Group
A Paramount Communications Company

© Ellis Horwood Limited, 1991

All rights reserved. No part of this publication may be reproduced, stored in a retrieval system, or transmitted, in any form, or by any means, electronic, mechanical, photocopying, recording or otherwise, without the prior permission, in writing, of the publisher

Typeset in Times by Ellis Horwood Limited
Printed and bound in Great Britain
by Bookcraft (Bath) Limited, Midsomer Norton, Avon

British Library Cataloguing in Publication Data

Cartwright, A. C.
 Pharmaceutical product licensing: Requirements for Europe. —
 (Ellis Horwood series in pharmaceutical technology)
 I. Title. II. Matthews, Brian. III. Series.
 615.0917
ISBN 0-13-662883-4

Library of Congress Cataloging-in-Publication Data available

Table of Contents

PREFACE 21
References to the European Communities texts — *The rules governing medicinal products in the European Community* 24

1 INTRODUCTION AND HISTORY OF PHARMACEUTICAL REGULATION
Anthony C. Cartwright
  1.1 Introduction....................................29
  1.2 A brief history of pharmaceutical regulation 29
      1.2.1 Early history to the nineteenth century 29
      1.2.2 The early twentieth century in the UK: beginnings of regulation 31
      1.2.3 The early twentieth century in the USA: early regulation 31
      1.2.4 Thalidomide..............................32
      1.2.5 Thalidomide: the regulatory aftermath 33
      1.2.6 Thalidomide: implications for chirality requirements 34
  1.3 The European Community: regulation of proprietary medicinal products (1965 to 1987)..................................34
      1.3.1 Introduction 34
      1.3.2 Directive 65/65/EEC: definitions and requirements 35
      1.3.3 Directive 75/318/EEC: the 'norms and protocols' Directive ...36
      1.3.4 Directive 75/319/EEC: legal and administrative provisions ...36
      1.3.5 Decision 75/320/EEC: the Pharmaceutical Committee 37
      1.3.6 Directive 78/25/EEC: approved colouring matters 37
      1.3.7 Commission Communication of 6 May 1982: parallel importation of medicinal products 38
      1.3.8 Directive 83/570/EEC: amending Directive 39
      1.3.9 Council Recommendation 83/571/EEC: 'guidelines'.......39
      1.3.10 Directive 87/19/EEC: the regulatory committee procedure ...40
      1.3.11 Directive 87/21/EEC: abridged applications for 'copy products' and protection of innovation 40

Table of contents

   1.3.12 Directive 87/22/EEC: the high technology/biotechnology procedure 41
 1.4 The *European Pharmacopoeia* 41
 1.5 Publication of the Community rules for product registration in 1989 42
 1.6 Other measures designed to eliminate the remaining barriers to the establishment of a Single European Market in pharmaceutical products 43
 References 44

2 THE EUROPEAN COMMUNITY: ITS STRUCTURE, INSTITUTIONS, AND REGULATION
Anthony C. Cartwright
2.1 Introduction 46
2.2 The Treaty of Rome 46
2.3 The Member States of the European Economic Community 46
2.4 The Community institutions 47
  2.4.1 The Commission of the European Communities 47
  2.4.2 The Council of Ministers 47
  2.4.3 The European Parliament 49
  2.4.4 The Economic and Social Committee 49
  2.4.5 The European Court of Justice 49
2.5 The legal instruments of the Community 50
  2.5.1 Regulations 50
  2.5.2 Directives 50
  2.5.3 Decisions 51
  2.5.4 Recommendations 51
  2.5.5 Opinions 51
  2.5.6 Communications 51
2.6 The Single European Act and the Single Market 51
2.7 The European Free Trade Association .52
2.8 The Nordic Council 52
Reference 53

3 NEW CHEMICAL ACTIVE SUBSTANCE PRODUCTS: QUALITY REQUIREMENTS
Brian R. Matthews
3.1 Introduction 54
3.2 Sources of information 54
3.3 Requirements relating to the format of the application 55
3.4 Part I: The summary of the dossier 56
  3.4.1 Introduction 56
  3.4.2 Administrative information 57
  3.4.3 Summary of product characteristics 58

		3.4.4	Expert Reports 59

- 3.5 Part II: The chemical, pharmaceutical, and biological documentation 60
  - 3.5.1 Introduction 60
  - 3.5.2 Description of analytical methods and analytical validation ... 61
  - 3.5.3 Part IIA: Composition 62
  - 3.5.4 Part IIB: Method of manufacture of the dosage form 63
  - 3.5.5 Part IIC: Control of the starting materials 64
    - 3.5.5.1 New active ingredients 64
      - (a) Identity of the material 64
      - (b) Manufacture of the active ingredient 65
      - (c) Quality control during synthesis 65
      - (d) Development chemistry 65
      - (e) Impurities 66
      - (f) Active ingredient specification 66
      - (g) Batch analyses 67
    - 3.5.5.2 Radiolabelled compounds 67
    - 3.5.5.3 Other ingredients 67
  - 3.5.6 Part IID: Control tests applied at an intermediate stage of the manufacturing process 68
  - 3.5.7 Part IIE: Control tests on the finished product 68
  - 3.5.8 Part IIF: Stability 69
    - 3.5.8.1 Active ingredients 70
    - 3.5.8.2 Finished product 70
- 3.6 Part V: Special particulars 72
  - 3.6.1 Part VA: Dosage form 72
  - 3.6.2 Part VB: Samples 73
  - 3.6.3 Part VC: Manufacturer(s) authorisation(s) 73
  - 3.6.4 Part VD: Marketing authorisation(s) 73
- 3.7 Product labelling 73
- References 75

4 NEW CHEMICAL ACTIVE SUBSTANCE PRODUCTS: PRECLINICAL REQUIREMENTS
James C. Ritchie

- 4.1 Introduction 76
- 4.2 Pharmacodynamics 77
  - 4.2.1 EC requirements 77
  - 4.2.2 EC guidelines 78
- 4.3 Pharmacokinetics 78
  - 4.3.1 EC requirements 78
  - 4.3.2 EC guidelines 78
- 4.4 Toxicology 79
  - 4.4.1 EC requirements 79
  - 4.4.2 EC guidelines 79
    - 4.4.2.1 Single dose toxicity 79

            4.4.2.2   Repeat dose toxicity 80
    4.5   Reproductive toxicology 80
            4.5.1   EC requirements 80
            4.5.2   EC guidelines 81
    4.6   Mutagenicity studies. 81
            4.6.1   EC requirements 81
            4.6.2   EC guidelines 82
    4.7   Carcinogenicity studies 83
            4.7.1   EC requirements 83
            4.7.2   EC guidelines 83

5   **NEW CHEMICAL ACTIVE SUBSTANCE PRODUCTS:
    CLINICAL REQUIREMENTS**
    J. Alex Nicholson
    5.1   Introduction 85
    5.2   Clinical trials 85
            5.2.1   National requirements for the regulation of clinical drug trials .85
            5.2.2   Good clinical practice 86
            5.2.3   Clinical guidelines 89
    5.3   The clinical documentation 89
            5.3.1   Introduction 89
            5.3.2   The index 89
            5.3.3   Part IVA: Clinical pharmacology 89
            5.3.4   Part IVB: Clinical experience 90
            5.3.5   Overall summary 90
    5.4   The Clinical Expert Report 91
    5.5   Conclusion 91

6   **ABRIDGED APPLICATIONS**
    Anthony C. Cartwright
    6.1   Introduction 93
    6.2   Abridged applications before July 1987 93
            6.2.1   Directive 65/65/EEC 93
            6.2.2   Directive 83/570/EEC 94
    6.3   Directive 87/21/EEC 94
            6.3.1   The objectives of the new Directive 94
            6.3.2   Protection of pharmaceutical innovation 94
            6.3.3   Harmonisation of the rules for products which are
                    copies of established medicinal products 95
            6.3.4   Harmonisation of the rules for combination products 96
    6.4   Requirements for information on second applicant products 96
    6.5   Evidence of ten year authorisation and marketing 96
    6.6   Essential similarity 97
            6.6.1   The Smith Kline and French judicial review 97
            6.6.2   Essential similarity and the active ingredient 97
            6.6.3   Essential similarity and the finished product 99

	6.6.4	Essential similarity and the clinical indications 99
6.7		Second applicant products by detailed reference to the published scientific literature — Article 4(8)(a)(ii) of 65/65/EEC 99
6.8		Chemistry and pharmacy of abridged applications. 100
	6.8.1	Composition/container/development pharmaceutics. 100
	6.8.2	Method of preparation 101
	6.8.3	Control of starting materials. 101
	6.8.4	Control tests on intermediate products 101
	6.8.5	Control tests on the finished product 101
	6.8.6	Stability of the active ingredient and the finished product . . .102
6.9	Pharmacotoxicological data 102
6.10	Clinical data. 102
6.11	Bioavailability and bioequivalence data 103
	6.11.1	Verifiability of bioavailability and bioequivalence studies . . 104
References 104

7 DRUG MASTER FILES
Brian R. Matthews

- 7.1 Introduction. 106
- 7.2 What is a drug master file and when may one be used? 106
  - 7.2.1 In the United Kingdom 106
  - 7.2.2 In the European Community 107
  - 7.2.3 Comparison with United States Food and Drug Administration DMFs. 107
- 7.3 Assessment procedures for DMFs in the United Kingdom 108
  - 7.3.1 Introduction 108
  - 7.3.2 Data requirements 109
  - 7.3.3 Experience with DMFs in the United Kingdom. 110
- 7.4 The European drug master file procedure 110
  - 7.4.1 Introduction 110
  - 7.4.2 The European drug master file procedure 111
  - 7.4.3 Related matters. 112
- References 113

8 RADIOPHARMACEUTICAL PRODUCTS
Brian R. Matthews

- 8.1 Introduction. 114
- 8.2 Radiopharmaceutical and related definitions 115
  - 8.2.1 UK definitions. 115
    - 8.2.1.1 The Medicines Act 1968 115
    - 8.2.1.2 The Medicines (Radioactive Substances) Order 1978 115
  - 8.2.2 Relevant *European Pharmacopoeia* definitions. 116
  - 8.2.3 Definitions from Directive 89/343/EEC. 116
  - 8.2.4 Definitions from Directive 65/65/EEC. 116
- 8.3 UK control of radiopharmaceuticals .117
  - 8.3.1 Introduction 117

	8.3.2	Basis of data expectations		117
	8.3.3	Expert Reports		118
	8.3.4	Pharmaceutical data requirements		118
		8.3.4.1	Composition	118
		8.3.4.2	Development pharmaceutics	118
		8.3.4.3	Manufacture	119
		8.3.4.4	Impurities	119
		8.3.4.5	Other constituents	119
		8.3.4.6	Control tests on the finished product	119
		8.3.4.7	Stability data	120
	8.3.5	Preclinical data requirements		120
	8.3.6	Clinical data requirements		120
8.4	EC involvement in the regulation of radiopharmaceutical products			121
	8.4.1	Introduction		121
	8.4.2	Predicted data requirements for radiopharmaceuticals under EC Directives		122
		8.4.2.1	Introduction	122
		8.4.2.2	Pharmaceutical, chemical, biological and microbiological data requirements	122
			(a) Qualitative particulars	122
			(b) Quantitative particulars	122
			(c) Development particulars	122
			(d) Method of preparation	122
			(e) Control of starting materials	123
			(f) Control tests on the finished product	123
			(g) Dosage form-related points	124
			(h) Stability testing	124
		8.4.2.3	Toxicological and pharmacological data requirements	124
			(a) General	124
			(b) Subacute toxicity studies	125
			(c) Mutagenic potential	125
			(d) Carcinogenic potential	125
			(e) Reproductive studies	125
			(f) Pharmacodynamics	125
			(g) Pharmacokinetics	125
			(h) Radiation dosimetry	125
		8.4.2.4	Clinical data requirements	125
	8.4.3	Labelling and instruction leaflets		126
		8.4.3.1	Introduction	126
		8.4.3.2	Directive 89/343/EEC specific requirements	126
		8.4.3.3	*European Pharmacopoeia* requirements	126
		8.4.3.4	Instruction leaflet	127

9 MEDICATED DEVICES
Brian R. Matthews
9.1 Introduction 129

9.2	The development of the medical device Directives		129
	9.2.1	Introduction	129
	9.2.2	The present EC market for medical devices	129
	9.2.3	Control of medical devices in the Member States of the EC	131
9.3	Ideal characteristics for a new system of controls for medical devices		133
9.4	'Old approach' and 'New approach' Directives		134
	9.4.1	The role of CEN and CENELEC	134
	9.4.2	The consultative processes in the EC in the development of a Directive	136
	9.4.3	Constituent parts of a 'new approach' Directive	137
9.5	Contents of the active implantable medical device Directive		138
	9.5.1	Article 1: Application, definitions, provision re: medicinal products, reference to Directive 89/336/EEC	138
	9.5.2	Article 2: Marketing of custom-made and investigational devices	139
	9.5.3	Article 3: Compliance with essential requirements	139
	9.5.4	Article 4: Member States' obligations and rights	139
	9.5.5	Article 5: Role of harmonised standards	140
	9.5.6	Article 6: Unsatisfactory harmonised standards; implementation and practical application of the Directive — the role of the Standing Committees	140
	9.5.7	Article 7: Removal of products from the market	140
	9.5.8	Article 8: Records of adverse events and withdrawals from the market	141
	9.5.9	Article 9: Conformity assessment options	141
	9.5.10	Article 10: Clinical investigation provisions	141
	9.5.11	Article 11: Appointment and withdrawal of notified bodies	141
	9.5.12	Article 12: Application of the CE mark and notified body's logo to products	141
	9.5.13	Article 13: Inappropriate application of the CE mark	142
	9.5.14	Article 14: Refused or restricted marketing provisions	142
	9.5.15	Article 15: Confidentiality	142
	9.5.16	Article 16: Effective dates	142
	9.5.17	Article 17: Addressees	142
	9.5.18	Annex 1: Essential requirements	142
		9.5.18.1 Introduction	142
		9.5.18.2 General requirements	142
		9.5.18.3 Requirements regarding design and construction	143
	9.5.19	Annex 2: Declaration of conformity (full quality system)	144
	9.5.20	Annex 3: EC type-examination procedure	145
	9.5.21	Annex 4: EC verification procedures	146
	9.5.22	Annex 5: Assurance of production quality in connection with the EC declaration of conformity to type	147
	9.5.23	Annex 6: Custom-made devices and devices intended for clinical investigations	148

		9.5.24 Annex 7: Clinical evaluation. 148

- 9.5.24 Annex 7: Clinical evaluation. 148
- 9.5.25 Annex 8: Minimum criteria for inspection bodies to be notified 149
- 9.5.26 Annex 9: CE mark 149
- 9.6 The draft Directive on medical devices 149
  - 9.6.1 Introduction 149
  - 9.6.2 Definitions 149
  - 9.6.3 Products containing medicinal substances 151
  - 9.6.4 Classification of medical devices 151
  - 9.6.5 Provisions which differ from the active implantable medical devices Directive 152
  - 9.6.6 Provisions in common with the active implantable medical devices Directive 153
  - 9.6.7 Essential requirements 154
    - 9.6.7.1 General requirements 154
    - 9.6.7.2 Design and construction 154
  - 9.6.8 Conformity assessment procedures 156
  - 9.6.9 Statement concerning devices intended for special purposes . 156
  - 9.6.10 Classification decision criteria 157
    - 9.6.10.1 Non-active medical devices 157
    - 9.6.10.2 Active medical devices 159
  - 9.6.11 Clinical evaluation 159
  - 9.6.12 Criteria to be met with designating inspection bodies to be notified 159
  - 9.6.13 CE mark of conformity 159
- 9.7 Comments on the medical devices Directives 159

10 CONTACT LENS PRODUCTS AND INTRAUTERINE CONTRACEPTIVE DEVICES
Brian R. Matthews

- 10.1 Introduction 162
- 10.2 Contact lens care products 162
  - 10.2.1 Contact lenses and contact lens care products in the UK . . 162
  - 10.2.2 Controls in the EC 163
  - 10.2.3 Requirements in the UK 163
    - 10.2.3.1 General requirements 163
    - 10.2.3.2 Chemical and pharmaceutical documentation . . 164
    - 10.2.3.3 Experimental and biological studies 165
    - 10.2.3.4 Studies in humans 165
    - 10.2.3.5 Product literature 165
- 10.3 Intrauterine contraceptive devices 166
  - 10.3.1 Introduction 166
  - 10.3.2 Data requirements in the UK 166
    - 10.3.2.1 Chemical and pharmaceutical documentation . . 166
    - 10.3.2.2 Experimental and biological studies 166
    - 10.3.2.3 Studies in humans 167

Table of contents

11 EXPERTS AND EXPERT REPORTS IN MARKETING AUTHORISATION APPLICATIONS
Anthony C. Cartwright

- 11.1 Introduction 168
- 11.2 Why are Expert Reports needed? 169
  - 11.2.1 To comply with the requirements of Articles 1 to 3 of Directive 75/319/EEC 169
  - 11.2.2 To be used in the compilation of assessment reports (for multistate and concertation applications) 169
  - 11.2.3 To provide a summary and overview of the product for any subsequent action by the authorities on the authorisation 170
  - 11.2.4 To identify the major issues raised by the data in the dossier for its subsequent consideration nationally or in the Committee for Proprietary Medicinal Products 170
  - 11.2.5 To ensure that all marketing authorisation applications have had critical review 171
  - 11.2.6 To provide the core of the Evaluation Report in the Product Evaluation Report scheme 171
  - 11.2.7 To provide the core of the assessment/evaluation report in the future in a wider European or global application . . . 172
- 11.3 The Expert — legal definitions and practical requirements (training, position, and experience) 172
  - 11.3.1 Legal definitions (Directive 75/319/EEC) 172
    - 11.3.1.1 The analyst 172
    - 11.3.1.2 The pharmacological/toxicologist 172
    - 11.3.1.3 The clinician 172
    - 11.3.1.4 Legal requirements as to qualification of Experts 172
  - 11.3.2 The practical requirements as defined in the 1989 edition of the 'Notice to Applicants' 173
- 11.4 The three Experts: further exploration of their roles 173
  - 11.4.1 The pharmaceutical Expert 173
  - 11.4.2 The pharmaco-toxicological Expert 173
  - 11.4.3 The clinical Expert 174
  - 11.4.4 The three Experts: their role in defining the applicability of published references (for abridged applications) 175
- 11.5 The Experts: who should they be? 175
  - 11.5.1 Single versus multiple Experts 175
  - 11.5.2 The consultant Expert 176
  - 11.5.3 The 'foreign' Expert versus national Expert 176
- 11.6 The flow of information — raw data in the laboratory to the Expert Report and the product profile 177
- 11.7 Links between the three Experts 177
- 11.8 The duties of the Experts 178
  - 11.8.1 To provide the Expert Report 178

- 11.8.2 To provide a justification for the acceptance of a product in List B ('high technology' procedure of Directive 87/22/EEC)... 179
- 11.8.3 To be available for consultation with the authorities 180
- 11.8.4 To participate in appeals. 180
- 11.9 The pharmaceutical Expert Report: structure, format, and content. 180
  - 11.9.1 Structure of the pharmaceutical Expert Report 180
  - 11.9.2 Contents of the pharmaceutical Expert Report 181
  - 11.9.3 Evaluation section of the pharmaceutical Expert Report 182
- 11.10 The pharmacotoxicological Expert Report: structure, format, and content 185
  - 11.10.1 Structure of the pharmacotoxicological Expert Report 185
  - 11.10.2 Contents of the pharmacotoxicological Expert Report 185
  - 11.10.3 Conclusions of the pharmacotoxicological Expert Report 185
- 11.11 The clinical Expert Report: structure, format, and content 186
  - 11.11.1 Structure of the clinical Expert Report............. 186
  - 11.11.2 Contents of the clinical Expert Report 186
  - 11.11.3 Conclusions of the clinical Expert Report 187
- 11.12 Miscellaneous issues in relation to Expert Reports.......... 187
  - 11.12.1 Products outside the Directives................. 187
  - 11.12.2 Clinical trial approval applications.............. 188
  - 11.12.3 Cross-referral marketing authorisation applications..... 188
- References.......... 188

12 DEFECTS IN APPLICATIONS — AN ANALYSIS
David B. Jefferys, Brian R. Matthews, and James C. Ritchie

- 12.1 Introduction 190
- 12.2 The clinical dossier................ 192
  - 12.2.1 Introduction 192
  - 12.2.2 Structure of the dossier................ 192
  - 12.2.3 The clinical Expert Report 193
  - 12.2.4 Overall summary 195
  - 12.2.5 Clinical pharmacology 195
  - 12.2.6 Reports of individual clinical trials 196
- 12.3 The pharmaceutical dossier 198
  - 12.3.1 Introduction 198
  - 12.3.2 Analysis of deficiencies in UK applications 199
    - 12.3.2.1 Deficiencies relating to the drug substance 199
    - 12.3.2.2 Deficiencies relating to the finished product.... 201
    - 12.3.2.3 Points of general applicability............. 203
  - 12.3.3 Deficiencies in applications referred to CPMP 204

        12.3.4   Objections remaining after consideration by advisory
                 committees 205
                 12.3.4.1 Introduction 205
                 12.3.4.2 The outcome of additional data consideration
                           of applications routed *via* the CPMP 205
                 12.3.4.3 Applications considered by the CSM 205
   12.4 The preclinical dossier...208
        12.4.1   Introduction 208
        12.4.2   Pharmacology 210
        12.4.3   Pharmacokinetics 210
        12.4.4   Toxicology 210
        12.4.5   Reproduction studies 211
        12.4.6   Mutagenicity 211
        12.4.7   Carcinogenicity 212
   References 212

13 CPMP AND THE PHARMACEUTICAL COMMITTEE
   Anthony C. Cartwright
   13.1 The Committee for Proprietary Medicinal Products (CPMP)
        and its activities..213
        13.1.1   The original functions of the CPMP 213
        13.1.2   The chairmanship and vice-chairmanship of the CPMP ...213
        13.1.3   The current role of the CPMP 214
        13.1.4   The future role of the CPMP 214
        13.1.5   The CPMP working parties 215
        13.1.6   The Commission working parties 217
   13.2 The Pharmaceutical Committee 217
   13.3 The Committee for the Adaptation to Technical Progress 218

14 CPMP MULTISTATE PROCEDURE
   Anthony C. Cartwright
   14.1 Introduction 220
   14.2 The former CPMP procedure 221
   14.3 The new rules of the multistate procedure 222
   14.4 What authorisations can be used in the multistate procedure? 222
   14.5 What authorisations cannot be used in the multistate procedure? ...223
   14.6 Suitability of products for the multistate procedure 224
   14.7 Second applicant (abridged) products..........................225
   14.8 Changes to the original authorisation ('variations') 226
   14.9 Multistate applications for products whose authorisations were
        granted in the originating (outgoing) Member State some years
        previously 226
   14.10 The multistate procedure and timing 227
   14.11 The role of the rapporteur and co-rapporteur.................229
   14.12 The assessment report..230
   14.13 Labels and leaflets 230
   14.14 Samples of the starting materials and dosage-form............230

Table of contents

    14.15 Applications to Portugal 231
    14.16 The format and language of multistate applications 231
    14.17 Hearings 231
    14.18 The 'Euro-SPC' 232
    14.19 Analysis of multistate applications (1986 to 1989) 233
    Reference 234

15 THE CONCERTATION (HIGH TECHNOLOGY/BIOTECHNOLOGY) PROCEDURE
Anthony C. Cartwright
    15.1 Introduction 235
    15.2 Protection of innovation 235
    15.3 Early evaluation of the procedure 236
    15.4 Biotechnology products — an obligatory procedure 236
    15.5 Exemption from the obligatory biotechnology procedure 237
    15.6 The high technology procedure .237
    15.7 The concertation timetable. 238
    15.8 Appeals 239
    15.9 The Summary of product characteristics 240
    15.10 Changes to the marketing authorisation ('variations') 240
    15.11 Experience with the biotechnology procedure 240
    15.12 Experience with the high technology procedure 241

16 REGULATORY STRATEGY: THE EC, EFTA, THE PER SCHEME
Anthony C. Cartwright
    16.1 Regulatory strategy 242
        16.1.1 Regulatory strategy in national applications 243
    16.2 Regulatory strategy in concertation applications for biotechnology products 244
        16.2.1 Quality of the dossier .244
        16.2.2 Choice of the rapporteur country 244
        16.2.3 Liaison with the rapporteur 245
        16.2.4 Choice of the Experts for the Expert Report 245
        16.2.5 Quality of the written response to questions 245
        16.2.6 Choice of the Experts for hearings 245
        16.2.7 Response to remaining 'subject to' points 245
    16.3 Regulatory strategy in high technology applications 245
    16.4 Regulatory strategy in the multistate procedure 246
    16.5 Overall regulatory strategy for the product 246
    16.6 The PER scheme 247
    Reference 248

17 THE UNITED KINGDOM'S SYSTEM FOR LICENSING PHARMACEUTICAL PRODUCTS
Brian R. Matthews
    17.1 Introduction 249

17.2	Sources of information		249
17.3	Product licences and clinical trial certificates for pharmaceuticals for use in humans		250
	17.3.1	Introductory remarks	250
	17.3.2	Purpose of an application	251
	17.3.3	Application forms	251
	17.3.4	Before submitting the application	252
	17.3.5	Submitting the application and supporting data	252
	17.3.6	Registration	252
	17.3.7	Validation	253
	17.3.8	Professional assessment	255
	17.3.9	Reference to advisory bodies	256
	17.3.10	Other appeal procedures	260
	17.3.11	The issue of a product licence or clinical trial certificate	261
	17.3.12	Processing of applications routed *via* the Committee for Proprietery Medicinal Products	261
17.4	The clinical trial exemption scheme		262
	17.4.1	The scope of the scheme	262
	17.4.2	How the procedure works	262
17.5	Changes to licences, certificates, and exemptions		263
	17.5.1	Scope	263
	17.5.2	The procedures	263
17.6	Renewals		263
	17.6.1	Scope	263
	17.6.2	The procedures	264
17.7	Legal status and related topics		264
	17.7.1	Introduction	264
	17.7.2	Proposed method of sale	264
	17.7.3	Prescription only medicines	265
	17.7.4	General sales list products	265
	17.7.5	The determination of legal status	266
	17.7.6	Changing legal status	267
	17.7.7	Examples of special cases	268
		17.7.7.1 Radiopharmaceuticals	268
		17.7.7.2 Breathing gases	269
		17.7.7.3 Surgical materials	269
		17.7.7.4 Contact lenses and contact lens care products	269
		17.7.7.5 Topical hydrocortisone creams and ointments	270
	17.7.8	An outline of the legal status position in the EC	270

18 THE OTHER NATIONAL AUTHORITIES IN THE EC
Anthony C. Cartwright

18.1	Introduction	280
18.2	The EC Member States	280
18.3	The organisation of the assessment of marketing authorisation applications	282

Table of contents

- 18.4 The role of the national committees of independent experts 283
- 18.5 The appeals procedures 287
- 18.6 The national control laboratories and their involvement in the premarketing testing of samples of active ingredients, intermediates, and finished products. 288
- 18.7 The names and addresses of national authorities in the EC Member States 290
- Reference 293

19 EEC GUIDELINES — QUALITY, SAFETY, EFFICACY, AND BIOTECHNOLOGY
Anthony C. Cartwright
- 19.1 Introduction 294
- 19.2 The purpose of guidelines 295
- 19.3 Status of guidelines. 295
- 19.4 Working parties and their membership 295
- 19.5 Procedure for drawing up guidelines. 295
- 19.6 Revision of existing guideline texts. 296
- Reference 296

20 THE NEW GENERAL DIRECTIVE, IMMUNOLOGICALS, ETC. DIRECTIVES
Anthony C. Cartwright
- 20.1 Introduction 297
- 20.2 Directive 89/341/EEC. The new general Directive 297
  - 20.2.1 Implementation date 297
  - 20.2.2 Objectives of the Directive 298
  - 20.2.3 Change of terminology. 298
  - 20.2.4 New categories of exemptions from the Directives 298
  - 20.2.5 Amendment to the Summary of product characteristics (SPC) requirements. 298
  - 20.2.6 Amendment to the labelling requirements 299
  - 20.2.7 Labelling of ampoules: batch number added 299
  - 20.2.8 Replacement of term 'proprietary medicinal product' by 'medicinal product' in Directive 75/318/EEC 299
  - 20.2.9 Testing of samples. 299
  - 20.2.10 Mandatory package leaflet 299
  - 20.2.11 A manufacturing authorisation required even for export only products 299
  - 20.2.12 Inspections and good manufacturing practice 300
  - 20.2.13 Exports and export certificates. 300
  - 20.2.14 Communicating the results of GMP inspections between the authorities 300
  - 20.2.15 Notification of suspensions and revocations. 300

20.3 Directives 89/342/EEC (Immunogicals), 89/343/EEC
      (Radiopharmaceuticals), and 89/381/EEC (Blood Products) 301
Reference 301

21 THE SINGLE MARKET AFTER 1992: NEW DIRECTIONS
Anthony C. Cartwright
- 21.1 Introduction 302
- 21.2 The consultation process 302
- 21.3 Review and adoption of the future system legislative proposals . . . 303
- 21.4 The proposals for procedures after 1992 303
- 21.5 Phasing and transitional arrangements for the new procedures 304
  - 21.5.1 National applications 304
  - 21.5.2 Centralised applications 304
- 21.6 Products authorised nationally before 1993 304
- 21.7 The objectives of the new institutions and procedures 305
  - 21.7.1 Public health 305
  - 21.7.2 Industrial policy 305
  - 21.7.3 EC interests 305
- 21.8 The European Medicines Evaluation Agency 306
  - 21.8.1 Managerial and administrative support 306
  - 21.8.2 Administrative board 307
  - 21.8.3 Scientific and technical support for the EMEA 307
  - 21.8.4 The scientific and technical committees 307
  - 21.8.5 The Scientific Council 307
- 21.9 The centralised procedure 308
  - 21.9.1 Products eligible for the procedure 308
  - 21.9.2 The working of the centralised procedure 309
  - 21.9.3 Appeals in the centralised procedure 309
- 21.10 The decentralised procedure 310
  - 21.10.1 Products eligible for the decentralised procedure 310
  - 21.10.2 The working of the decentralised procedure 310
  - 21.10.3 Appeals in the decentralised procedure 311
- 21.11 The 'regulatory mechanism' — turning Opinions into Decisions . . 312
- 21.12 The supervisory authority 312
- Reference 313

APPENDIX: ABBREVIATIONS AND ACRONYMS 314

INDEX 318

Preface

The authors have written this book to provide a comprehensive reference text of information as to how to obtain a marketing authorisation (product licence) for human pharmaceutical medicinal products in the various countries in the European Community EC and beyond.

The objectives
The objectives of the book are to describe the current requirements and procedures in the European Community to obtain a marketing authorisation for a medicinal product. The multistate and concertation procedures are described in detail, as well as the more familiar process of applying individually for separate national authorisations in the EC Member States.

The book includes requirements for some of the special products — radiopharmaceuticals, medicated devices, and contact lens products.

In view of the background of the authors, they have drawn particularly on their long experience with the United Kingdom's Medicines Control Agency as a model to describe the process of obtaining a national marketing authorisation. However, Chapter 18 describes the different features of the other major authorities in the EC Member States, so that the reader is given a clear idea of the major differences he might expect to encounter in trying to register a product in those countries.

It is from these current procedures that the future system for registering pharmaceuticals in 1993 will develop and evolve. The national agencies will still provide the assessors and Experts to carry out the assessment, provide the rapporteurs, etc. The development of the future system will be phased, and initially it will only be for limited categories of product for which applications will be able to be made directly to the new European Medicines Evaluation Agency. The knowledge of the current system, its highways and byways, will help to provide a route-map for these future systems.

The readership
The book is intended for all of those who are involved or interested in the development and registration of pharmaceutical products — whether directly as discovery chemists, toxicologists, pharmacologists, analytical chemists, pharmaceutical research and development staff, clinicians, and statisticians; or indirectly as educators and students of the biomedical sciences.

It is also hoped that it may be of interest to those concerned with the use of medicinal products — clinicians, pharmacists, nurses, consumer interests, and even patients. It is felt that the book should give this wider readership some insight into the complex nature of the regulatory process, particularly the inevitable balancing of the risks attendant on taking any efficacious product with the clinical benefits to be obtained.

The contents of the book
Given the complexity of the subject, it would need an encyclopaedia, not a single book, to cover all facets of the development of medicinal products, their regulation and in-use monitoring. This book is therefore only concerned with the process of obtaining an approval to market a medicinal product in countries in Europe. It is not concerned, at least directly, with pharmacovigilance (adverse drug reaction monitoring and post-marketing surveillance). Neither is it concerned with the detail of the scrutiny of the adequacy of manufacturing premises, equipment, and personnel (Good Manufacturing Practice). Readers should refer elsewhere for information on these topics.

The economic importance of the European market for pharmaceutical products
The EC now consists of 320 million people in its 12 Member States. It is the largest pharmaceutical market in the world, bigger than the USA (with 240 million) or Japan (with 122 million). The economic value of total sales in 1986 in these markets was $32 500 millions in the EC, $20 000 millions in the US, and $20 500 in Japan.

The development of harmonised European Community requirements
The first European Directive on pharmaceuticals (65/65/EEC) was adopted in 1965. In the subsequent 25 years, the European Member States have been slowly harmonising their requirements. The process of harmonisation has covered the requirements for safety, quality, efficacy, and in the field of biotechnology. It has also extended to the format and contents of an application for a marketing authorisation. In 1989 these requirements were published in the five volumes entitled *Rules governing medicinal products in the European Community.*

Acceptance of these largely harmonised requirements in a wider Europe
The above requirements are also accepted by the six European Free Trade Area (EFTA) countries — Austria, Norway, Finland, Sweden, Iceland and Switzerland. These countries comprise a total market of another 33 million people. It also seems very likely that many of these requirements will also be accepted by the new, more

liberal, governments in Eastern Europe. In 1989, in advance of the (October 1990) reunification, the then Communist authorities in the German Democratic Republic announced their intention to do so.

The development of the Single European Market
The Single European Act was adopted in December 1985 by the European heads of government. It amended the Treaty of Rome which had set up the European Community. The Single European Act stated the objective of establishing a single market by 31 December 1992. The internal market is defined as comprising 'an area without internal frontiers in which the free movement of goods, services, and capital is ensured in accordance with the provisions of this treaty'.

The future European system for registering pharmaceuticals
In relation to the development of the Single Market in pharmaceuticals after 31 December 1992, the Pharmaceutical and Veterinary services of the Internal Market and Industry Directorate-General (DG III) of The Commission of The European Communities (CEC) published a Discussion Document in February 1990 on the future system. This proposed an evolution from the present multistate and concertation procedures to new 'centralised' and 'decentralised' procedures. It proposed the creation of a new European Medicines Evaluation Agency, which would not be a European Food and Drug Administration, but based firmly on the use of the existing assessors and Experts from the Member States of the EC. The new system would be phased in at different rates for different categories of products. The new procedures will evolve from the present procedures. It is therefore very important that regulatory staff and others within the pharmaceutical industry understand and use the present system, since the future one will evolve from it.

The development of an international dossier
The increased pace of harmonisation in the EC has led many in the industry and the authorities to the realisation of the possibility of an international dossier. This would be a single format and set of requirements for a marketing authorisation application in any developed country in the world.

For the future, the fifth International Conference of Drug Regulatory Authorities (ICDRA) held in Paris in October 1989 was invited by the International Federation of Pharmaceutical Manufacturers Associations (IFPMA) to accept a proposal for a joint international conference in November 1991 to discuss the question of harmonisation of requirements. The EC held fruitful bilateral talks in September 1988 and October 1989 with the Japanese authorities, and in November 1989 with the FDA on the subject of harmonisation of requirements. These talks are important, in that harmonised requirements would reduce the costs of the industry — and perhaps produce lower costs to the national health services. The harmonisation is also important to prevent unnecessary repetition of animal tests or clinical trials in man.

Since the most detailed and comprehensive requirements are those already accepted by the eighteen EC and EFTA countries, it may not be an overstatement to suggest that the European requirements could form the core of such an international marketing authorisation application.

A disclaimer
The contents of this book represent the views of its authors. They do not commit the Medicines Control Agency in the UK, the Department of Health, or the EC Committee for Proprietary Medicinal Products (CPMP).

Acknowledgements
The authors wish to thank all those who have helped with the publication of this book. The idea arose from the use of various materials in training courses devised and presented by the editors and others. Professor M. H. Rubinstein (the Series Editor) originally suggested that this material could be developed into a book, and this is the result.

Many in the UK Medicines Control Agency (MCA), in the other Member States, and in the EC (DG III/C-3), have helped with information or ideas which form part of this book. They are too numerous to mention by name; we can only express our very grateful thanks for all their help. However, particular thanks are due to Mr Sandy Stewart (a former Deputy Chief Pharmacist) who read and commented on the text.

The authors and the editors
This book is the work of a number of authors:

Chapters 1, 2, 6, 11, 13, 14, 15, 16, 18, 19, 20, and 21 were written by Mr Anthony (Tony) C. Cartwright.

Chapters 3, 7, 8, 9, 10, and 17 were written by Dr Brian. R. Matthews.

Chapter 4 was written by Dr James C. Ritchie.

Chapter 5 was written by Dr Alex Nicholson.

Chapter 12 was written by Dr David B. Jefferys, Dr James C. Ritchie and Dr Brian R. Matthews.

The joint editors were Tony Cartwright and Brian Matthews.

REFERENCES TO THE EUROPEAN COMMUNITIES TEXTS — *THE RULES GOVERNING MEDICINAL PRODUCTS IN THE EUROPEAN COMMUNITY*
Introduction
References will be made throughout the text of this book to the EC texts entitled *The rules governing medicinal products in the European Community.*

Inevitably, each of the individual chapter authors has referred to these texts. For convenience, and to save having to include references to them in the list of references for each individual chapter, they are listed in this introductory note.

The texts of the EC Directives, the EC content and format for marketing authorisation applications, the specific technical guidelines, the good manufacturing practice guide, and the veterinary products guide were all published as a five-volume set in 1989 by the Office for Official Publications of the European Communities in Luxembourg. The series title is *The rules governing medicinal products in the European Community*. The individual volumes are as follows:

Volume I *The rules governing medicinal products for human use in the European Community.*
English edition: ISBN 92-825-9563-3
Editions also in Spanish, Danish, German, French, Italian, Dutch, and Portuguese.

Volume II *Notice to applicants for marketing authorization for medicinal products for human use in the Member States of the European Community.*
English edition: ISBN 92-825-9503-X
Editions also in Spanish, German, French, and Italian.

Volume III *Guidelines on the quality, safety, and efficacy of medicinal products for human use.*
English edition: ISBN 92-825-9619-2
Editions also in Spanish, German, French, and Italian.

Volume IV *Guide to good manufacturing practice for medicinal products.*
English edition: ISBN 92-825-9572-2
Editions also in Spanish, Danish, German, Greek, French, Italian, Dutch, and Portuguese.

Volume V *The rules governing medicinal products for veterinary use in the European Community.*
English edition: ISBN 92-825-9643-5
Editions also in Spanish, Danish, German, Greek, French, Italian, Dutch, and Portuguese.

Volume I is the text of the Directives. For convenience, these are collated so that the texts of the later amendments replace the earlier text. It does not include the text of some of the later Directives (e.g. 89/341/EEC, 89/342/EEC), and these are described in Chapter 21.

The addendum to Volume III. *Guidelines*
An addendum to Volume III. *Guidelines on the quality, safety, and efficacy of medicinal products for human use*, was published in December 1990 (English edition: ISBN 92-826-0421-7; Spanish; German, and French editions are to be published in 1991). This contains the following guidelines (with their date of adoption by the CPMP in parentheses):

- Analytical validation (July 1989)

- European drug master file procedure for active ingredients (July 1990)
- Production and quality control of cytokine products derived by means of biotechnological processes (February 1990)
- Production and quality control of human monoclonal antibodies (July 1990)
- Good clinical practice for trials on medicinal products in the European Community (July 1990)
- Clinical testing of prolonged action forms with special reference to extended release forms (July 1990)
- Evaluation of anticancer medicinal products in man (July 1990)
- Medicinal products for the treatment of epileptic disorders (revision of earlier version of guideline, December 1989)
- Data sheets for antibacterial medicinal products (revision, November 1989).

Date of application of guidelines

It should be noted that guidelines are now given a date on which they should be applied, since they often represent a considerable change to existing practices. This is normally six months from the date of adoption by the Committee for Proprietary Medicinal Products (CPMP) and the issue of the guideline to the European pharmaceutical industry associations. The date of application of a particular guideline is not the date of publication of the volume of a collection of guidelines — the volume is merely provided for the convenience of users. In the case of the guidelines on the European Drug Master File (DMF) procedure and on good clinical practices (GCP) a more extended timescale of introduction and application is envisaged, since both will need further legal instruments (e.g. a Commission Directive in the case of the European DMF procedure) to enable them to be fully introduced.

Availability of these publications

All of these publications are available from sales points/distributors/bookshops selling the official publications of the European Community.

In the USA these publications are available from:

> UNIPUB
> 4611 F Assembly Drive
> Lanham
> MD 20706-4391 USA
> Tel: (800) 274 4888

In Japan these publications are available from:

> Kinokuniya Company Ltd
> 17-7 Shinjuku 3-Chome
> Shinuku-ku
> Tokyo 160-91
> Tel. (03) 354 0131

For other countries (outside the EC) the publication may be ordered through:

Office des publications officiels des Communautés européennes
2, rue Mercier
L-2985 Luxembourg
Tel. 49 92 81

1

Introduction and history of pharmaceutical regulation

1.1 INTRODUCTION

Any book written about a subject which is rapidly changing necessarily represents a 'snapshot' in time — the author's attempts to describe the current situation, and to predict what might be the state of things when the book is published. In the case of this book, the speed of change is rapidly increasing as the European Community (EC) nears 31 December 1992, the target date which the Single European Act defines as that by which a Single Market in products should be established.

The pharmaceutical and technical requirements for a marketing authorisation (MA) in the EC have developed from the existing national systems, largely as a response to the thalidomide disaster. They have been particularly concerned with eliminating the existing national requirements and replacing them by Community ones. New EC procedures for registering products (multistate, and concertation) have been set up alongside the existing systems in the Member States for obtaining marketing authorisations. In particular, the role of the Committee for Proprietary Medicinal Products (CPMP) has been crucial in providing a central forum for discussing the different views of the Member States on particular products, and for devising harmonised requirements which all of the EC Member States can adopt in relation to safety, quality, and efficacy of medicinal products.

In any description of a rapidly evolving system, it is helpful to try to place the present procedures and requirements and the new proposals for the future into their historical perspective. Thus, this first chapter is devoted to a short account of the history of regulation and control of medicinal products. As the Spanish/American philosopher and writer George Santayana (1863–1952) said in *The life of reason*: 'Those who cannot remember the past are condemned to repeat it'.

1.2 A BRIEF HISTORY OF PHARMACEUTICAL REGULATION

1.2.1 Early history to the nineteenth century

Penn (1979) claims that the state control of medicines dates back 3000 years to the early Greeks and Egyptians. He documents the controls exercised by the mutsahib in mediaeval Muslim countries on the syrup manufacturers who made medicinal products. These controls included the unannounced inspection of their premises. Quality was regarded as important, and tests were laid down to detect adulteration in drugs.

Penn documents the code of quality control exercised on imported drugs and spices by the Guild of Pepperers of Soper Lane in London in 1316. Their ordinances forbade the mixing of wares of different quality and price, or of the adulteration of goods.

From the Middle Ages onwards, another technique used to control drug quality was to issue an authoritative list of drugs, their preparation, and their uses — a pharmacopoeia. The earliest was probably the *New compound Dispensatory* of 1498 issued by the Florentine guild of physicians and pharmacists. Other cities followed — Barcelona published a pharmacopoeia in 1535, Nuernberg in 1546, Cologne in 1565, Rome in 1583, and London in 1618.

The first *London Pharmacopoeia* was superseded by the second in 1650, and further editions were issued until 1851. The *Edinburgh Pharmacopoeia* was issued in 1699, and that of Dublin in 1807. The first *British Pharmacopoeia* was published in 1864. In words which will strike a chord with all who now struggle to agree harmonised international quality standards, the editors of the 1864 *British Pharmacopoeia* describe the difficulties associated with their task thus: '... the Committees in London, Edinburgh, and Dublin who had to execute the difficult task, which had been previously attempted in vain, of reducing to one standard the processes and descriptions of three different pharmacopoeias, and, what was still more difficult, of reconciling the various usages in pharmacy and prescriptions of the people of these three countries hitherto separate and independent'.

The monographs of the 1864 *British Pharmacopoeia* often included a section called 'Characters and tests'. This section included the following tests — appearance, odour, boiling point, specific gravity, solubility in water or other solvents, and colorimetric identification tests.

An interesting feature of one of the monographs in the 1885 *British Pharmacopoeia* is its very modern controls on impurities in quininae sulphas (quinine sulphate), where there are separate gravimetric estimations for cinchonidine, cinchonine, quinidine, and cupreine (cardiotoxic components), and a limit for the total impurity content. In the late 1980s there was considerable discussion in the US in the *United States Pharmacopeia's* (USP) journal *Pharmacopeial Forum*, and in Europe in the European Pharmacopoeia Commission's journal *Pharmeuropa* on this question of control of impurities in active ingredients. A century earlier the compilers of the *British Pharmacopoeia* had clearly anticipated the need for this type of control.

As Mann (1989) has pointed out, as the nineteenth century developed, the character of medicinal products changed. In the early years of the nineteenth century, medicines were mainly botanical in origin. Inhalation anaesthetics were introduced in the middle years, and the early analgesics and barbiturates in the later part. These changes encouraged the development of the early pharmaceutical industry.

1.2.2 The early twentieth century in the UK: beginnings of regulation

Many of the modern concepts of pharmaceutical regulation were included in the UK Therapeutic Substances Act of 1925. Paul Ehrlich (1853–1915) had discovered the anti-syphilitic drug Salvarsan which was commercialised in 1911. Penn (1979) points out that although Salvarsan was synthetic, it contained highly toxic arsphenamine impurities which could only be detected by biological testing. Each batch used in the UK was submitted to the Medical Research Council for approval prior to release for marketing.

This requirement for biological testing and/or standardisation for substances whose purity and potency could not be measured by purely chemical means, led to the Therapeutic Substances Act of 1925. The Act applied to vaccines, sera, toxins, antitoxins, antigens, arsphenamines (such as Salvarsan), insulin, pituitary hormone, and catgut surgical sutures.

The Therapeutic Substances Act provided for a licensing system administered by the Ministry of Health, for inspections of the factory premises (for the suitability of the employees and the manufacturing premises themselves). Records of sale had to be kept by the manufacturers for each batch of the controlled products. The Act also laid down labelling requirements for the container, to identify the manufacturer and the batch. The system of batch release by an independent state laboratory (e.g. by the National Institute for Biological Standards and Control in the UK, by the Paul Ehrlich Institut in the Federal Republic of Germany, by the Institut Pasteur in France), is followed to this day in many countries of the EC.

1.2.3 The early twentieth century in the USA: early regulation

Young (1967) documents the crusade in the United States of America (USA) against patent medicines which led to the provisions of the 1906 US Pure Food and Drugs Act against misbranding. This required certain named ingredients (alcohol, opiates, chloral hydrate, acetanilide) to be stated on the label. Products were also regarded as adulterated if their strength or purity 'fell below the professed standard under which it is sold'. The Act went on to forbid 'any statement design or device' which was 'false or misleading in any particular'. The 1906 Act was administered by the Bureau of Chemistry in the Department of Agriculture of Washington. A Drug Control Laboratory was created in 1923.

In 1927 the Food Drug and Insecticide Administration was created. In 1930 the title was amended to delete 'Insecticide'.

In 1937, the Samuel Massengill Company, a small pharmaceutical manufacturer in Tennessee, started distributing a sulfanilamide elixir containing the solvent diethylene glycol. The solvent was not named on the label. 107 people (many of them children) died as a result of ingesting the elixir containing this toxic solvent. The Food and Drug Administration (FDA) was able to take action under the 1906 Act, since according to the *United States Pharmacopeia* an elixir must contain alcohol. The US Congress was pressed to strengthen the 1906 Act, and in June 1938 the Food Drug and Cosmetic Act was passed.

The 1938 Act contained stronger provisions against misbranding — not only against false labelling but also against failure to indicate when the medicine might be dangerous. The Act forbade the sale and supply of any medicine dangerous to health when used according to its recommended dosage. It required the names of all active ingredients to be stated on the label. Any new medicinal product (such as the Massengill sulfanilamide elixir) could not be marketed until the FDA approved it as safe.

1.2.4 Thalidomide

In 1946, the West German soap and cosmetic company of Dalli-Werke, Mäurer, and Wirtz formed a new pharmaceutical subsidiary named Chemie Grünenthal. In 1956 Grünenthal test marketed a combination product called Grippex containing thalidomide in Hamburg. This product was indicated for the treatment of respiratory infections.

In 1957 thalidomide tablets were marketed in West Germany under the trade mark Contergan. Grünenthal also sold thalidomide combination products with aspirin (acetylsalicylic acid), phenacetin, quinine, aminopyrine, bacitracin, dihydrostreptomycin, and secobarbitone on the West German market for a variety of conditions including colds, coughs, nervousness, migraine, and asthma (Sjöström & Nilsson 1972).

Other companies acquired marketing or distribution rights for thalidomide products from Grünenthal. Distillers (Biochemicals) Ltd in the UK sold it as Distaval. In Canada, Frank W. Horner marketed it as Talimol and the William S. Merrell Co. as Kevadon. The marketing publicity for the thalidomide products gave special emphasis to its claims to complete atoxicity — since it showed a lack of acute toxicity by single dose injection. In 1959, in a letter which Sjöström and Nilsson document, Grünenthal claimed that with 'prolonged medication the drug's effectivenesss is not impaired by unwanted side-effects'.

From August 1959, reports in West Germany and elsewhere started to flow in to the Grünenthal company of peripheral neuropathy in patients — paraesthesia and numbness in the toes, feet, and ankles, spreading later to the fingers. After some time the patients experienced severe muscular pains and cramps, weakness of the limbs, and ataxia. Other toxic effects on the central nervous system included twitching of the facial muscles, muscle trembling, speech difficulties, and double vision. In the UK Florence (1960) described four cases of thalidomide polyneuritis, and this was the first description in the medical literature. By May 1961 the UK licensees had reported 75–90 cases of polyneuritis.

In October 1960 Drs Koserow and Pfeiffer in Münich showed infants with a new gross deformation (phocomelia – sealed limbs) to a paediatric congress.

In November 1961 a meeting of West German paediatricians in Dusseldorf had noted a dramatic increase in the incidence of phocomelia, and Dr. Widukind Lenz suggested that this was due to the intake of a new drug.

In May 1961 Dr. William McBride of Sydney saw his first case of phocomelia. In October he saw other cases, and he published his observations in December 1961 in the *Lancet*.

On 27 November 1961 Chemie Grünenthal withdrew the products containing thalidomide from the German market. The West German Ministry of Health issued a statement that Contergan was suspected as the major factor in causing phocomelia.

The drug was withdrawn from the UK market on the same day as a result of this teratogenicity (i.e. causing congenital malformations in children).

In March 1962 the product was withdrawn from the Canadian market by William S. Merrell Co. and Frank W. Horner.

In the USA, William S. Merrell made an application in September 1960 to market thalidomide tablets under the proprietary trade name Kevadon. However, the reviewing medical assessor in FDA (Dr. Frances O. Kelsey) had doubts about the safety of the product, and in particular about the incidence of peripheral neuritis. The marketing authorisation was still unapproved when the company withdrew the product from the German market.

1.2.5 Thalidomide: the regulatory aftermath

The near-disaster in the US forced the passage of the Kefauver-Harris Drug Amendments to the Food Drug and Cosmetic Act in October 1962. For the first time the new law required evidence of efficacy in the proposed indications. FDA was also required to approve all plans for clinical trials of new drugs — the Investigatory New Drug Application (IND) was introduced. Adverse drug reactions were required to be notified to FDA. Manufacturers were required to operate according to good manufacturing practice (GMP).

In the UK, a voluntary arrangement to scrutinise the safety of new products was set up by Health Ministers. The new Committee on Safety of Drugs (CSD) was chaired by Sir Derrick Dunlop and consisted of eleven scientists, physicians, and pharmacists assisted by a small secretariat. Their advice was only concerned with what Dunlop (1973) termed 'reasonable safety for its intended purpose'. Dunlop continues 'Although the safety and efficacy of medicines are often inextricably intertwined, efficacy *per se* was not the function of the Committee'. This voluntary arrangement worked well, with excellent cooperation from the industry.

In 1968 the UK Parliament approved the Medicines Act, which became operative in September 1971. The main Committee advising the Licensing Authority was renamed the Committee on Safety of Medicines (CSM), with policy advice to the Licensing Authority and recommendations on final appeals being given by the Medicines Commission. Other advisory committees were subsequently appointed — including the Committee on the Review of Medicines (CRM) and the Committee on Dental and Surgical Materials (CDSM) for human medicines, the Veterinary Products Committee (VPC) for veterinary products, and the British Pharmacopoeia Commission. The new Act required the assessment of the evidence for the safety, quality, and efficacy of all medicinal products. Fuller details of the working of the UK authority (now called the Medicines Control Agency — MCA) are given in Chapter 17 of this book.

In the Netherlands in 1958, a new Bill was approved by Parliament which created a new system for registration of pharmaceuticals. Teijgeler (1989) has documented the establishment of the College ter Beoordeling van geneesmiddelen (Committee for the Evaluation of Medicines) which took place in 1963. Its main objectives are the evaluation and registration of medicines — based on the criteria of safety, quality, and efficacy. In 1978 an amendment to the Dutch Medicines Act introduced a new requirement for registration of generic products. The Dutch committee is unique in the EC since it is an executive one — it takes the decision whether to approve a marketing authorisation application or not. In other EC Member States (such as the UK) the registration committees (such as the CSM) are advisory, although in practice their advice is very seldom disregarded.

In the Federal Republic of Germany the first German Drug Law of 1961 (AMG 1961) set up the Federal Health Office (Bundesgesundhheitsamt), made manufacture of products approvable by the authorities in the Länder (local authorities), and made registration of proprietary products obligatory. Schmitt-Rau (1988) summarised the changes made by the Drug Law of 1976. This introduced the need for approval of products in terms of safety, quality, and efficacy, risk-monitoring of approved drugs, supervision of clinical trials, manufacture, quality control, and importation and marketing of pharmaceutical preparations.

1.2.6 Thalidomide — implications for chirality requirements

Recently, interest has been expressed in the use of single enantiomers where previously a racemic mixture or racemate had been used. Also, single enantiomers are increasingly being developed from the 'discovery chemistry' stage of the development of a new chemical active substance — synthetically, biosynthetically, or by a resolution or separation process. The 'eutomer' (the desired isomer) can then be tested without any biological interference from the 'distomer' (the unwanted isomer). Some authors have suggested that (R)-thalidomide is a safe sedative and hypnotic, whereas (S)-thalidomide is a potent teratogen. The active substance sold in the 1950s was a racemic mixture (i.e. a mixture of the R and S isomers). If this hypothesis is true, it is perhaps the most vivid illustration of the need for companies to define and justify the use of a racemate, by investigating and reporting the toxicological and pharmacological properties of the individual stereoisomers in a racemate.

1.3 THE EUROPEAN COMMUNITY: REGULATION OF PROPRIETARY MEDICINAL PRODUCTS (1965 TO 1987)

1.3.1 Introduction

In 1965 the EC consisted of six Member States — France, the Federal Republic of Germany, Italy, Belgium, the Netherlands, and Luxembourg. After the withdrawal of thalidomide products from the major European markets in November 1961, there was clearly a need for legislation to regulate the marketing of pharmaceutical products and to supersede national controls with a more comprehensive EC system. The first of the pharmaceutical Directives (65/65/EEC) was drawn up and adopted by the Council of Ministers on 26 January 1965; eighteen months were allowed for its implementation.

In 1973 the UK, Denmark, and Ireland joined the EC. In 1981 Greece joined, followed by Spain and Portugal in 1986. Greece, Spain, and Portugal have transitional arrangements in respect of some of the requirements of the Directives while they adapt their national procedures and review the older licensed products. The differences in requirements in this transition period to 1992 will be indicated where appropriate.

1.3.2 Directive 65/65/EEC: definitions and requirements

The preamble to this Directive states the objectives for this and indeed all future pharmaceutical legislation. It defines the primary purpose as being to 'safeguard public health'. It goes on, however, to state that 'this objective must be attained by means which will not hinder the development of the pharmaceutical industry or trade in medicinal products within the Community'.

This Directive has the following principal features:

- the definition of a medicinal product (Article 1),
- the requirement for the Member States to issue authorisations for medicinal products (Article 3),
- the need for documents and particulars to accompany an application for a marketing authorisation (Article 4),
- the obligation on the authorities to refuse an application for a product if it is 'harmful in its normal conditions of use' or lacking in therapeutic efficacy; if efficacy is insufficiently shown; or if its qualitative or quantitative composition is not as declared (Article 5),
- the time allowed for the authorities to process applications — 120 days with exceptionally another 90 days (Article 7),
- the period of validity of marketing authorisations (5 years),
- the requirement for the authorities to revoke or suspend an authorisation where the product is harmful in its normal conditions of use, is inefficaceous, or its quantitative composition is not as declared (Article 11),
- container and outer package labelling requirements (Articles 13 to 20).

It should be noted that although the current (1991) definition of a medicinal product is that of 65/65/EEC, this will change on 1 January 1992 when Directive 89/341/EEC comes into force (see Chapter 19). The current definition (in Article 1 of 65/65/EEC) of a 'proprietary medicinal product' is:

'any ready-prepared medicinal product placed on the market under a special name and in a special pack'

It is further defined as:

'Any substance or combination of substances presented for treating or preventing disease in human beings or animals. Any substance or combination of substances administered to human beings or animals with a view to making a medical diagnosis or of correcting or modifying a physiological function in human beings or animals...'

The following section is a brief summary of some of the major provisions of some of the subsequent Directives. It does not attempt to provide a complete authoritative guide and interpretation to the Directives. The reader is referred to the text of the

EC publication *The rules governing medicinal products in the European Community*, Volume I, *Rules governing medicinal products for human use in the European Community*. This is an invaluable but unofficial version of the legal texts where the amendments of the text made by later Directives is interpolated and amends the earlier legal requirements. It is a 'scissors and paste' version produced for the convenience of the lawyer and non-lawyer alike.

1.3.3 Directive 75/318/EEC: the 'norms and protocols' Directive

This was adopted on 20 May 1975 and implemented within 18 months.

Directive 65/65/EEC had indicated that 'documents and particulars' shall accompany an application for a marketing authorisation (MA). Article 4 defined these 'documents and particulars' as follows:

- Article 4(7) description of the control methods . . . .
- Article 4(8) results of physicochemical, biological, or microbiological tests; pharmacological and toxicological tests and clinical trials.

The second Directive (75/318/EEC) is the agreed statement by the EC Member States of their harmonised view of what information should be supplied in these 'documents and particulars'. These harmonised standards and requirements (the 'norms and protocols') are given in the Annex to the Directive:

Part 1: Physicochemical, biological, or microbiological tests
Part 2: Toxicological and pharmacological tests
Part 3: Clinical trials.

These requirements have formed the basis for all of the subsequent technical requirements and the technical guidelines. As science and technology have advanced, this Directive has been amended by later Directives. For example, Directive 83/570/EEC introduced the requirement for development pharmaceutics and process validation as well as the requirements for mutagenicity and bioavailability testing.

There is a partial relaxation of the clinical requirements for active ingredients used to treat rare diseases where it would be unreasonable to ask for the complete clinical data package needed for a more common disease. This provides the European equivalent of the 'orphan drug' provisions in the USA. Such an authorisation is granted on the following conditions (Chapter III of Part 3 of the Annex to the Directive):

- that the product is only supplied on medical prescription and may need to be administered under medical supervision (e.g. in a hospital or clinic),
- that the package leaflet and medical information (e.g. data sheet in the UK) draws attention to any inadequacies in the data supplied to the authorities.

1.3.4 Directive 75/319/EEC: legal and administrative provisions

This Directive was adopted on 20 May 1975. It sets out the legal and administrative framework for the authorities in the Member States. It concerns:

Sec. 1.3] **The EC: regulation of proprietary medicinal products** 37

- the submission and processing of marketing authorisation applications (Articles 1 to 7), including the requirement for three 'Experts' to draw up the application (see Chapter 11),
- the establishment of a new European Committee (the CPMP) to consider questions referred to it related to approval, refusal, suspension, or revocation of marketing authorisations (Articles 8 to 15),
- the requirements for the inspection of manufacturers, issue of manufacturing authorisations, and the need for a 'Qualified Person' who is responsible for ensuring that the manufacture is in accord with the marketing authorisation (Articles 16 to 24),
- the need for the national authorities to inspect manufacturing and contract test laboratories to ensure that testing is carried out as laid down in the marketing authorisation (Articles 25 to 27),
- an exemption from the Directives for immunologicals, radiopharmaceuticals, homoeopathics, and blood products (Article 34)
- the need for a review of old medicinal products already licensed in accordance with previous provisions (i.e. earlier national requirements (Article 39)).

The creation of the CPMP in 1975 was an important step. In 1975 its legal role was seen mainly as arbitration (where there were disagreements between the Member States on whether to authorise, or to suspend or revoke an authorisation). It could also provide an Opinion when a company submitted an application in five Member States after first obtaining an authorisation in one of the other Member States. This procedure was called the 'CPMP procedure' and was the precursor of the current 'multistate' procedure.

Since 1975 the work of the CPMP has become increasingly important (see Chapter 13), and the proposals for the future system for 1993 (see Chapter 21) envisage a strengthened CPMP as being the central decision-making and arbitration body in the various pan-European licensing arrangements.

1.3.5 Decision 75/320/EEC: the Pharmaceutical Committee

This Decision was adopted on 20 May 1975. It created a new body — the Pharmaceutical Committee. This consists of the Directors of Pharmacy (or their equivalents) in each of the Member States. It is chaired by a representative of the CEC (from Directorate-General III — the Internal Market Directorate). It considers any proposals relating to new Directives (or to amend existing Directives) from the CEC. It also considers the broad policy issues in relation to the control of medicinal products.

The Pharmaceutical Committee normally meets once or twice a year, depending on the legislative workload.

1.3.6 Directive 78/25/EEC: approved colouring matters

This Directive was adopted on 12 December 1977, and it created an EC list of colouring matters which may be used in medicinal products. The approved colouring matters list is in the Annex to the Directive and is identical to those approved for use in food.

The EC approved colouring matters list includes natural colourants (e.g. beetroot red, alpha-carotene), inorganic colourants (e.g. titanium dioxide, iron oxides and hydroxides, silver), and synthetic organic dyes and their lakes (e.g. erythrosine, tartrazine).

The Directive refers back to an earlier Directive of October 1962 on food colouring matters (as amended by Directive 76/399/EEC) for the specifications for these colouring matters.

1.3.7 Commission Communication of 6 May 1982: parallel importation of medicinal products

Parallel importation of products in the EC is their importation and distribution using systems parallel to those conventionally used by the manufacturer and his wholesaler/retailer network. The importation is from a country where the price charged is low, to one where the price is much higher. Parallel imports can be of any type of product — automobiles, human medicines, veterinary medicines, pesticides, electrical goods, etc. For pharmaceuticals the large importing countries have been the UK, the Netherlands, and the Federal Republic of Germany. Products come from the low labour cost countries (e.g. Greece) or countries where the national reimbursement price of pharmaceuticals has been kept low (e.g. Belgium).

The trade in parallel imports is a substantial one. The Office of Health Economics estimated the 1987 value of imported pharmaceuticals into the UK as being between £209 million and £216 million ($340 to $350 million). This represented 10 to 13% of the UK National Health Service pharmaceuticals bill.

Parallel importation of pharmaceuticals started in the EC about seventeen years ago with the Dutch wholesaler Centrapharm. They started to import products licensed elsewhere in the EC and sell them on the Dutch market in competition with what they considered to be the same product already being distributed through normal channels. The actions of the Dutch authorities in trying to regulate the trade (by requiring the importers to produce batch records) led to a reference to the European Court of Justice under Article 177 of the Treaty of Rome. Their judgement (the De Peijper judgement) interpreted the provisions of Articles 30 to 36 of the Treaty of Rome.

In June 1980 the CEC brought forward proposals for a parallel import Directive. The European Parliament voted against this proposal on 16 October 1981. The CEC then withdrew this proposal and instead issued the Commission Communication of 6 May 1982.

The main elements of this Commission Communication (a guideline for the authorities in regulating this trade) reflected the findings of the European Court of Justice in the De Peijper case. This guidance has been adopted by all the national authorities to regulate parallel importation.

The main aspects of the Communication are:

- The authorities should ask the parallel importer to provide information to verify that the imported product is covered by a marketing authorisation.
- The authorities should make enquiries to find out whether the product is produced in several variants in the EC Member States. (It is very common for this to be the

Sec. 1.3]   **The EC: regulation of proprietary medicinal products**   39

case, from the UK experience.) If these differences would have therapeutic effect, the products should not be treated as the same (i.e. the application for a parallel import licence should be refused).
- The products must be manufactured under good manufacturing practice (GMP).
- Wholesalers and importers should be licensed and approved, and they should preserve documents relating to the imported batches of products.
- The parallel importer should provide specimens or mock-ups of the product to be marketed.
- The parallel importer should keep a register of the origins, quantity, and batch numbers of the product.
- Batch control reports can be made available to the authorities either from the manufacturer directly, from the authorities in the Member State concerned, or by other means (e.g. requiring that the importer test the product himself, or having it tested at his expense in the state national control laboratory).

1.3.8 Directive 83/570/EEC: amending Directive
This Directive was adopted on 26 October 1983. It amended the first three Directives.

One of the most important changes introduced by 83/570/EEC is the requirement for the applicant to produce a draft Summary of Product Characteristics (SPC) as part of his documentation. This is then reviewed by the authorities, and the applicant is given the revised and accepted version when he receives his marketing authorisation. The wording of the SPC is then used by the applicant as the basis of the product 'data sheet', and in the subsequent advertising and promotion of the product.

The Summary of Product Characteristics comprises:

- the product name,
- the qualitative and quantitative composition in terms of the active ingredients and those of the excipients which the physician, pharmacist or patient needs to know for the proper use of the product,
- the pharmaceutical form (e.g. tablets),
- the pharmacological properties and relevant pharmacokinetic particulars,
- the clinical particulars (indications, contraindications, warnings, etc.),
- the pharmaceutical particulars (incompatibilities, shelf-life, special storage precautions etc.).

1.3.9 Council Recommendations 83/571/EEC: 'guidelines'
The first series of CPMP Notes for Guidance were adopted by the Council of Ministers on 26 October 1983. These related to repeated dose toxicity, reproduction studies, carcinogenic potential, pharmacokinetic and metabolic studies in the safety evaluation of new drugs in animals, and to fixed combination products.

These Notes for Guidance provide an authoritative but non-mandatory interpretation of the requirements of the 'norms and protocols' Directive — 75/318/EEC. They provide an agreed interpretation for the industry to use, and also represent the harmonised views of the national authorities when considering the dossier which accompanies a marketing authorisation application.

These first Notes for Guidance were adopted after a complex legislative process (involving the Economic and Social Committee, the European Parliament, and the Council of Ministers). They have now been included with some other guidelines on safety, quality, and efficacy in Volume III of the *Rules governing medicinal products in the European Community*. These later guidelines (see Chapter 18) have been adopted by the CPMP after consultation with the European pharmaceutical industry but without the need for cumbersome formal consultation of the European legislative machinery.

1.3.10 Directive 87/19/EEC: the regulatory committee procedure

This Directive was adopted on 22 December 1986 and implemented on 1 July 1987. It introduces a new rapid procedure for adapting the technical requirements in the 'norms and protocols' Directive (75/318/EEC) for the dossier to be submitted with a marketing authorisation.

A new Committee for the Adaptation to Technical Progress of the Directive on the Removal of Technical Barriers to Trade in the Proprietary Medicines Sector has been set up to consider the proposed amendments to 75/318/EEC. A CEC representative acts as Chairman, the Committee will work by a qualified majority vote of the Member States. In qualified majority voting the Federal Republic of Germany, France, Italy and the UK have 10 votes; Spain has 8 votes; Belgium, Greece, the Netherlands, and Portugal have 5 votes; Denmark and Ireland have 3 votes; Luxembourg has 2 votes.

The concept behind this procedure is to rapidly elaborate new technical requirements or amendments to 75/318/EEC. These will be produced as technical (Commission) Directives

1.3.11 Directive 87/21/EEC: abridged applications for 'copy products' and protection of innovation

This Directive was adopted on 22 December 1986, and implemented on 1 July 1987. Greece, Spain, and Portugal, however, will not implement the Directive until 1 January 1992.

It amended Article 4(8) of Directive 65/65/EEC — the statement of the documents and particulars which must accompany any application for a marketing authorisation in an EC Member State. It defines much more precisely the cases in which the results of pharmacological and toxicological tests do not have to be provided for a product which is 'essentially similar' to an already authorised originator's product.

As a result of this Directive, any application submitted in the EC Member States must be complete (i.e. unabridged) except where:

- the authority of the first applicant is provided to refer to the relevant toxicology/pharmacology and clinical data,
- or, detailed references to published literature on the pharmacology/toxicology and clinical data are provided,

- or, the product is 'essentially similar' to the first (originator's) product, more than ten years have elapsed (six years in the case of Denmark, Ireland, and Luxembourg) since the date of first authorisation in the EC, and the original product is marketed in the Member State concerned.

Before this section of Directive 65/65/EEC was amended, the EC Member States pursued different approaches to the requirements for 'second applicant' products (such as generic products). Some (such as the Federal Republic of Germany) insisted on the formal submission of data, others (such as the UK) recognised well-established uses of the active ingredient and approved in many cases without formal submission of bibliographic or other data.

1.3.12 Directive 87/22/EEC: the high technology/biotechnology procedure

This Directive was adopted on 22 December 1986 and implemented by 1 July 1987.

The Directive introduced the concertation procedure (i.e. a procedure to obtain a mutual agreement on the authorisation) for the products defined in the Annex to the Directive.

List A of the Annex defines biotechnology products (the recombinant DNA technology, monoclonal antibodies, and products purified by using monoclonal antibodies). If an applicant wishes to make an application for a marketing authorisation for such a product, then use of the procedure is compulsory.

List B of the Annex describes the product categories which can be put into the procedure if the applicant requests it and the authorities agree that the product complies with the requirements. The List B products all have to satisfy the authorities as to the significance of their therapeutic interest, their innovation, or their novelty.

This procedure represents the first EC procedure when the same MA application dossier is reviewed by all of the concerned Member States without a previous authorisation being granted in one of them. It is thus the first pan-European licensing procedure. The 'centralised procedure' in the proposed future system from 1 January 1993 is modelled closely on the existing concertation procedure (sometimes called the 'high tech' procedure).

The procedure is described in detail in Chapter 15.

1.4 THE *EUROPEAN PHARMACOPOEIA*

The European Pharmacopoeia Convention was signed in 1964 by six Member States of the Council of Europe. There are currently nineteen countries which are signatories to the Convention. They include all of the EC countries and a number outside the EC (e.g. Switzerland, Sweden).

From the beginning of the implementation of Community-wide pharmaceutical controls, standardisation of quality specifications for active ingredients, excipients, and finished products has been of vital importance. The 'norms and protocols' Directive (75/318/EEC) requires that the *European Pharmacopoeia* monographs apply to both active ingredients and excipients. It states 'the monographs of the *European Pharmacopoeia* shall be applicable to all substances appearing in it'.

In relation to the general monographs for dosage forms (tablets, capsules, etc.) Directive 75/318/EEC was amended to state that 'if general monographs on pharmaceutical forms appear in the *European Pharmacopoeia* or, failing this, in the national pharmacopoeias of the Member States, finished products must meet the requirements contained therein'.

There has been an increasing dialogue between the CPMP (particularly its Quality Working Party) and the European Pharmacopoeia Commission on the requirements of the national authorities concerned with marketing authorisation approvals. This has included discussions on concerns about impurity controls in pharmacopoeial active ingredient monographs, the need for one or two additional general monographs, and specific requirements for particular products or groups of products.

In 1989 the negotiations with the Council of Europe to allow the EC itself to become a contracting party to the European Pharmacopoeia Convention were successful. The changes to the Convention have now been ratified by nearly all of the European countries concerned. This will herald an era of increasing collaboration by the EC in the activities of the European Pharmacopoeia Commission.

The monographs and requirements set out in the *European Pharmacopoeia* have influence in a far wider forum than the EC and a wider Europe. The monographs are reprinted in national European pharmacopoeias (the *Deutsches Arzneibuch* (DAB), the *Pharmacopeé Française*, the *Farmacopeia Ufficiale della Republica Italiana* (Italian pharmacopoeia), and the *British Pharmacopoeia*). Often the standards of these national pharmacopoeias are accepted by countries with historic links with them (e.g. Commonwealth countries with the UK).

1.5 PUBLICATION OF THE COMMUNITY RULES FOR PRODUCT REGISTRATION IN 1989

Throughout the present book, reference will be made to the texts of the EC Directives, the European guidelines on format of marketing authorisation applications and the content of the dossier, and the specific technical guidelines. These were all published in 1989 as a 5 volume set by the Office for Official Publications of the European Community in Luxembourg. The series title of all of the volumes is *The rules governing medicinal products in the European Community*. The individual volumes are as follows:

Volume I *The rules governing medicinal products for human use in the European Community.*

Volume II *Notice to applicants for marketing authorization for medicinal products for human use in the Member States of the European Community.*

Volume III *Guidelines on the quality, safety, and efficacy of medicinal products for human use.*

Volume IV *Guide to good manufacturing practice for the manufacture of medicinal products.*

Volume V   *The rules governing medicinal products for veterinary use in the European Community.*

Volume I is the text of the Directives. For convenience these have been collated so that the texts of the later amendments replaces the original texts. An unofficial Addendum has been published in October 1989 containing the texts of the so-called 'extension Directives'. These are described in Chapter 21.

This five-volume set of texts forms part of the essential library for the researcher, the research and development pharmacist, the toxicologist, the pharmacologist, and the clinician engaged in organising clinical trials. They are equally necessary for the regulatory affairs professionals who submit marketing authorisation applications in Europe. The present book is designed to complement these official texts.

1.6 OTHER MEASURES DESIGNED TO ELIMINATE THE REMAINING BARRIERS TO THE ESTABLISHMENT OF A SINGLE EUROPEAN MARKET IN PHARMACEUTICAL PRODUCTS

In its 1985 White Paper on the Completion of the Internal Market, the CEC identified 300 measures needed to remove obstacles to the establishment of a real internal market by 31 December 1992. Thirteen specific measures for the pharmaceutical sector were identified. New Directives (a general Directive amending the definition of a medicinal product; making certain patient information mandatory; establishing a legal basis for good manufacturing practice; Directives on immunological products, blood products, radiopharmaceutical products) were adopted in 1989, but these will not be implemented until 1 January 1992. These Directives (89/341/EEC, 89/342/EEC, 89/343/EEC, and 89/381/EEC) are described in Chapter 20.

Other draft Directives and a Regulation will (after discussion and amendment by the European Parliament, the Economic and Social Committee, Council of Ministers Expert Working Party, the Committee of Permanent Representatives of the EC Ambassadors (COREPER), etc.) form the legal basis of the post-1992 future system to be adopted by the Council of Ministers. These are discussed in Chapter 21.

One area of harmonisation, not strictly within the remit of this book, is that of pricing. However, the economics of selling products in a Single European Market is crucial, and the acceptability of any future system proposals will depend on an acceptable system of pricing being agreed in the Community which will limit the drug bill in the national Member States on the one hand, but provides a fair return on capital on the other hand for an innovative industry with a huge research investment made in Europe. A brief mention needs therefore to be made of pricing.

The majority of the European Member States have adopted national systems to control the costs of human pharmaceutical products — by controlling price and/or by limiting the range of products reimbursable under national health insurance schemes. As we have seen earlier, these national price differences lead to parallel importation of products from one country to another.

On 21 December 1988 the Council of Ministers adopted Directive 89/105/EEC on the 'transparency' of national price/reimbursability controls. The objective is to ensure that the national systems by which the price/reimbursability are set are objective and clear (i.e. 'transparent') to those concerned. The Directive lays down requirements for the time limit for decisions on pricing etc., rights of appeal, and publication of decisions.

It is likely that further measures on EC cooperation on pricing/reimbursability will be needed, since it is difficult to envisage a Single European Market without some attempt to reduce existing price differentials and to start to establish a common basis for pricing/reimbursability.

Other measures on the harmonisation of controls on advertising and promotion were proposed in 1989, and will be adopted as a Directive in 1991. These are seen as increasingly important with (for example) sophisticated cross-border advertising of over-the-counter (OTC) products by national television and by cable and satellite television.

A new Directive on the legal status of pharmaceutical products (prescription or OTC sale) will also be adopted in 1991.

In 1988, the European Council of Health Ministers had a request from the European Parliament to include a package insert in all medicinal products. This was accepted, and Directive 89/341/EEC will make this obligatory after 1 January 1992. The CEC consulted an *ad hoc* group of consumers, clinicians, pharmacists, and industry representatives on the way in which patient information should be provided, and new proposals will be issued on this point in due course.

REFERENCES

Addendum 1989 to Volume I of the *Rules governing medicinal products for human use in the European Community*. III/8272/89-EN.

Dunlop, Sir Derrick (1973). *Medicines in our time.* Nuffield Provincial Hospital Trust, London.

Florence, A. L. (1960) Is thalidomide to blame? *Brit. Med. J.*, 2, 1954.

Mann, R. D. (1989). The historical development of medicines regulations. *International medicines regulations: Proceedings of Centre for Medicines Research Workshop.* Ciba Foundation, London 20/21 September 1988. Edited by Walker, S. R. and Griffin, J. P. Kluwer Academic, London.

McBride, W. G. (1961) Thalidomide and congenital abnormalities *Lancet*, 2, 1358.

Penn, R. G. (1979). The state control of medicines: the first 3000 years. *Brit. J. Clin. Pharmac.* 8, 293–305.

Preface to the *British Pharmacopoeia* 1864. The General Council of Medical Education and Registration of the United Kingdom. Spottiswode and Company, London.

Santayana, G. *The life of reason.* Volume I. Reason in common sense (cited in Bartlett's Familiar Quotations).

Schmitt-Rau, K. (1988). The drug regulatory affairs system in the Federal Republic of Germany. *J. Clin. Pharmacol.* 28, 1064–1070.

Sjöström, H. & Nilsson, R. (1972). *Thalidomide and the power of the drug companies.* Penguin Books, Middlesex, England.

Teijgeler, C. A. (1989). Objectives and achievement of regulation in the Netherlands. *International medicines regulations: Proceedings of Centre for Medicines Research Workshop.* Ciba Foundation, London 20/21 September 1988. Edited by Walker, S. R. & Griffin, J. P. Kluwer Academic, London.

Young, J. H. (1967). *The medical messiahs. A social history of health quackery in twentieth century America.* Princeton University Press, Princeton, USA.

2

The European Community: its structure, institutions, and regulation

2.1 INTRODUCTION

The present and future arrangements for registration of pharmaceutical products in Europe must be understood against the changing European economic and political structures. Indeed, it is likely that they will become more important as moves are made towards economic, monetary, and political union in the Community. Also, there are increasing links with the newly liberalised governments of Eastern Europe.

This chapter sets out some of the more important of the European institutions, and mentions in particular their relevance to the pharmaceutical sector.

2.2 THE TREATY OF ROME

The European Economic Community (EEC) was founded in 1957 by six countries (Belgium, France, the Federal Republic of Germany, Italy, Luxembourg, and the Netherlands). The Treaty of Rome was signed on 25 March 1957.

2.3 THE MEMBER STATES OF THE EUROPEAN ECONOMIC COMMUNITY

The United Kingdom (UK), Denmark, and the Republic of Ireland joined the EEC in 1973 and completed a transition period to full membership in 1977. Greece joined the EC in May 1979. Portugal and Spain joined on 1 January 1986.

The twelve Member States (countries) of the EC currently comprise 320 million people (with approximately another 17 million with the German Democratic Republic fully integrated with the Federal Republic of Germany). The Member States are listed in Table 2.1.

The main official languages are recorded in Table 2.1. In Belgium German is also an official language. In Luxembourg Luxemburgish is also official and widely used.

2.4 THE COMMUNITY INSTITUTIONS

2.4.1 The Commission of the European Communities

There are seventeen Commissioners appointed by the twelve Member States for a renewable term of four years. They are pledged to be independent of national and particular interests. The current President of the Commission (second term) is M. Jacques Delors.

The Commissioners act as the policy-making body of the Community. Their staffs are in the twenty-two Directorates-General (Table 2.2).

Pharmaceutical and veterinary regulation is included in DG III (Internal Market). The services responsible are DG III/C-3. Veterinary matters are also a part responsibility of DG VI (Agriculture) — particularly the feed premix products (growth promoters, hormones, etc.).

DG III/C-3 (current Chef de services M. Fernand Sauer) is responsible for:

- producing proposals for pharmaceutical and veterinary legislation,
- servicing and running the Committee for Proprietary Medicinal Products (CPMP),
- servicing and running the Committee for Veterinary Medicinal Products (CVMP),
- servicing and running the Pharmaceutical Committee.

2.4.2 The Council of Ministers

The Council of Ministers meets to discuss and decide on specific issues according to their portfolios. For the most important political and strategic issues it will meet as a Council of Prime Ministers (and equivalents) of the Member States. For trade issues it meets as a Council of (Trade) Ministers, for health issues as a Council of (Health) Ministers, for agricultural questions as a Council of (Agriculture) Ministers etc.

The Council of Ministers may decide on particular issues by majority vote, by qualified majority vote, or by unanimity — depending on the issue.

The Commission of the European Communities (CEC) can propose a variety of legal instruments to the appropriate Council of Ministers, and, after consultation with the Economic and Social Committee and the European Parliament, they may be adopted. The available legal instruments are Regulations, Directives, Decisions, Recommendations, and Opinions. The characteristics of each type of legal instrument is discussed later in relation to the current and future legislation in the pharmaceutical sector.

Draft measures are examined by the Council — firstly by expert Working Groups of officials, then by the Committee of Permanent Representatives of the EC Ambassadors in Brussels (COREPER). If there is agreement in COREPER, the measure will normally be adopted by the Council of Ministers.

Table 2.1 — The EC Member States

Country	Population (millions)	Language(s)
Belgium	10	French/Flemish
Germany (West)	62	German
Italy	57	Italian
United Kingdom	56	English
France	54	French
Spain	38	Spanish
Netherlands	14	Dutch (Flemish)
Portugal	10	Portuguese
Greece	10	Greek
Denmark	5	Danish
Ireland	3	English
Luxembourg	0.5	French

Table 2.2 — The Directorates-General

DG I	External Relations
DG II	Economic and Financial Affairs
DG III	Internal Market and Industry
DG IV	Competition
DG V	Employment, Social Affairs, Education
DG VI	Agriculture
DG VII	Transport
DG VIII	Development
DG IX	Personnel and Administration
DG X	Information and Culture
DG XI	Environment, Consumer Protection, Nuclear Safety
DG XII	Science and Research
DG XIII	Telecommunications, Information Industries, Innovation
DG XIV	Fisheries
DG XV	Financial Institutions and Company Law
DG XVI	Regional Policy
DG XVII	Energy
DG XVIII	Credits and Investment
DG XIX	Budgets
DG XX	Financial Control
DG XXI	Customs Union and Indirect Taxation
DG XXII	Coordination of Structural Instruments

The Presidency of the Council of Ministers is a rotating one, each country (in an alphabetical sequence) having a six-month period. In 1990 there was an Irish presidency followed by an Italian one. In 1991 they will be succeeded by the Luxembourg presidency, etc.

The Council of Ministers meets in Brussels for nine months of the year. For the other three months (April, June, and October) it meets in Luxembourg.

2.4.3 The European Parliament
The first Parliament had 142 members, and this has been increased to 518 as more EC Member States have acceded to the Treaty of Rome. The last elections were held in June 1989.

Members of the European Parliament (MEPs) exercise joint control with the Council of Ministers on non-obligatory expenditure (i.e. all except farm support).

The 1985 Single European Act amended the Treaty of Rome and gave the Parliament greater powers. In particular, under the 'co-operation procedure' the Council of Ministers adopts a common position on a bill taking into account the Parliament's opinion. The Parliament then has three months to accept the proposals (or not); if it accepts the proposals it passes and becomes law. Under the 'assent' procedure Parliament has a final say in commercial agreements between EC and non-EC countries, and on the admission of new Member States. (Turkey applied in 1987.)

2.4.4 The Economic and Social Committee
This is an advisory body which brings together industrialists, trades unionists, and other sectors of EC opinion.

2.4.5 The European Court of Justice (ECJ)
This is the final court of appeal against decisions in the national Member States. The ECJ exists to safeguard Community law, and it is the final court of appeal where there are difficulties in the interpretation or application of Community law. An example in the pharmaceutical sector is the judgement in the 'De Peijper' case in 1976 where a dispute between a Dutch wholesaler and the Dutch authorities on requirements to be applied to parallel imported pharmaceutical products was referred to the ECJ under Article 177 of the Treaty of Rome. This judgement gave the Commission an interpretative ruling on the application of the Treaty to the free movement of pharmaceutical products, and in particular on the provisions of Articles 30 to 36 of the Treaty of Rome. This interpretation is stated in the Commission communication on parallel imports of 6 May 1982, which is now used as the basis for all the national schemes to regulate parallel pharmaceutical imports in the EC.

There are thirteen judges and six advocate-generals who serve the ECJ. They serve a six-year term. The Court is situated in Luxembourg.

The stages in an ECJ case are:

- written complaint and defence,
- oral hearing in front of the judges,

- opinion by the advocate-general,
- verdict (by majority vote).

2.5 THE LEGAL INSTRUMENTS OF THE COMMUNITY

In the pharmaceutical sector, the majority of legal instruments have been Directives and Recommendations. A Council Decision was used (75/320/EEC) to establish the Pharmaceutical Committee on 20 May 1975.

The legal instruments used to set up the post-1992 future system will be a Regulation and three Directives.

The characteristics of the various types of instrument are as follows.

2.5.1 Regulations

These have a general scope and have a mandatory effect in the Member States. They bind the Member States and have the force of law without the need of transformation into national legislation or of confirmation by their legislative assemblies (national parliaments). A regulation cannot be overriden by national legislation which is incompatible with it. Regulations have to be published in the *Official Journal of the European Communities*. They become binding on the date specified or, in the absence of such a specified date, on the twentieth day following their publication. Regulations are designed to act as an instrument to achieve conformity in the Community. However, some aspects may have to be left to the Member States — such as fees, levies and national penal sanctions.

2.5.2 Directives

These can be issued by the Council or the Commission. Unlike Regulations, which are binding in their entirety, Directives are binding as to the result to be achieved upon each EC Member State. The choice of the method is left to the State concerned. Thus Directives do not have uniformity as their objective, but instead the approximation of national laws. The text of the Directives themselves usually sets a time limit upon implementation of the Directives. Even so, the Member States may not always comply promptly with the agreed timetable for implementation. Like Regulations, Directives have to be based on the powers in the Treaty of Rome. If national laws are inconsistent with the Directives, it is usually assumed that the Directive has an overriding effect.

Most of the pharmaceutical sector legislation has been Directives emanating from the Council of Ministers. Some of the more recent Directives (e.g. 89/341/EEC, 89/342/EEC, 89/343/EEC) have created a Committee for Technical Adaptation, which will look at some of the technical details required in (say) marketing authorisation applications for particular products. These will be 'technical' Directives. The Directives which created these new powers, and which brought (for example) new categories of product into the Directives, are often referred to as 'framework Directives', i.e. they created a framework on which the more detailed provisions could be based. The technical Directives are likely to be Commission Directives.

2.5.3 Decisions

A Decision of the Council or the Commission is binding in its entirety on those to whom it is addressed. It may be addressed to Member States, to individuals, or to companies. It must be notified to those to whom it is directed, and it takes effect on such a notification.

In the pharmaceutical sector, a Council of Ministers Decision was used to establish the Pharmaceutical Committee on 20 May 1975.

It is also proposed as part of the future system proposals (Chapter 21), that the CEC would have powers to issue Decisions on individual marketing authorisation applications after receiving the opinion of the Committee for Proprietary Medicinal Products (CPMP) for human pharmaceutical products) or the Committee for Veterinary Medicinal Products (CVMP) (for veterinary products). These Decisions would be addressed to both the applicant company and the Member States.

2.5.4 Recommendations

These have persuasive force on those addressed. Many of the early guidelines on various aspects of testing of pharmaceutical products to provide information for a marketing authorisation application were Council Recommendations. In more recent times the CPMP itself has directly issued guidelines without involving the Council of Ministers.

2.5.5 Opinions

These also have persuasive but not binding force.

2.5.6 Communications

These again have persuasive but not binding force. The CEC issued the text of a Communication on parallel imports on 6 May 1982 setting out guidance for the Member States as to how to regulate this trade. The Communication took into account the precedents set by the various European Court judgments — such as the De Peijper case in 1976.

2.6 THE SINGLE EUROPEAN ACT AND THE SINGLE MARKET

The Single European Act was adopted in December 1985, and it amends the Treaty of Rome. Its provisions include:

- the adoption by the Community of the means to establish the Single Market by 31 December 1992. It defines this as 'an area without internal frontiers in which the free movement of goods, services, and capital is ensured in accordance with the provisions of this Treaty',
- deregulation for small/medium businesses,
- progressive realisation of monetary union,
- help for the poorer EC regions,
- the European Parliament given a new 'co-operation procedure',
- encouragement of technological research,
- action to improve the environment,

2.7 THE EUROPEAN FREE TRADE ASSOCIATION (EFTA)

EFTA was formed on 3 May 1960 as a reaction to the EEC. The six current EFTA countries are Austria, Finland, Iceland, Norway, Sweden, and Switzerland. They have a total population of about 33 million.

The EFTA countries have privileged access to the EC in terms of trade, and there is a programme of multilateral cooperation on trade matters and removal of technical barriers to trade. This common trading area of the EC and EFTA is sometimes referred to as the 'European Economic Space'.

From 1990, the EFTA countries have observers on the main technical working parties of the CPMP, and they are particularly concerned with development of new guidelines.

The EFTA countries all accept the same format for applications as laid down in the 'Notice to Applicants', the same requirements for Expert Reports, and the same technical guidelines.

2.8 THE NORDIC COUNCIL

The Nordic Council on Medicines is a joint Nordic organisation comprising Denmark (an EC Member State), Finland, Iceland, Norway, and Sweden. It was established in 1975 by the Nordic Council of (health and social services) Ministers. The objective is to promote the harmonisation of legislative and administrative procedures in the Nordic countries. The Council consists of two representatives from each of its Member States appointed by national governments and including medical, pharmaceutical, and legal experts. The Council has an advisory and coordinating function and is not a supranational body.

The Council has issued Nordic guidelines on subjects such as:

- labelling of proprietary medicinal products,
- registration of allergen preparations,
- clinical trials,
- drug applications,
- evaluation reports,
- bioavailability studies in man,
- radiopharmaceuticals.

Other duties of the Nordic Council include the coordination of statistics on medicines, adverse drug reaction reporting, drug information, and pharmacopoeial requirements.

From 1990 the Nordic Council has also had an observer on each of the main working parties of the CPMP.

REFERENCE

The 'De Peijper' case. Court of Justice of the European Communities 20 May 1976, Case 104/75, Page 613, 1976 Report.

3
New chemical active substance products: quality requirements

3.1 INTRODUCTION

This chapter discusses the chemistry and pharmacy data requirements applying to new chemical active ingredient-containing pharmaceutical products intended for use in humans. In this context a new chemical active substance is an active ingredient prepared by chemical synthesis which has not been previously assessed by the regulatory authority to which an application for a product licence (marketing authorisation) is submitted. The data requirements for such chemicals are demanding.

It should be noted that it is possible for the term 'new active ingredient' to apply to materials used widely outside the geographical limits of the authority to which an application is made if that authority has not previously approved the material concerned. An example came to light recently where a material included in the *United States Pharmacopeia* (USP) was included in an application to the United Kingdom (UK) regulatory authority which had not been previously licensed in the UK: it was treated as a new chemical active substance.

If a novel pharmaceutical excipient (that is part of the non-active component of the formulated product) is used in a product it is possible for it to be treated in the same way as a new active ingredient in terms of data requirements, especially if it is significantly absorbed. New salts, esters, or molecular compounds of known active ingredients may also be treated as new active ingredients.

The framework of the European Community (EC) pharmaceutical Directives is common to the whole of the EC, as are the guidance notes and the Notice to Applicants produced by the Committee for Proprietary Medicinal Products (CPMP). These form the basis for the data expectations for all Member States. The contents of this chapter reflect the interpretation put on these documents in the UK in the summer of 1990.

3.2 SOURCES OF INFORMATION

The main sources of information are the EC pharmaceutical Directives (Table 3.1), the notes for guidance produced by the CPMP (Table 3.2), and the 1989 edition of

Table 3.1 — The EC pharmaceutical Directives

Directive	Date of adoption
65/65/EEC	26 January 1966
75/318/EEC	20 May 1975
75/319/EEC	20 May 1975
83/570/EEC	26 October 1983
87/19/EEC	22 December 1986
87/21/EEC	22 December 1986
87/22/EEC	22 December 1986
89/341/EEC	3 May 1989
89/342/EEC	3 May 1989
89/343/EEC	3 May 1989
89/381/EEC	14 June 1989

Table 3.2 — CPMP guidance notes on quality

Guidance notes: quality matters
Development pharmaceutics and process validation
Chemistry of active ingredients
Stability tests
Herbal remedies
Analytical validation[†]
European drug master file procedures for active ingredients[‡]

[†] Adopted and circulated to trade associations.
[‡] Adopted summer 1990.

the Notice to Applicants, also produced by the CPMP. In addition there are a number of national guidelines for areas not yet covered by EC guidance; those in use in the UK are given in Table 3.3.

3.3 REQUIREMENTS RELATING TO THE FORMAT OF THE APPLICATION

The EC Notice to Applicants includes a standardised format for applications. The application is divided into five parts which are listed in Table 3.4.

The number of copies of the dossier required varies from country to country, with different requirements for different parts of the dossier. Up to four copies of the complete dossier are requested (the highest number being required by Germany),

Table 3.3 — UK national guidelines on quality matters current summer 1990

UK national quality and related guidelines	
Medicines Advice Leaflet (MAL)	Topic
2	Sterilisation processes and validation
	Radiopharmaceuticals
	Sustained release theophylline products
	Over-the-counter hydrocortisone products
	Construction of pharmaceutical trade marks
	Contact lens care products
2(PI)	Parallel imports
4	Data requirements for clinical trial certificate and clinical trial exemption applications
39	Herbal ingredients (now largely replaced by CPMP guideline with respect to quality aspects)
41	Biological medicinal products
61	Intrauterine contraceptive devices

Note: A full list of currrent MALs is included in Appendix 2 of Chapter 17.

with up to seventeen copies of the pharmaceutical section (by the UK). Most countries require additional copies of the summaries (Parts I and V and Expert Reports), with fifty copies required by France. Full details of the numbers of copies required according to the 1989 edition of the Notice to Applicants are reproduced in Table 3.5.

In principle, all Member States require applications to be submitted in their own national language(s). In practice, most will allow submission of some or all parts of the dossier in alternative languages. The effect of this is that the greater part of the dossier can be submitted in English across the EC. With respect to the pharmaceutical aspects of the application and the Expert Reports, the only exception to this is in Spain for both Part II and the Expert Report, and France and Portugal for the Expert Report (both of whom will accept French).

In this chapter the information requirements of Parts I, II, and V are discussed, with some consideration of the interplay between Part II and Parts III and IV.

3.4 PART I: THE SUMMARY OF THE DOSSIER

3.4.1 Introduction

This part of the application includes necessary administrative information, the summary of product characteristics (which becomes the basis of the marketing authorisation), and the Expert Reports. Each of these sections is discussed in turn.

Table 3.4 — Standard format for EC applications for marketing authorisation for pharmaceutical products

Part		Content
I		Summary of the dossier
	IA	Administrative data
	IB	Summary of product characteristics
	IC	Expert Reports (chemical and pharmaceutical; toxicopharmacological; clinical)
II		Chemical, pharmaceutical, and biological documentation
	IIA	Composition
	IIB	Method of preparation
	IIC	Control of starting materials
	IID	Control on intermediate products
	IIE	Control tests on the finished product
	IIF	Stability
	IIQ	Other information
III		Pharmacotoxicological documentation
	IIIA	Single dose toxicity
	IIIB	Repeated dose toxicity
	IIIC	Reproduction studies
	IIID	Mutagenic potential
	IIIE	Oncogenic/carcinogenic potential
	IIIF	Pharmacodynamics
	IIIG	Pharmacokinetics
	IIIH	Local tolerance (toxicity)
	IIIQ	Other information
IV		Clinical documentation
	IVA	Clinical pharmacology
	IVB	Clinical experience
	IVQ	Other information
V		Special particulars
	VA	Dosage form
	VB	Samples
	VC	Manufacturers authorisation(s)
	VD	Marketing authorisation(s)

Note: Parts II to V are preceded by a Table of Contents.

3.4.2 Administrative information

This part of the application includes basic information on the name of the pharmaceutical product and its active ingredient(s) (using the international nonproprietary names (INNs) where these are available) and describing the pharmaceutical form of

Table 3.5 — Numbers of copies of parts of the dossier required in EC Member States

Country	Full dossier	Part II	Additional summaries Parts I, V
Belgium†	1	+2	5
Denmark	1	—	1
Germany	4	—	10
Greece	1	—	5
Spain‡	2	+3	12
France§	2	+3	50
Ireland	1	—	3
Italy	2	—	10
Luxembourg	1	+2	1
Netherlands¶	2	+1	3
Portugal	2	+1	4
UK	3	+17	—
CPMP	1	—	2

Notes: † Belgium: 2 additional copies of Part IVA. Clinical pharmacology may be requested.
‡ Spain: 1 additional copy of Part III Toxicology required.
§ France: 1 additional copy of Part III Toxicology required. 8 additional copies of Part II. Pharmaceutical required for concertation applications.
¶ Netherlands: 1 additional copy of part IVA Clinical pharmacology required. 1 additional copy of Part II Pharmaceutical required for concertation applications.

All member States and CPMP require 2 copies of consolidated responses except Germany, who requires 4 copies.

the product (such as tablet, injection, solution), route of administration, and the amount of active ingredient(s) present.

The names and addresses of any company holding a marketing authorisation are stated, as is the name of the person or company who submitted the specific application. The person responsible for marketing the product in the Member State is stated where this differs from the applicant. Manufacturer(s) of the active ingredient are stated, together with an indication of what stages of the synthesis they undertake. Importers and distributors are also named.

The signature of the applicant and the date of the application are required. In addition, the content and number of volumes of supporting data provided are stated. Where an application is submitted through the multistate procedure (which is discussed in detail in Chapter 14) the applicant is required also to identify any differences in the files that have been submitted, compared with the data provided to the Member State which issued the first marketing authorisation on which the multistate application is based.

3.4.3 Summary of product characteristics

This is a key document, since the information contained in it determines the basis for the assessment of the application, and, once a marketing authorisation has been gained, controls the claims that can be made for the product. The advertising material and the information provided to practitioners (for example in data sheets in the UK) has to be in line with the information in the approved summary of product characteristics. Within the CPMP high technology and multistate procedures there is an increasing desire to arrive at a common summary of product characteristics throughout the EC for a given product. This is likely to increase as proposed new CPMP/EC procedures are progressively introduced. (This is discussed further in Chapters 14, 15, and 21.)

This part of the dossier contains information on the name of the medicinal product and qualitative and quantitative particulars of its composition in terms both of the active ingredient(s) and the excipients. Where they exist, INNs are used to describe the ingredients, or in their absence appropriate common names or chemical descriptions (or botanical descriptions where necessary). The pharmaceutical form and route of administration are stated.

Where useful for therapeutic purposes, information on the pharmacological properties of the active ingredient is included together with the clinical indications, contraindications, precautions, and special warnings associated with the use of the product. The dosage (described in the Notice of Applicants as 'posology') for adults, the elderly, and children are differentiated as necessary, and information included on the symptoms, appropriate emergency procedures, and any antidotes to overdoses. Any special considerations relating to use in pregnancy or lactation or effects on the ability to drive or operate machinery are stated.

Information on known clinical interactions (with other medication or any other factor) or pharmaceutical incompatibility is included. Additional pharmaceutical information is included in the summary of product characteristics on the type and contents of the container, the shelf life, and storage precautions for the product (and if necessary for the reconstituted product).

3.4.4 Expert Reports

Each application includes Expert Reports. Three such reports are required in the case of applications for products containing new chemical active ingredients. These are on the chemical, pharmaceutical, and biological documentation; on the toxicological and pharmacological documentation; and on the clinical documentation. While each Expert Report is self-standing it is important to realise that the Experts should be familiar with all relvant aspects of the application: there are certain areas of common interest, such as the relevance of the purity profile of the active ingredient used in the preclinical safety studies compared with that of the material to be marketed, and in certain aspects of the bioavailability testing, for example. It is expected that such common areas will be discussed by all relevant Experts.

The subject of Expert Reports is discussed fully in Chapter 11. In the present chapter discussion is limited to the necessary qualifications of the author of the pharmaceutical Expert Report and what is expected of him in general terms.

The pharmaceutical Expert for a chemical new active ingredient, according to the Notice of Applicants, should hold a formal qualification in pharmacy and have had practical experience in research and development, manufacture, or physicochemical, biological, or microbiological control of medicinal products. In the UK consideration will be given to the acceptability of Expert Report authors who do not hold these qualifications, but the use of such Experts has to be fully justified on each occasion they are used.

The pharmaceutical Expert Report should consist of three sections. The first is a short product profile, consisting of a one or two page summary which extracts key information from the summary of product characteristics. This should include information on the type of application, the chemical and pharmacokinetic properties of the active ingredient, and relevant characteristics of the dosage form. Clinical indications, pharmacological and therapeutic classification of the active ingredient(s), and their mode(s) of action are included. The product profile also includes significant precautions and warnings associated with the use of the product. In the case of a product already on the market, the countries in which authorisation has been obtained are stated and a list of post-marketing surveillance studies provided.

The second section of the Expert Report, which can be particularly useful, consists of a critical evaluation of the methods, results, and conclusions based on the data submitted. The suggested sequence of the data closely follows the recommended format for applications, with the addition of a conclusion, a reference list, and information on the expert. The Expert is expected to take a position on the basis of the information included in the dossier which he can defend in the light of current technical and professional knowledge. This section is not normally expected to be more than ten pages long.

The Notice to Applicants includes suggested formats for the concise but accurate summaries of the supporting data which form the basis of the third part of the Expert Report. These 'formats' are not obligatory and are not 'forms' to be completed slavishly. They are a useful *aide mémoire* to the type of information that is often included in an application, but the detail will vary with specific cases. The omission of data from major sections of the formats should, however, be justified.

Where a drug master file has been referred to in connection with an application for a marketing authorisation it is necessary for the applicant and the drug master file provider to ensure that, between them, all relevant information has been submitted. This may involve the pharmaceutical expert discussing matters of common interest with the author of the drug master file Expert Report.

3.5 PART II: THE CHEMICAL, PHARMACEUTICAL, AND BIOLOGICAL DOCUMENTATION

3.5.1 Introduction

This is the main section of the application with respect to pharmaceutical data. In it all the relevent information is provided. The following comments take into account the data requirements in the EC pharmaceutical Directives (particularly the Annex to Directive 75/318/EEC) which are obligatory, and the relevant EC and national (in this case UK) guidance notes as well as the CPMP Notice to Applicants (the latter two sets of documents being advisory).

3.5.2 Description of analytical methods and analytical validation

Increasing emphasis is being placed on adequate descriptions being included of the analytical methods used in applications. They should be described in sufficient detail to enable the regulatory authority to repeat the methods on samples of the ingredient or product. In order to do this it is necessary to provide details of the test conditions, reagents, reference materials used, and any special precautions necessary in carrying out the test. It is often necessary for system suitability tests or other verification procedures to be included in the information provided. Where necessary, the formulae used to calculate the results are also included.

Full details are required where non-commercially available equipment is used in a particular procedure. Where possible, comparative data on the performance of similar commercially-available equipment should be included.

The provision of adequate analytical validation data is becoming increasingly important. In the case of pharmacopoeial methods applied to monograph materials validation may not be required where the relevance of the method to the source of material can be demonstrated.

Analytical validation of a method may need to take into account the following factors: specificity, precision (both repeatability and reproducibility), accuracy, linearity, range, sensitivity, limit of detection, limit of quantitation, and robustness. Which of these need to be established in a particular case depends on the intended use of the analytical procedure.

The interpretation of 'specificity' varies according to the use to which the analytical procedure is to be put. In an identity or impurity test it relates to the ability of the method to identify an individual analyte, which might be the active molecule or a related substance, organic solvent, heavy metal, etc., depending on the purpose of the test. In an assay the specificity relates to the measurement of the signal from the wanted analyte and the lack of interference from excipients, degradation products, or impurities. For routine assays specificity may not be an absolute requirement; it is more important in stability test assays.

'Accuracy' is the closeness of agreement of the determined value with the true value or with an accepted reference value (for example, compared with a pharmacopoeial reference material with an assigned purity). The determination of the accuracy of a method may involve a comparison of the method to be used with one of a defined accuracy such as a standard pharmacopoeial procedure for a class of active ingredients, or may involve the addition of known quantities of the analyte to matrix of the usual excipients found in a formulated product.

The determination of 'precision', or the closeness of agreement of a series of measurements, requires two series of experiments. One of these determines the repeatability of the method, using the same analysts and apparatus over a short time interval and using identical reagents. The second series of experiments involves different laboratories, using different reagent sources, different analysts, and different equipment manufacturers, with determinations carried out over a longer period.

The limit of detection is the lowest amount of an analyte that can be detected (but not quantified exactly). The limit of quantitation is the lowest amount of analyte that can be determined with a defined level of precision and accuracy under the stated conditions.

Linearity of a method relates to the range of concentrations of the analyte over which test results are obtained which are directly proportional to the concentration of the analyte. The range of the method is the interval between the upper and lower concentrations of the analyte over which acceptable precision, accuracy, and linearity are demonstrated. The sensitivity of a procedure is its ability to record small variations in the concentration of the analyte.

The need for appropriate validation of analytical methods is not restricted to the pharmaceutical parts of the dossier. The methods of analysis applied to the samples of biological origin in the preclinical and clinical sections of the application should also have been validated.

3.5.3 Part IIA: Composition

In this part of the application information is included on the qualitative and quantitative composition of the product, on the containers and closures, and on any different formulae used during clinical trials. An account of the pharmaceutical development of the product is included in this section.

The names (ideally INNs) of all active and other ingredients are stated, together with an appropriate unit or percentage formula. The function of each ingredient in the formulation is stated briefly, and a statement made concerning the standard applied to each ingredient. This may relate to in-house standards or to pharmacopoeial specifications. Where there is a *European Pharmacopoeia* (Ph Eur) specification this should be used.

A brief statement is included on the fabric of the container and the closure, with fuller details included elsewhere (Part VA). The method of opening and closing the container is stated. In the UK particular attention is paid to the tamper-evident nature of closures for products which are supplied sterile — for example, ophthalmic multi-dose preparations, multi-dose vials for injectable products — although tamper evidence is a useful safety feature against unauthorised tampering with any product before it is used. Some products — such as aspirin and paracetamol tablets and capsules for general sales — need to be in child resistant containers.

Where different formulations from those proposed for marketing have been used in the clinical trials these are discussed in this section. The pharmaceutical Expert Report should include a discussion of the possible effects of the differences in formulation on bioavailability, bioequivalence, and stability profile in appropriate cases.

The development pharmaceutics information included in this section of the dossier is the applicant's opportunity to show how the formulation was developed. It is not unusual for the development of a formulation to be fraught with problems: the development pharmaceutics section of the application is the company's chance to show what problems were encountered and overcome in arriving at the final product.

Consideration of the compatibility of the active and the inactive components of the formulation and of the excipient components with each other is discussed in this section. The physical characteristics of the active ingredient (such as crystal size and shape, solvation, or polymorphism) that affect the performance of the finished product are discussed. Factors affecting physical properties of the formulated product such as dispersibility, rheological properties, and the need for additives such as antioxidants or antimicrobial preservatives are included. Compatibility with other products with which the product may be co-administered (for example intravenous solutions used as solvents for the product) is discussed. In the case of intravenous solutions, data are required in some cases on compatibility with giving sets, for example where adsorption may be a problem.

In this section a justification is advanced for any claimed overages in the product with an explanation for their need (such as manufacturing loss or instability on storage).

In the case of solid dosage forms some data are normally included on the dissolution performance of the formulated product, with justification for the dissolution medium and conditions chosen and the acceptance limits proposed. Where different test procedures have been applied at different stages of the development of the product their equivalence is usefully discussed. The use of unusual dissolution media such as those containing non-aqueous solvents or surfactants is also justified in this section.

Depending on the stability profile and the batch to batch variability of the manufactured product it is sometimes possible to justify the omission of routine dissolution controls from the finished product specification based on such data.

The homogeneity of distribution of the active ingredient in the finished product is discussed; this is particularly relevant in products containing less than 2 mg of active ingredient per dosage form and where the concentration of active ingredient is 2 percent m/m or less of the total.

The inclusion of unusual constituents in a product — for example, the matrix of a modified release product, new antimicrobial preservative — is discussed in this section. It should be borne in mind that the use of a novel excipient may require additional data on the safety of that material. New uses for known excipients may also result in the need for additional safety data, especially where significant systemic exposure results.

The choice of the container system in terms of integrity and potential interaction with the product (either sorption or leaching) is justified in this section. In appropriate cases the applicant provides data to demonstrate the reproducibility of the dose when using the proposed marketing system, especially where this is critical.

3.5.4 Part IIB: Method of manufacture of the dosage form

In this section the applicant includes information on the manufacturing batch size and formula, the manufacturing process, and its validation. Information is also included on in-process controls and the assembly process.

Where a number of different batch sizes are to be used for the manufacture of the product an indication of the reasons behind the different options is usefully included in this section. The actual figures quoted for the percentage formula and the batch formula should be in agreement but surprisingly are often at variance.

The essential stages of the manufacturing process are described in sufficient detail. Where a specialised piece of equipment is required this is normally stated, but it is not normally necessary the stipulate the make or model of machinery used for standard operations. Any special unit operations are described in sufficient detail, and the process controls applied are discussed. Any sterilisation or disinfection processes applied should be stated. Where these are not generally accepted or pharmacopoeial processes additional information may be required. For products made outside the geographical limits of the Member State to which the application is directed additional information on the manufacturing process and environment are sometimes required; this is true also for products made outside the EC.

The validation of the manufacturing process should be discussed in sufficient detail. The aim of this information is to demonstrate that the process is capable of producing an adequate yield of in-specification material on a routine basis. The use of nonstandard methods of manufacture (or if certain processes are crucial to the production of material of adequate safety) may require additional data. Examples of such cases include the use of nonstandard sterilisation processes (for example, F_0 values of less than 8 minutes, or gamma-irradiation doses of less than 25 kGy) and the manufacture of controlled release products where the manufacturing process contributes significantly to the characteristics of the product.

The information on the in-process controls applied to the manufacturing process indicates what is tested regularly and from what stage of the process the tested material is taken.

The assembly operation is described in outline in this section.

3.5.5 Part IIC: Control of starting materials

The information required in this section depends on whether the material being discussed is novel or not. In the case of a new chemical active ingredient full details are required. For a pharmacopoeial excipient less information is usually required. The following sections consider the information required for different types of ingredient separately.

3.5.5.1 *New active ingredients*

(a) Identity of the material

This section includes details of the nomenclature, tests, and procedures to confirm the identity of the material. This includes its nomenclature, identity, chemical structure, and physical characteristics.

Nomenclature. The nomenclature of the ingredient is described in terms of its INN, any EC national approved name (such as the British Approved Name or BAN), or the United States Adopted Name (USAN). Failing this, the IUPAC systematic chemical name(s), laboratory codes, or proprietary names may be used.

Description. This includes some information on the physical form of the material and the structural and molecular formulae. Stereochemical designations are included, using accepted conventions. The molecular formula and relative molecular mass are included, including those of the therapeutically active part of the molecule. Where such information cannot be provided, some other acceptable detailed description of the material is included.

The appearance is briefly described, following the style of the *European Pharmacopoeia* statements.

(b) Manufacture of the active ingredient

Information is included on the manufacturing sites used to synthesise the active material and on the synthetic or manufacturing route(s) used. This includes a description of the process in general terms as well as details of the solvents, reagents, catalysts, and any critical conditions of reaction used. Information is provided on any isolated or purified intermediates, and particular attention is paid to the final purification stage, including the nature and specification of the solvents used. An annotated flowchart is a useful means of summarising information, and data on the scale of manufacture and the yields obtained are sometimes useful.

Where alternate pathways, reagents, or solvents are used in the synthesis adequate information is provided to demonstrate that the end-product is not significantly different whichever production technique is used.

(c) Quality control during synthesis

The controls applied to the starting materials contributing significantly to the final structure of the chemical are described. These controls normally include identity tests and quality specifications including controls on isomeric and other impurities, especially where these can result in the presence of unwanted impurities or related substances in the finished material. Specifications for solvents which may find their way into the finished material are stated. Acceptance or rejection criteria are stated for all key materials.

For isolated intermediates the controls applied are discussed, as are any control checks carried out at each stage of the synthesis. Acceptance and rejection criteria are stated for each stage of the synthesis, as appropriate.

(d) Development chemistry

This section of the application provides an insight into the development of the synthetic route and proof of the structure of the material to be marketed. The information generated in the development of the synthesis is used when considering what control tests are necessary to ensure batch-to-batch consistency of the material.

Evidence of the chemical structure and potential isomerism are provided. Proof of structure, configuration conformation, and potential isomerism of the material are considered to be important. The stereochemical properties of the compound are of particular significance; a justification for the use of a racemate is necessary. This needs to be discussed by the pharmaceutical, the pharmacotoxicological, and the clinical Experts in their Reports. The introduction of a single isomer of a marketed racemate may be treated as a new substance in its own right.

Details are included of the structure of key intermediates, with elemental analyses of the finished compound and spectral evidence obtained by using techniques such as infrared spectrophotometry, proton and ^{13}C-carbon nuclear magnetic resonance spectrometry, ultraviolet spectrometry (including evidence of pH-dependent shifts), mass spectra, X-ray crystallography, etc., as well as diagnostic chemical reactions and optical rotation values as supporting data. One practical problem often encountered is poor quality reproduction of spectral evidence. Applicants should check carefully that the copies of the spectra are actually legible and that they are accompanied by accurate interpretations. It has not been unknown for the interpretation of a mass spectrum to be a few units of mass out throughout the range!

Other physicochemical attributes of the chemical are discussed, especially where these might have a bearing on the bioavailability of the finished product. The information in this section can include solubility in a range of solvents including the dissolution medium used in development studies and, particularly in the case of topical formulations in the component parts of the basis proposed for use, crystallinity, particle size and shape, solvation, pH, pK_a, melting or boiling point, and potential polymorphism.

Full characterisation details of any primary reference material are provided, together with information on any secondary or working standards. Analytical development and validation are adequately discussed.

(e) Impurities

The purpose of this section of the application is to demonstrate the adequacy of the test procedures proposed for impurity control. Particular attention is again paid to analytical validation, especially the limit of detection and limit of quantification of the methods.

The impurities to be considered are those which may arise as synthetic by-products (including products of side reactions, impurities carried through from the starting materials, and isomers formed during synthesis), residual reagents or catalysts, residual solvents, and even degradation products. The potential impurities that could be present on theoretical grounds are derived from pH, light, moisture, or heat stress studies on the material are discussed. These should be compared with those impurities actually found in practice. Wherever possible, impurities are identified and quantified. Where the identities of impurities are not known they are still reported and quantified as far as possible.

Actual results of impurity levels found in a number of recently manufactured batches of material prepared by the proposed synthetic route are required. Statements such as 'complies with the limit' are not helpful in this context. Data are also provided on the levels and the nature of impurities present in batches used for toxicity testing. All available data should be used to formulate a proposed impurity control specification for the material. This should be justified in the pharmaceutical Expert Report. Particular attention will be paid during assessment to differences between the purity of preclinical and marketing material. Adequate discussion of this is usefully included in the pharmaceutical and the pharmacotoxicological Expert Reports.

Where chromatographic methods are used to monitor impurities, legible copies of the chromatographs are provided. In the case of thin-layer chromatographic methods, photographs of typical plates can be useful. It should be remembered that photographs do not photocopy well. Where it is necessary to use photographs, originals are best provided with each copy of the application.

(f) Active ingredient specification

A specification is proposed which includes adequate controls on the physical and other relevant characteristics of the material, its identity (including each part of the molecule in the case of a salt or ester), and standards for its potency. Assays need not necessarily be specific provided that the identity of the material is adequately controlled by other means. Purity controls for individual and total named impurities and adequate controls over individual and total unknown impurities are required. Full details of analytical methods are required, together with validation data.

(g) Batch analyses
It has already been indicated that impurity profiles are required for a number of active ingredient batches of the materials prepared by the synthetic route proposed for marketing. Ideally, data are provided on at least five consecutive, full-scale, recently-manufactured lots, although it might be possible to provide data on full-scale manufacture on an on-going basis. Similar data for batches used in toxicity testing and clinical trials are also required. The analytical data cover all aspects of the proposed specification for the material, and actual results should be provided. The proposed methods of analysis should have been used to generate these data.

Batch analysis reports normally include details of the date and place of manufacture, the batch size and number, the use to which the batches were put, and the actual analytical results. Where the tests carried out or the methods of analysis used differ from those proposed for the marketing authorisation an explanation is provided of the significance of the differences.

Where an optically active compound is involved, data are provided on the batch-to-batch constancy of the isomeric ratio. This information is taken into account by the three Expert Report authors in discussing the toxicological, pharmacological, pharmacokinetic, and clinical significance of any variability.

The application includes a discussion of the results, with particular attention being paid to any inconsistencies or anomalies apparent in the data.

3.5.5.2 *Radiolabelled compounds*
The information expected for these materials is similar in many respects to that described for new active ingredients. Particular attention may need to be paid to the stability of the radiolabel. The metabolic stability of the radiolabelling will need to be addressed in the pharmacotoxicology section of the dossier.

3.5.5.3 *Other ingredients*
Where there is a pharmacopoeial specification in the *European Pharmacopoeia* or the pharmacopoeia of a Member State of the EC, then the monograph specification is to be applied. It might be necessary for the applicant company to demonstrate that the specification is relevant with regard to the adequacy of the monograph in controlling impurities likely to be present for material from the stated manufacturing source. There may be some instances where a pharmacopoeial monograph is considered to be inadequate for the intended use of the material. In such cases additional tests may be required.

If it is wished to use the monograph of a non-EC Member State full justification is required. A translation of the monograph and any associated analytical methods is required unless the original is in an acceptable language, and the adequacy of the specification for the control of the material to be used may have to be demonstrated.

Where the material is not the subject of a pharmacopoeial specification, information of the kind expected for a new active ingredient may be expected. The amount of data required depends on factors such as the amount of material likely to be systematically absorbed and the period over which the material will be administered. The specification proposed for the material is expected to include adequate controls on its characteristics and description, its identity, its purity, its potency, and other relevant evaluations which may include performance standards.

3.5.6 Part IID: Control tests applied at an intermediate stage of the manufacturing process

This section includes information on any testing carried out to ensure that the production process results in a consistent product. This type of testing may be of particular importance in cases where analytical techniques are not available for monitoring the content of particular ingredients in the finished product. It may also be used where the manufacturing process confers a key property to the finished product — for example, modified release — which is best monitored as part of the production process.

Details are also included in this section of any control tests carried out on intermediate products, such as testing of the cores of tablets which are subsequently coated.

3.5.7 Part IIE: Control tests on the finished product

The proposals for control tests on the finished product take into account current technical and scientific developments in the relevant field. All methods are adequately described, especially if they are not described in a phamacopoeia and are not otherwise well known. The requirements of the general monographs of the *European Pharmacopoeia* are to be applied to all relevant dosage forms, even in the absence of a specific monograph. Any additional requirements of a Member State's national pharmacopoeia monograph that apply to a particular product are to be complied with.

The tests falling under this heading include those for mechanical and physical properties and pharmaceutical tests such as disintegration tests and dissolution tests, and those for relevant microbiological attributes such as compliance with a permitted total viable count of microorganisms and/or absence of named pathogens, or compliance with the requirements of a sterility test. Controls on average weights, or in the case of products containing small amounts of active ingredients, the uniformity of content, and permitted deviations from these are included if appropriate.

The finished product specification also includes relevant tests for organoleptic properties (appearance, smell, taste in appropriate cases, clarity, density, pH, refractive index, etc.) and identity of active ingredients and certain excipients such as antimicrobial preservatives and antioxidants as well as permitted colours. Some Member States require at least identity tests for the components of the excipient.

Quantitative determinations of active ingredients and important excipients such as antioxidants and antimicrobial preservatives (which must have at least an upper assay limit, but which in practice should usually have upper and lower limits) are normally required as a minimum. The assay limits for active ingredients at the time of manufacture are normally expected to be within ±5 per cent of the nominal content unless wider limits can be appropriately justified. Release limits for other constituents may be rather wider if justified. Where it is not possible to assay for each component of a complex mixture of active ingredients (each present at a relatively low concentration) it may be allowable to omit assays for some of the components provided that adequate in-process controls are applied. In such cases it is a normal requirement that suitable analytical methods be available for monitoring the product for composition after it has been released for sale, if the need arises.

Any excipient which potentially affects physiological function or affects the bioavailability of the product is adequately controlled.

Where it is not possible to carry out a chemical or physicochemical assay for the active ingredient it is a requirement that an assay for biological activity be used. If it is necessary to undertake routine tests for abnormal toxicity or local tolerance in animals to ensure the quality of the product, this is stated.

Where stability considerations require wider shelf life specification limits than those proposed for the time of release, a shelf life specification is proposed under the Stability section of the application.

The application should differentiate between those tests carried out as a matter of routine and those carried out on a (stated) periodic basis. If parametric release is requested this is fully justified in the application. Particular attention is paid in such cases to the adequacy of the manufacturer's quality (assurance) system.

Batch analyses of several (at least five) consecutive full-scale production batches of the finished product are preferred. The information provided includes the date and place of manufacture, the batch size, the use to which the batch was put, and the actual results obtained. The method of manufacture should be that proposed in the application. If such information is not available, then any information to hand should be submitted and an undertaking provided to submit the additional information on an on-going basis.

The pharmaceutical Expert Report includes a justification for the proposed release and, if different, check or shelf life specifications in the light of all the information available.

3.5.8 Part IIF: Stability

In the case of a product containing a new active ingredient stability data are required for both the active ingredient and the finished product. The purpose of stability testing is to provide information to enable the applicant to put forward a retest interval for the active ingredient and one or more shelf lives for the dosage form(s). Both are intended to ensure the continued quality, safety, and efficacy of the materials concerned. In order to do this it is necessary to monitor the quality of the material as a function of time under a variety of environmental conditions. The design of stability studies in an individual case is influenced by information gained from the development pharmaceutics, chemical development, and analytical development and validation stages of the development of the product.

3.5.8.1 Active ingredients

In the case of active ingredients which are novel it is necessary to generate stability data in all cases. In the case of known active ingredients, data from the scientific literature may suffice provided that the route of synthesis has not been amended significantly from that already approved by the regulatory authorities. If the route differs in any important way, additional experimental data may be required. Where several sources of raw material are requested, additional comparative stability data may be required.

Data from a minimum of two batches of each novel active ingredient are reported. The batch numbers, date and place of manufacture, and batch size are stated. Material synthesised by the process described in the product licence application is used in the studies unless any alternative can be fully justified. The fabric of the containers used for the stability study is stated, and the relevance of this to normal production, shipping, and storage containers may need to be discussed by the pharmaceutical Expert in his Report.

The test conditions employed are determined by the known physical and chemical properties of the active material, and particularly its sensitivity to light, air, temperature, and moisture. The storage conditions and duration of test are recorded.

Details of the analytical methods and their validation are required. The ability of the analytical methods to detect and quantify both the intact drug and its degradation products are demonstrated. It is also demonstrated that the methods are themselves stable for the duration of the test. In the case of chromatographic tests it might be necessary to include adequate routine system suitability tests, for example.

The stability data are presented with actual numerical test results. It is of little use to indicate that a particular result is in compliance with a limit when part of the purpose of the study is to justify the setting of the limit in the first place. The data are used by the pharmaceutical Expert in discussing the suitability of the proposed active ingredient specification. From the data presented the most appropriate storage conditions for the active ingredient are proposed together with the maximum interval between retests for compliance with the specification.

The pharmaceutical Expert and pharmacotoxicological Expert should both discuss the significance of the levels of decomposition products found in the stability study, particularly with respect to the potential toxicity of the materials found.

3.5.8.2 Finished product

The purpose of stability studies on the dosage form is to establish the product's expected shelf life under stated conditions of storage. With the publication of the guidance note on stability testing by the CPMP the basis of the test's purpose has been somewhat modified; the aim now includes the establishment of the shelf life and storage conditions that can be applied throughout the EC.

The design of stability studies for dosage forms is based on a knowledge of the properties of the active ingredient and the results obtained in the pharmaceutical development studies. The properties of the chosen formulation and the recommendations for the use of the product are also to be taken into account. The detail of the

Sec. 3.5] Part II: Chemical, pharmaceutical and biological documentation

design is also influenced by the proposals included in the CPMP guidance note on stability testing.

It is recommended that real time stability studies be undertaken at 25°C. The mean temperature and the range of temperatures and humidities actually used in the study are recorded. The minimum period over which data are collected for submission with the application is six months, at a mean temperature of 25°C. It is expected that this, taken together with the results from accelerated studies at elevated temperatures, will enable the shelf life at 'room temperature' throughout the EC to be estimated. Labelling statements regarding special storage temperatures (to be stated in °C) are required only for products that will not withstand a temperature of 30°C.

Other conditions suggested in the guidance note for stability tests use accelerated studies to emphasise any potential degradation. The actual conditions used in a particular case depend on the properties of the product concerned but might include elevated temperatures (up to, say, 40°C) or low temperatures (down to, say, −15°C, or at 2° to 8°C, or using a freeze–thaw cycle) or elevated humidity (for example up to 75 per cent relative humidity) or combinations of elevated temperature and humidity (such as 40°C and 75 per cent relative humidity). Additional stress is added by using natural or artificial light in appropriate cases, and the presence or absence of air is another factor to consider.

The product under test is adequately defined. The formulation, container, and manufacturing method are ideally those proposed for the marketed product. Other packaging systems might provide useful supporting data, but data relating to the proposed marketing combination are of greatest relevance. Normally a minimum of three batches are reported, unless the stability of the product is known to be particularly high in which case a minimum of two batches are reported. The active ingredient used is ideally taken from different lots for each batch of finished product. The composition; date, place of manufacture, and name of the manufacturer of the dosage form; batch number; batch size; and lot numbers of the active ingredient are reported. As far as possible the batches are manufactured at full scale, using the proposed manufacturing process, although data from the first two or three production batches may be provided on an on-going basis. Details are included of the packaging system used.

It should be borne in mind that there can be more than one shelf life for a particular product. A freeze-dried injection has a shelf life in the dry state and another after reconstitution. Similarly, a bulk container of a liquid pharmaceutical for dispensing purposes can have a limited shelf life once the pack is opened (possibly due to the effects of air on the stability of the active ingredient or an excipient, or to the potential effects of microbial contamination during use). It is necessary to address each of the potential shelf lives in the stability studies.

The stability study is intended to monitor any aspect of the product that might be affected on storage. This normally includes all those characteristics monitored in the release specification, but additional items may need to be determined in the stability trial if they are likely to provide useful additional information.

In the case of solid dosage forms the dissolution of the active ingredient is monitored during the stability study even if it is proposed that this not be included specifically in the routine testing specification. The characteristics studied normally extend to organoleptic properties of the formulated product and its physical properties (for example, tablet hardness, emulsion stability, resuspendability of suspensions, crystal size, and shape). The antimicrobial preservative efficacy over the proposed shelf life of the product is monitored by using a suitable protocol which enables a kill-curve to be generated over the recommended period of repeat dosing of the product. Antimicrobial preservative efficacy requirements are related to the route of administration and the frequency of use of the product. Multi-dose injections and ophthalmic products are likely to be expected to have greater antimicrobial efficacy activity than, say, an oral mixture or a topical cream used on intact skin.

The chemical stability of the dosage form is also monitored, including assays for the active ingredient and for decomposition products. The content of materials such as antimicrobial preservatives and antioxidants is reported. The possibility of product–container interaction is considered and reported.

Numerical results are presented and discussed, including initial results (that is those at the time of manufacture). An attempt to effect a mass balance (by adding together the total amounts of active ingredients and degradation products over the period of the study) is useful, with any shortfall explained as far as possible. Trends in stability data are analysed. Extrapolations from accelerated studies are explained and justified by the pharmaceutical Expert.

Where different batches of product have different patterns of stability the results are discussed fully. In many cases it is appropriate to set the shelf life of the product based on the least stable batch of material, especially where limited real time data are submitted.

The stability data are used to justify any differences between the release and the shelf life specifications. They also help to justify the inclusion of overages in the formula if the reason for their inclusion is claimed to be limited stability of the product. However, it is important that the pharmaceutical Expert and the pharmaco-toxicological Expert discuss the significance of any degradation products in relation to their potential concentration and toxicological properties.

The note for guidance indicates that additional stability test data from comparative accelerated or real time studies may be required in the case of significant changes being introduced into the formulation, packaging materials, or method of manufacture of the product.

It should be borne in mind that data are also expected on the stability of drugs incorporated in feed or water for use in toxicity studies. A case was recently found where the interpretation of the toxicity data had been compromised because it had not been realised that the drug under test isomerised in the feed.

3.6 PART V: SPECIAL PARTICULARS

3.6.1 PART VA: Dosage form

This part of the dossier contains information on the packaging together with at least a draft of the labelling and any package insert.

3.6.2 Part VB: Samples

Samples of the product are required for applications submitted to Belgium, Spain, Greece, Ireland, Italy, Luxembourg, the Netherlands, and Portugal. For Spain, Greece, Ireland, Luxembourg, and the Netherlands the sample provided is required to be large enough to permit the assay to be repeated and the other control methods to be verified. In the case of applications to Denmark, West Germany, France, and the UK, samples are provided only when requested by the regulatory authority concerned.

3.6.3 Part VC: Manufacturer(s) authorisation(s)

Copies should be provided of the authorisations of each manufacturer of the finished product to make the class of products concerned. Where necessary a translation of the authorisation should be provided with a copy of the original.

3.6.4 Part VD: Marketing authorisation(s)

Where appropriate the application includes a copy of the marketing authorisation from the Member State of origin and a copy of the approved summary of product characteristics. Copies are also provided of the marketing authorisations of any other Member States and from any other country in which the product is sold.

3.7 PRODUCT LABELLING

Directive 65/65/EEC includes requirements for information that appears on the product labelling. This relates to the container and outer packaging.

The name of the product and a qualitative and quantitative statement of the active ingredient(s) present is included, using the INN or, if none is available, the common name of the active material(s). A code by which the batch may be identified and the marketing authorisation number are stated. The names of the person or company responsible for the manufacture of the product and for placing it on the market are required. The method of administration is stated, together with the expiry date (in plain language) and any special storage conditions. The pharmaceutical dosage form and the contents are stated on the outer package.

For ampoules the normal information requirements apply to the outer package, but the container need state only the name of the product, the quantity of the active ingredients, the route of administration, and the expiry date. Small containers other than ampoules carry the normal information requirements on the outer package only.

National labelling requirements also apply, and compliance with any relevant pharmacopoeial recommendations is likely to be expected. In the UK the relevant general labelling requirements are included in the Medicines (Labelling) Regulations, the Medicines (Labelling) Amendment Regulations, and the Medicines (Labelling) Amendment (No. 2) Regulations.

The Commission of the European Communities services have recently been considering the labelling requirements for pharmaceuticals, and has issued a preliminary draft of a proposed new Council Directive. This includes some interesting changes to the existing requirements. The following notes consider some of these. It should be noted that the final version of the labelling Directive — if it is agreed — may not include all of the matters discussed and may contain new points.

The outer packaging, or if there is none, the immediate container, will probably need to state much of the information currently required. A special warning that the product should be stored out of the reach of children may also be required.

Consideration is being given to a requirement for the inclusion of a list of excipients in the product, and a requirement that any special precautions to be observed in the disposal of the unused product be stated.

The existing requirements for the name and address of the person placing the product on the market and, where different, the manufacturer of the product and a manufacturing reference number seem likely to be continued.

The immediate packaging of the product (except for single dose presentations which are too small to carry the information) is likely to be required to carry the name of the product, the names and quantities of active constituents, the route of administration, the expiry date, and the batch number.

Provision may be included for the grouping of related information within a field of view, and for national or multiple language labelling. Clarity and legibility of the labels is likely to be a requirement. Price information and reimbursement conditions may appear on the labelling.

The provision of a user leaflet within the package may be made a requirement. Equivalent information may be allowed on the label instead. The information to be included in this leaflet may include the name of the product, and qualitative and quantitative information concerning the active ingredient(s) together with the name and address of the marketing authorisation holder and, if necessary, the manufacturer. The therapeutic indications may be required unless the regulatory authority concerned decides that these should not be mentioned owing to potential disadvantage for the patient, together with information such as contra-indications, precautions for use, possible interactions with other medicines, food, alcohol or tobacco, and any special warnings. Excipients may need to be discussed where knowledge of their presence is of relevance to the safe and effective use of the product.

Instructions for the proper use of the medicine will probably be required, taking into account the usual and maximum doses; the method, route, and frequency of administration; what action should be taken if a dose is missed; what action is necessary in the case of an overdose (including the symptoms, any antidote and emergency procedures); the recommended duration of therapy; and the manner in which treatment should be stopped.

Side effects of the medicine in normal usage may need to be described. Where the product is new, the patient may be invited to report any side effects to his physician or pharmacist.

The expiry date on the label may have to be referred to in the leaflet, with a recommendation that the product not be used beyond that date.

It is likely that the leaflet will be required to be written in plain language, using the national languages of the Member States concerned. If multi-language leaflets are used then the text of each language will have to contain the same information. All information will have to be in in line with the approved summary of product characteristics.

REFERENCES

Cartwright, A. C. (1989) Stability tests on active substances and finished products: new European guideline, *Drug Development and Industrial Pharmacy*, **15**(10) 1743–1757.

Dobson, K. (1990) Analytical validation, *BIRA Journal* **9**(3) 9–12.

Matthews, B. R. (1990) CPMP chemistry and pharmacy guidelines: Stability testing, *BIRA Journal* **9**(3) 13–15.

Morris, J. M. (1990) Development pharmaceutics and process validation, *BIRA Journal* **9**(3) 6–8.

Morris, J. M. (1990) Development pharmaceutics and process validation, *Drug Development and Industrial Pharmacy*, **16**(11) 1749–1759.

Stewart, A. G. (1988) The pharmaceutical expert report — UK regulatory viewpoint, *BIRA Journal* **7**(3) 15–16.

4

New chemical active substance products: preclinical requirements

4.1 INTRODUCTION

The toxicology and pharmacology requirements for a new active substance clearly depend upon the nature and proposed clinical use of the medicinal product. The requirements for a drug which may be used long-term in young patients for comparatively minor conditions will, for example, require more extensive testing than a drug given on a single occasion to elderly patients with quite severe disease. Thus, the philosophy that has been promulgated by regulatory authorities is that the package of preclinical safety and pharmacology studies presented to support an application for marketing authorisation should be individually tailored to suit the particular circumstances of the medicinal product's intended use.

To help drug developers to come to a rational and relevant package of preclinical studies, the European Community's (EC) Committee on Proprietary Medicinal Products (CPMP) has over the years published a number of guidelines in the various areas of preclinical testing. Guidelines are now available on single-dose toxicity (published 1987), repeated-dose toxicity (1983), reproduction studies (1983), testing of medicinal products for their mutagenic potential (1987), carcinogenic potential (1983), pharmacokinetics and metabolic studies in the safety evaluation of new drugs in animals (1983), and preclinical biological safety testing of medicinal products derived from biotechnology (1988).

Further guidelines on local tolerance testing, general pharmacodynamics, development of non-clinical testing strategies, and stereoisomerism may emerge in due course.

Other texts which are important to consider in the context of preclinical testing requirements are Council Directive 87/18/EEC (on the harmonisation of laws, regulations, or administrative provisions relating to the application of the principles of good laboratory practice and the verification of their application for tests on chemical substances), Council Directive 88/320/EEC (on the inspection and verification of good laboratory practice), and Council Directive 86/609/EEC (on the approximation of laws, regulations, and administrative provisions of the Member States regarding the protection of animals used for experimental and other scientific purposes).

It is important to emphasise that the guidelines are simply that — sources of guidance, and not recipe books for studies to perform in order to obtain a marketing authorisation (or product licence). They are intended to guide the pharmaceutical industry in designing a package of studies which will investigate fully only those areas of potential toxicity which are relevant to the proposed clinical use of the product. Thus, it is hoped, overextensive as well as inadequate or inappropriate testing will be minimised.

In designing and interpreting a package of preclinical studies it is vitally important to consider the interface between the pharmaceutical data and the preclinical studies. Issues such as impurity profile, stability, isomerism, and dosage forms all may have a bearing on the conduct or interpretation of the preclinical studies. One common example relates to the problems caused by performing toxicology studies with batches of drug substance that have different impurity profiles from those intended for clinical use. If a particular impurity present in the production material was not present in the material tested in toxicity studies, then, obviously, no reassurance can be obtained from these studies as to the safety of the material containing that impurity when used clinically.

It is also critical that the findings in the preclinical package are properly followed up in the clinical trial programme. For example, if the product has been shown to produce cataracts in animal toxicity studies, then it would be appropriate for adequate ophthalmological monitoring to be performed in man.

Furthermore, some of the preclinical data, for example data on teratogenic potential in animals, may need to be included in the product information on use of the drug in pregnancy.

Applications for marketing authorisation should contain discussions of these issues as they pertain to the particular medicinal product in question. Generally, the most appropriate place for these considerations is the preclinical Expert Report. This should be a critical document which evaluates all the available information on the product, much in the way that a regulatory authority would assess an application. High quality, critical Expert Reports do much to speed the assessment process for regulatory approval by highlighting the important issues in an application.

In the following sections the current EC requirements for each area of preclinical testing are outlined.

4.2 PHARMACODYNAMICS

4.2.1 EC requirements

Directive 75/318/EEC (Annex, Part 2, Chapter 1, Section F) describes, in general terms, the requirements for preclinical pharmacodynamic studies. It states that there are two distinct aspects of the pharmacodynamic profile of a product which require consideration.

The first is the pharmacology of the new medicinal product that is directly relevant to the proposed therapeutic use. Data should be presented to establish the mechanism of action of the product in validated model systems. Where the product is a member of a group of substances which share a common mechanism of pharmacological action, a comparison should be made between the activity (including potency, specificity, duration of effect, etc.) of the new product against others in the class.

The second aspect of the product's pharmacological activity to be considered is its secondary pharmacology (that is, pharmacological activity unrelated to its desired therapeutic use). This set of studies is sometimes referred to as the 'safety pharmacology' since adverse effects seen in patients may be related to the secondary pharmacological properties of a product.

Ideally, a new medicinal product possesses no secondary pharmacological activity, the drug being entirely specific for its proposed therapeutic use. In practice, however, virtually all medicinal products have some secondary activity, and this needs to be elucidated and defined.

To this end, a general pharmacological profile of the substance is required, with particular attention being paid to the major body systems (central nervous system, autonomic system, cardiovascular system, etc.). Where secondary pharmacological effects occur at doses/concentrations approaching those for the desired primary activity, further careful investigations, concentrating on dose/effect relationships, are warranted.

Where combinations of active substances are proposed, the pharmacodynamic consequences of such a combination should be adequately investigated.

4.2.2 EC guidelines
There are currently no EC guidelines on preclinical pharmacodynamic testing of pharmaceutical products. In practice this causes few regulatory problems since drug developers are very well aware of the need to fully characterise the pharmacodynamic profiles of new medicinal products.

4.3 PHARMACOKINETICS

4.3.1 EC requirements
The EC requirement for pharmacokinetic studies was published in 1975 in Directive 75/318/EEC (Annex, Part 2, Chapter 1, Section G). The Directive gives only very generalised comments on the need for these studies. More detailed suggestions on the type and extent of the studies required are given in the Note for Guidance on pharmacokinetic studies, published in 1983 (Council Recommendation 83/571/EEC).

4.3.2 EC guidelines
The primary purpose of the preclinical pharmacokinetic studies is to generate a package of data which validates the toxicity studies and allows the clinical relevance of any toxic effects seen in these studies to be assessed. Pharmacokinetic data are therefore required from all the species and strains used in toxicity studies. These

data, together with human pharmacokinetic data, should enable an assessment to be made of the comparative exposures to drug and/or metabolites.

A helpful way of expressing this data is for applicants to submit comparative pharmacokinetic tables consisting of data from species used in pivotal to toxicity studies and data from man. This type of table enables a rapid assessment to be made of the relationships between dose, systemic exposure, target organ toxicity, and safety margins for man. Such tables are usually included in the preclinical Expert Report.

To perform these assessments the pharmacokinetic studies should be designed to obtain information on the absorption, distribution, metabolism, and excretion of the medicinal product. It may be important to consider issues which were identified in the pharmaceutical section of the application, for example, dosage form and absorption problems.

Studies should also be performed to investigate the extent of plasma protein binding and the possibility of enzyme induction/inhibition.

4.4 TOXICOLOGY

4.4.1 EC requirements

The EC requirements for animal toxicity studies were published in 1975 in Directive 75/318/EEC (Annex, Part 2, Chapter 1, Section B). The requirements are given in a fairly generalised manner in the Directive with more detailed guidance being given in the Notes for Guidance discussed below.

In the introduction to Chapter 1 of Part 2 of the Annex to Directive 75/318/EEC it is stated 'The toxicological (and pharmacological) tests must show: the potential toxicity of the product and any dangerous or undesirable toxic effects that might occur under the proposed conditions of use in human beings; these should be evaluated in relation to the gravity of the pathological condition being treated'. In this paragraph the important concept of risk to benefit ratio is introduced in terms of the toxicological testing of products. Clearly, in the evaluation of pharmaceutical products there is always the need to balance the risks elucidated from toxicity tests and clinical trials against the potential benefits of human exposure to the product.

4.4.2 EC guidelines

CPMP guidelines have been published on the conduct of both single and repeat dose toxicity studies. The Note for Guidance on single dose studies was published in 1987 (Council Recommendation 87/176/EEC), and the Note for Guidance on repeat dose studies in 1983 (Council Recommendation 83/571/EEC).

4.4.2.1 Single dose toxicity

Single dose toxicity studies are performed to give some indication of the likely effects of acute overdosage in man, and may be useful for the design of the repeat dose toxicity studies. The usual EC requirement is for single dose studies on at least two mammalian species of known strain, using equal numbers of both sexes. Generally, two routes of administration are investigated, one being the clinical route and the other a route ensuring adequate systemic exposure to the unchanged drug. Signs of acute toxicity should be revealed and the mode of death determined.

It is important to state that the guidelines do not require a high level of precision in the determination of lethal dose-effect relationships.

4.4.2.2 Repeat dose toxicity

Repeat dose toxicity studies are normally performed in two species, one a rodent and one a non-rodent (most commonly dog), using the route of clinical administration and dose levels sufficient to reveal target organ toxicity.

The durations of repeat dose toxicity studies are determined by the proposed duration of use in man: the longer the duration in man, the longer the duration of the toxicity studies. The suggested duration of these studies in the guidelines is as in Table 4.1.

The primary purpose of these studies is to elucidate the target organ toxicity for

Table 4.1 — Suggested duration of repeat dose toxicity studies

Duration of human treatment	Suggested duration of toxicity test
One or several doses in one day	2 weeks
Repeated doses up to 7 days	4 weeks
Repeated doses for up to 30 days	3 months
Repeated doses beyond 30 days	6 months

the new medicinal product. Depending on the nature, severity, and dose–effect relationships of the toxicological findings, decisions will be made on the nature and degree of the human exposure to the product both in clinical trials and in widespread clinical use after registration. Further considerations relating to the design and interpretation of these studies are described in detail in the guidelines, and do not need further discussion here.

4.5 REPRODUCTIVE TOXICOLOGY

4.5.1 EC requirements

The EC requirements for testing medicinal products for toxic effects on the reproductive process are described in Directive 75/318/EEC (Annex, Part 2, Chapter 1, Sections C and D) which was published in 1975. The Directive distinguishes between 'foetal toxicity' (Section C) and 'examination of reproductive function' (Section D).

The investigation of foetal toxicity is stated to comprise 'a demonstration of the toxic and especially the teratogenic effects observed in the issue of conception when the substance under investigation has been administered to the female during pregnancy'. It is suggested that these tests be performed in at least two animal species; rabbits and either rats or mice are suggested, but other species may be appropriate in certain circumstances.

Under 'examination of reproductive function' the Directive merely states 'If the results of other tests reveal anything suggesting harmful effects on progeny or impairment of male or female reproductive function, this shall be investigated by appropriate tests'.

4.5.2 EC guidelines

The CPMP Note for Guidance on reproduction studies was published in 1983 (Council Recommendation 83/571/EEC). It states that 'The study of drug effects on reproduction should be conducted on all new drugs in such a manner as would reveal the presence of any effect on mating behaviour and of any effect which might result in fetal loss, fetal abnormality, and damage to the offspring in later life, e.g.:

(1) changes in fertility or in the production of abnormal young due to damage to the male and/or female gametes;
(2) interference with preimplantation and implantation stages in the development of the conceptus;
(3) toxic effects on the embryo;
(4) toxic effects on the fetus;
(5) changes in maternal physiology producing secondary effects on the embryo or fetus;
(6) effects on uterine or placental growth or development;
(7) interference with parturition;
(8) effects on postnatal development and suckling of the progeny, and on maternal lactation;
(9) late effects on the progeny'.

The package of studies which is normally performed to investigate this large number of toxicological end-points is a fertility study in one species (usually rat), a peri/post-natal study in one species (also usually rat), and embryotoxicity (teratogenicity) studies in two species (usually rat and rabbit). This package of studies is designed to cover all sections of the reproduction process so that an adverse effect on any part of the process will be revealed.

With a new medicinal product there will be little or no information on human experience in pregnancy or lactation, thus the available animal data (with all their limitations) have to be interpreted in terms of advice for the prescriber. These data and advice must be included in the product information for prescribers.

4.6 MUTAGENICITY STUDIES

4.6.1 EC requirements

A specific requirement for the study of the mutagenic potential of new medicinal products was first introduced in the EC in October 1985 under Article 2 of Directive 83/570/EEC (which amended the Annex to Directive 75/318/EEC regarding toxicological and pharmacological tests).

The amendment states 'The purpose of·the study of mutagenic potential is to reveal the changes which a substance may cause in the genetic material of individuals or cells and which may have the effect of making successors permanently and hereditarily different from their predecessors. This study is obligatory for any new substance. The number and types of results and the criteria for their evaluation shall depend on the state of scientific knowledge at the time when the application is lodged'.

4.6.2 EC guidelines

A Note for Guidance on 'The testing of medicinal products for their mutagenic potential' was published in February 1987 (Council Recommendation 87/176/EEC). These notes give general guidance on how a mutagenicity testing programme should be designed and conducted. However, for detailed guidance on protocols for individual tests, companies are advised to consult the current international scientific literature.

It is emphasised in the Note for Guidance that the procedure should be capable of detecting the three main classes of relevant genetic damage, namely gene mutation, chromosomal mutation, and genome mutation.

Other important considerations in designing a package of mutagenicity tests are that the tests should be, where possible, cheap and rapid; that the tests selected should have complementary end-points; and that the tests should take into account the effect of potential metabolism of the medicinal product in man.

A system using four categories of test is proposed in the Note for Guidance, whereby normally one test from each of the four categories should be performed:

(1) test for gene mutations in bacteria;
(2) test for chromosomal aberrations in mammalian cells *in vitro*;
(3) test for gene mutations in eukaryotic systems;
(4) test for genetic damage *in vivo*.

The Note for Guidance emphasises that the above is a suggested package, and other tests may be more appropriate in certain circumstances.

It is important that companies include in marketing authorisation applications a critical discussion of the reasoning behind the construction of the mutagenicity package, particularly when the package deviates from that recommended in the Note for Guidance. The most appropriate place for this discussion is generally the Expert Report.

The aim of performing these tests is to establish whether the product possesses mutagenic potential or not. Once this question has been settled, the quite separate issue of the significance of the obtained results in terms of a genetic hazard for man then follows. Issues to be considered in this context include the effect of metabolic activation, whether the mutagenic activity was seen *in vivo*, or only *in vitro*, and the effect of concentration/dose on the level of mutagenic activity. Further tests may be appropriate in order to investigate the significance of any positive results.

The final consideration as far as mutagenicity testing is concerned is the risk/benefit judgement for the individual medicinal product in its intended clinical use.

Sec. 4.7] **Carcinogenicity studies** 83

Potent mutagens (such as some anti-tumour agents) may still be useful human medicinal products as long as the benefit of using the product in the proposed indication outweighs the potential risks.

It is surprisingly common for one of the grounds for refusal of a marketing authorisation application to be an inadequate mutagenicity package. It is possible that this sometimes occurs because of confusion over the differing international requirements for mutagenicity testing.

To avoid these problems, it is stressed that the choice of tests submitted in the mutagenicity package should always be discussed and justified in the Expert Report, and that this is particularly important when the package differs from the one recommended in the EC guidelines.

4.7 CARCINOGENICITY STUDIES

4.7.1 EC requirements

Directive 75/318/EEC (Annex Part 2, Chapter 1, Section E), which was adopted in 1975, describes the conditions under which 'tests to reveal carcinogenic effects shall normally be required'. These are:

(1) where substances have a close chemical analogy with known carcinogenic or co-carcinogenic compounds;
(2) where substances have given rise to suspicious changes during the long-term toxicological tests;
(3) where substances have given rise to suspicious results in mutagenicity or short-term carcinogenicity tests.

The Directive states that carcinogenicity tests may also be required for substances likely to be administered regularly over a prolonged period of a patient's life.

No details are given in the Directive as to how these tests should be performed, but it is suggested that 'the state of scientific knowledge at the time when the application is lodged shall be taken into account when determining the details of the tests'.

4.7.2 EC guidelines

The CPMP Note for Guidance on carcinogenic potential was published in 1983 (Council Recommendation 83/571/EEC). The Note for Guidance discusses in detail the scientific basis of testing medicinal products for carcinogenic potential, gives some practical guidance for the conduct of these studies in animals, and gives slightly more detail on the circumstances where carcinogenicity studies would be required than is given in the Directive.

The Note for Guidance states that carcinogenicity studies will usually be required in the following circumstances:

(1) when the medicine is likely to be administered regularly over a substantial period of life (continuously during a minimum period of six months, or frequently in an intermittent manner so that the total exposure is similar); or

(2) where a substance has a chemical structure that suggests a carcinogenic potential; or
(3) where a substance causes concern due to
   (a) some specific aspect of its biological action (for example a therapeutic class of which several members have produced positive carcinogenic results);
   (b) its pattern of toxicity or long-term retention (of the drug or its metabolites);
   (c) the findings in mutagenicity/short-term carcinogenicity tests.

Animal carcinogenicity studies are at present considered the most satisfactory method of determining whether or not a new medicinal product presents a carcinogenic hazard in clinical use. However, it is recognised that these studies are extremely costly in terms of animal, human, and financial resources. Consequently they are only required in circumstances where the proposed clinical use of the drug is considered to justify them.

Carcinogenicity testing may not be regarded as necessary where the medicinal product will be used only in patients with a life expectancy shorter than that in which any carcinogenic hazard might be revealed, or for medicinal products which are insoluble and/or not absorbed into the body. When carcinogenicity studies are required, the guidelines suggest that they should normally be performed in two species (most commonly rat and mouse).

The design, performance, and interpretation of carcinogenicity studies are technically very complex. There are often difficulties in designing and performing adequate studies, and subsequently in establishing the significance of the findings from these studies for man. Consequently, the guidelines describe in considerable detail some important points to consider when performing these tests. These include species and strain selection, route and frequency of dosing, selection of dose levels, age of animals at commencement of study, duration of studies, number of animals per group, composition of diet, monitoring to be performed during the study, statistical design of the study, terminal investigations to be performed, and analysis of the data obtained. Full consideration should be given to the points raised in the CPMP guidelines on the conduct of these studies.

5

New chemical active substance products: clinical requirements

5.1 INTRODUCTION

The purpose of this chapter is to describe, in broad terms, the existing requirements for registering medicinal products based on new chemical active substances in the European Community (EC). The rules, details of the procedures, and extant guidelines have been published in three volumes issued by the Commission of the European Communities. These are: Volume I, *The rules governing medicinal products for human use in the European Community*; Volume II, *Notice to applicants for marketing authorisations for medicinal products for human use in the member states of the European Community*; and Volume III, *Guidelines on the quality, safety, and efficacy of medicinal products for human use*. References in this chapter to 'Vol. I', 'Vol. II', and 'Vol. III', are to these three volumes.

There is no point in reproducing the contents of the relevant sections of these three volumes here; it is assumed that readers will already have possession of the volumes. Rather, emphasis will be placed on impending new developments and on some aspects of the rules and guidelines which experience suggests may not be fully understood.

5.2 CLINICAL TRIALS

5.2.1 National requirements for the regulation of clinical drug trials

Currently, amongst the Member States of the EC, there are differences in the requirements for the regulation of clinical drug trials. These differences relate to notification, documentation, ethical requirements, and regulatory measures. The differences are listed in Volume III at page 131.

Notwithstanding these differences in the regulatory procedures, the rules governing the actual conduct of the clinical trials are set out in Part 3 of the Annex to Council Directive 75/318/EEC (Vol. I at page 43). In particular, clinical trials must always be preceded by adequate pharmacological and toxicological tests carried out on animals in accordance with the relevant requirements of the Directive. The clinician must acquaint himself with the conclusions drawn from the pharmacological and toxicological studies, hence the applicant must provide the clinician with the complete pharmacological and toxicological reports. Further guidance on the conduct, performance, and control of clinical trials can be found in the general clinical guideline, 'Recommended basis for the conduct of clinical trials of medicinal products in the European Community' (Vol. III at page 115). More recently, the Committee on Proprietary Medicinal Products (CPMP) has adopted a guideline on good clinical practice. This is discussed below.

5.2.2 Good Clinical Practice (GCP)

The definition of GCP is 'a standard by which clinical trials are designed, implemented, and reported so that there is public assurance that the data are credible, and that the rights, integrity, and confidentiality of subjects are protected.'

Much of the ground covered by the guideline will be familiar. On ethics, there is reaffirmation of the current revision of the Declaration of Helsinki as the accepted basis for clinical trial ethics; the consequential requirement for approval of clinical trial protocols by ethics committees; and the need for informed consent by trial subjects, their relatives, guardians, or legal representatives.

Next, the responsibilities of the sponsor (the individual or organisation which takes responsibility for the initiation, management, or financing of the trial), the monitor (a person appointed by the sponsor or a scientific body to which a sponsor may have transferred obligations), and the investigator, are addressed. Since the responsibilities of the sponsor are important and since the GCP guideline was not at the time of writing generally available, it is worth reproducing the relevant text in full.

The responsibilities of the sponsor are as follows:

- the sponsor must establish detailed standard operating procedures (SOP) to comply with good clinical practice, and is responsible for conducting an internal audit of the trial. The sponsor should agree with the investigator on the distribution of responsibilities;
- both the sponsor and investigator must agree on and sign the protocol as an agreement of the details of the clinical trial and the means of data recording (e.g. CRF). Any amendments to the protocol must have agreement of both sponsor and investigator before the amendment is implemented; any such agreement must be documented.

Particular responsibilities of the sponsor are:

(a) To select the investigator, taking into account the appropriateness and availability of the trial site and facilities, and be assured of the investigator's qualifications and availability for the entire duration of the study; to assure the investigator's agreement to undertake the study as laid down in the protocol, according to these guidelines of good clinical practice, including the acceptance of verification procedures, audit, and inspection.

(b) To inform the investigator of the chemical/pharmaceutical, toxicological, pharmacological, and clinical information (including previous and on-going trials), which should be adequate to justify the nature, scale, and duration of the trial, as a prerequisite to planning the trial and to inform the investigator of any relevant new information arising during the trial. All relevant information must be included in the investigator's brochure which must be supplemented and/or updated by the sponsor whenever new pertinent information is available.

(c) To submit notification/application to the relevant authorities (when appropriate) and to ensure submission of any necessary documents to the Ethics Committee, and to ensure communication of any modification, amendment, or violation of the protocol, if the change may impact on the subject's safety, and to inform the investigator and relevant authorities about discontinuation of the trial and the reasons for discontinuation.

(d) To provide the fully characterised investigational medicinal product(s) prepared in accordance with good manufacturing practice (GMP), suitably packaged and labelled in such a way that any blinding procedure is ensured.

Sufficient samples of each batch and a record of its analyses and characteristics must be kept for reference, so that there is the possibility for an independent laboratory to re-check the investigational products, e.g. for bioequivalence.

Records of the quantities of investigational medicinal products supplied must be maintained with batch/serial numbers. The sponsor must ensure that the investigator within his/her institution establishes a system for the safe handling, storage, and use of the delivered investigational products.

(e) To appoint, and ensure the on-going training of, suitable and appropriately trained monitors and their clinical research support personnel.

(f) To appoint appropriate individuals and/or committees for the purpose of steering, supervision, data handling, statistical processing, and trial report writing.

(g) To consider promptly, jointly with the investigator, all serious adverse events (AEs) and take appropriate measures necessary to safeguard trial subjects, and to report to appropriate authorities according to their requirements.

(h) To inform promptly the investigator of any immediately relevant information that becomes available during a trial and ensure that the ethics committee is notified by the investigator(s) where required.

(i) To ensure the preparation of a comprehensive final report of the trial suitable for regulatory purposes whether or not the trial has been completed. Safety updates may be required. For long-term trials an annual report may be required by the authorities.

(j) To provide adequate compensation/treatment for subjects in the event of trial related injury or death, and provide indemnity (legal and financial cover) for the investigator, except for claims resulting from malpractice and/or negligence.

(k) To agree with the investigator(s) on the allocation of responsibilities for data processing, statistical handling, reporting of the results, and publication policy.

The monitor, as the principal communication link between the sponsor and the investigator, has important responsibilities. He must work according to a predetermined standard operating procedure and visit the investigator before, during, and after the trial to control adherence to the protocol and assure that all data are correctly and completely recorded and reported, and that informed consent is being obtained and recorded from all subjects before their participation in the trial. He should also ensure that the trial site has adequate space, facilities, equipment, and staff, and that an adequate number of trial subjects is likely to be available for the duration of the trial. The other responsibilities of the monitor include checking the case report form entries with the source documents, assisting the investigator in reporting the trial data, and submitting a written report to the sponsor after each visit to the investigator and after all relevant telephone calls, letters, and other contacts with the investigator.

In the GCP guideline the responsibilities of the investigator are addressed in detail. The investigator must be thoroughly familiar with the properties of the investigational medicinal product. Information should be provided to all staff members taking part in the trial or with other elements of the patient's management. It is the investigator's duty to collect, record, and report data properly and to make all the data available to the sponsor and relevant authority (where required) for verification/audit/inspection purposes. The investigator must agree and sign the final report of the trial. Finally, the responsibilities of the investigator towards the subjects under his/her care are set out in detail. Appropriate, fully functional resuscitation equipment should be immediately available in case of emergency. The investigator must ensure that appropriate medical care is available throughout the duration of the trial and that it is maintained after the trial. All clinically significant abnormal laboratory values or clinical observations must be followed up to the subject's benefit after completion of the trial. The medical record should be clearly marked that the subject is participating in a clinical trial, and the family doctor should normally, with the subject's consent, be informed.

With respect to validation of the trial data, guidelines on data handling and archiving of data are included with particular reference to computerised systems. Use of such a system is acceptable when it is controlled as recommended in the EC guide to good manufacturing practice. Guidelines on the archiving specify that the investigator must arrange for the retention of the patient identification codes for at least fifteen years after the completion or discontinuation of the trial. The sponsor must retain all other documentation pertaining to the trial for the lifetime of the product. The protocol, documentation, approvals, and all other documents relating to the trial, must be retained by the sponsor in a trial master file. All data on adverse events must always be included in the trial master file. The final report must be retained by the sponsor for five years beyond the lifetime of the product. Any change of ownership of the data should be documented, and the new owner must retain the final report for five years beyond the lifetime of the product. All the data and documents should be made available if requested by a relevant authority.

Finally, general advice of the experimental design and statistical analysis of clinical trials is given, and a system of quality assurance outlined. More detailed statistical guidelines are being prepared by the CPMP.

Further towards an assurance of quality, particularly in relation to bioavailability and bioequivalence studies, the CPMP has adopted additional guidelines. Details of the laboratory conducting the study, the investigator, the coordinator, and the manufacturing site used for the manufacture of batches of experimental product are required. Copies of the certificates of analysis for batches of experimental products, the batch manufacturing record, and the results of *in vitro* dissolution studies will also be required. Applicants will need to state what steps they have taken to satisfy themselves about the testing laboratory, and a statement certifying the authenticity of the studies and the steps taken to ensure this should be included. Finally, the need for retention samples and access for inspection of investigational sites and to all data and documentation are addressed.

5.2.3 Clinical guidelines
Apart from the general guideline on the recommended basis for the conduct of clinical trials, Vol. III contains guidelines for the investigation of products in children and in the elderly, on the testing of drugs intended for long-term use, and on pharmacokinetic and bioavailability studies. The volume also contains guidelines for a number of therapeutic classes of drugs.

Recently, the CPMP has adopted new guidelines for the evaluation of anti-cancer products. At the time of writing (July 1990) guidelines on hypnotic agents are in a late stage of development, and it is expected that work on the drafting of statistical guidelines will commence soon.

5.3 THE CLINICAL DOCUMENTATION
5.3.1 Introduction
A table listing the various parts of the dossier which should accompany an application for marketing authorisation is at page 44 of Vol. II. Guidance on the presentation of part IV, The Clinical Documentation, is at pages 60 to 62. Some aspects of the documentation required, both in general and specifically in relation to applications made to the Medicines Control Agency in the UK, are discussed below.

5.3.2 The index
As is well known, there has been a steady increase in the size of applications for marketing authorisation, particularly the clinical sections. Accordingly, it is difficult to overstate the importance of a comprehensive and accurate index of the contents of the documentation as an aid to the assessment of the clinical data.

It is usually helpful to introduce the index with a brief description of the way in which the data have been organised and presented. Whatever method has been used to organise the data, it is obvious that an accurate and meaningful index can be constructed only if a coherent system for numbering the volumes and the pages has been adopted.

5.3.3 Part IVA: Clinical pharmacology
The pharmacological particulars are described in part 3, chapter II of the Annex to Council Directive 75/318/EEC (Vol. I at page 44). The documentation to be submitted is further described in Vol. II, pages 60–61. The content and general organisation of the documentation should follow these general guidelines, but the details of the content will vary according to the product and its indications.

For applications to the UK, applicants should include a pharmacokinetic table which allows comparison between the results seen in animals used in toxicity testing and those demonstrated in man. This is of value in predicting safety margins, and is one of the criteria used in considering the relevance and adequacy of the preclinical studies. A suggested format for the table has been published by the Medicines Control Agency in the 1989 edition of the Guidance Notes on applications for product licences, MAL 2 at page 27.

5.3.4 Part IVB: Clinical experience
The clinical particulars and general considerations are set out in part 3, Chapter II of the Annex to Council Directive 75/318/EEC (Vol. I, pages 44 to 46). The necessary documentation is described in Vol. II, pages 61 to 62.

Much of the ground covered in these sections of the two volumes relates to the presentation of individual studies. There are, however, clear advantages if a 'free standing' overall summary of the clinical documentation is submitted as part of the dossier. This is discussed below.

5.3.5 Overall summary
As an Appendix to the Expert Report on the clinical documentation, applicants are required to submit a tabular presentation of all clinical studies, and summaries of the most important and significant studies in tabular form (Vol. II at page 163). A written summary is considered as optional, but, in the UK, such a summary is regarded as a valuable aid to assessment. As in any document where complex information is being presented, tables and figures illustrating the data are useful additions to the narrative.

The overall summary, though providing summary descriptions of all studies, could be organised in such a way that attention is focused on those studies which are of pivotal importance. The main objective of the summary should be to bring together the data from the multiplicity of individual studies in such a way as to facilitate the assessment of the efficacy and safety of the product for each indication in relation to the recommended dosage range.

With respect to evidence of efficacy, the data for each indication should be summarised separately. The relative importance of each type of study should be addressed in a logical sequence (e.g. double-blind, placebo-controlled studies; active comparator-controlled studies; open uncontrolled studies). Particular attention should be given to those studies which can justify the recommended dosage range.

When possible, and particularly when there is a multiplicity of relatively small studies, consideration should be given to a pooled analysis of the studies. A justification for pooling is required, but the details of the pooled analysis should not be included in the summary. The necessary, comprehensive, details of the analysis of pooled studies should be documented in 'free standing' reports.

The overall summary of safety data should be organised in such a way that safety in relation to dosage, duration of exposure, age, sex, and special groups, both overall and for each particular indication, can be readily assessed. In these respects, the details of safety monitoring protocols, particularly when pooled data for the product are compared with data for comparators or placebo, should be outlined so that it is evident that like is being compared with like.

5.4 THE CLINICAL EXPERT REPORT

The general principles underlying Expert Reports are set out in Vol. II at pages 66 to 69. Details of the style and content of the Clinical Expert Report are at pages 158 to 175. Some aspects of the Expert Report are worthy of emphasis.

First of all, it is important to understand that failure to provide a properly prepared Expert Report constitutes grounds for refusing an application.

Apart from its essential nature, the report serves several important functions.

Following a dispassionate and critical review of the existing documentation, the Expert should be in a position to indicate to the applicant any inadequacies in the data which require either evidence from additional studies or modification of the claimed indications. Through this kind of interaction between Expert and applicant it was expected that the standard of licence applications would be improved. This can occur only if Experts, particularly external Experts, are involved at a relatively early stage of the development of the product and if they are familiar with all aspects of the documentation including the pharmaceutical and preclinical data.

Another important function of a well-prepared Expert Report is to facilitate assessment of the application so that the increasing burden placed on the regulatory authorities within the EC is lessened.

A third important aspect of the Expert Report is that, inasmuch as the Assessment Report used in the multi-state procedure is drawn up and derived from the Expert Reports included in the initial application, it is obvious that well-prepared reports will enhance the mutual recognition and harmonisation of licensing decisions throughout the EC.

Toward these ends, it is worth discussing the length, the style, and the content of the clinical Expert Report and its relationship to the documentation. The report should be contained in no more than 25 pages. This is possible because it is not intended that the report be a mere summary of the totality of the documentation. Rather, the report should be a dispassionate and critical review of the evidence for the safety and efficacy of the product used in the recommended dosage range for the specified indications. Due account must be taken of any issues arising from the pharmaceutical or pre-clinical data.

Because of the limitation in space, the overall summary discussed above provides a crucial link between the Expert Report itself and the volumes containing the clinical documentation. The Expert can focus on the most important issues in the knowledge that the totality of the clinical data has been accurately and comprehensively summarised.

There is no doubt whatever of the importance of the role that a well-prepared Expert Report plays in the determination of licence applications.

5.5 CONCLUSION

As the EC develops systems which further harmonise licensing decisions, it is likely that details of the extant regulatory procedures will alter. It should not be expected, however, that there will be any lessening of the quality of the clinical documentation required to obtain a marketing authorisation. Rather, new guidelines on the conduct of clinical trials for specific classes of drugs and on the statistical analysis of data will have the effect of setting new standards acceptable to the EC as a whole.

For applicants, the main advantage of common European standards is to facilitate the preparation of applications which will be recognised by all twelve Member States. A thorough knowledge of the rules, procedures, and guidelines is therefore required by all who wish their applications to be successful.

The clinical documentation, as one of the most important parts of the dossier, needs particular attention not only in respect of the format, but also in respect of its content. Ease of access to the contents of the many volumes of documentation which nowadays often accompany applications for a new chemical active substance will be considerably enhanced if the volumes are adequately indexed, and if care is taken in the preparation of an overall summary of the documentation and in the writing of the Expert Report.

6

Abridged applications

6.1 INTRODUCTION

A marketing authorisation application for a new chemical active substance (NCAS) product normally needs to include all of the information (documents and particulars) specified in Article 4 of Directive 65/65/EEC. In particular, it needs to include:

(a) a description of the control methods employed by the manufacturer, and
(b) results of physicochemical, biological, or microbiological tests; pharmacological and toxicological tests; and clinical trials.

However, for a well-known active ingredient in a conventional formulation (for example a tablet or capsule) indicated for therapeutic uses which are well established, it would obviously be both unethical and scientifically unnecessary to ask companies to repeat all of the pharmacological and toxicological tests in animals or the clinical trials in man. All EC Member States have therefore allowed the submission of 'abridged' or 'abbreviated' marketing authorisation applications — applications where some or all of the original animal data or human clinical trials data are omitted. In such cases, bibliographic references were often submitted in place of these data.

6.2 ABRIDGED APPLICATIONS BEFORE JULY 1987

6.2.1 Directive 65/65/EEC

The original text of Directive 65/65/EEC allowed the submission of references to the scientific literature on (animal) pharmacological and toxicological studies and human clinical trials in the following circumstances (Article 4(8) of Directive 65/65/EEC) in the following cases:

(a) (i) a proprietary product with an established use, which has been adequately tested in human beings so that its effects, including side effects, are already known and included in the published references;

(a) (ii) a new proprietary product in which the combination of active constituents is identical with that of a known proprietary product with an established use;
(a) (iii) a new proprietary product consisting solely of known active constituents that have been used in combination in comparable proportions in adequately tested medicinal products with an established use;
(b) in the case of a new proprietary product containing known constituents not hitherto used in combination for therapeutic purposes, references to published data may be substituted for the tests of such constituents.

6.2.2 Directive 83/570/EEC

Directive 83/570/EEC was adopted on 26 October 1983, and implemented by all of the Member States on 1 November 1985. This amended the English text to replace the words 'a list of published references' in Article 4(8)(a) of Directive 65/65/EEC with the words 'a bibliography'. The intention behind this change was to require the applicants to submit a complete list of all relevant references, not a selective one.

As Armstrong (1989) has reported, the Commission of the European Communities (CEC) wanted to amend this situation because not all Member States interpreted Article 4(8) in the same way. The published literature (or bibliography) was often incomplete or inappropriate, and there were differences between the Member States in the amount of information required. This state of affairs penalised the innovative company whose product was copied at low cost.

6.3 DIRECTIVE 87/21/EEC

6.3.1 The objectives of the new Directive

Directive 87/21/EEC was adopted by the Council of Health Ministers on 21 December 1986 and introduced into the EC Member States on 1 July 1987. It amended 65/65/EEC and had two main objectives — the protection of pharmaceutical innovation (particularly for biotechnology products), and to ensure greater harmonisation of all of the requirements for 'copy products' which are submitted without full pharmacotoxicological and clinical documentation.

The Directive was implemented in all Member States except for Greece, Portugal, and Spain, who have a derogation until 1992. In those countries applicants can apply under the old 'literature references/bibliography' requirements.

6.3.2 Protection of pharmaceutical innovation

As mentioned above, one of the objectives of this new Directive was to provide a certain form of 'market exclusivity' for high technology/biotechnology products. The CEC had felt that the protection offered by the patent law under the Münich convention to pharmaceutically innovative products was not always sufficient, because the theoretical twenty years patent term is always substantially eroded — both by the testing necessary to obtain a marketing authorisation and also by the process of obtaining the authorisation through the national authorities. In addition, for biotechnology products the patent law was not considered to provide adequate protection for innovation.

In nine out of the twelve of the EC Member States, this 'second applicant protection' period of ten years is applied to any new active substance (NAS) product. In Denmark, Ireland, and Luxembourg the period of second applicant protection is six years for an NAS product.

In all EC Member States a full ten years second applicant protection is given to any product submitted through the Directive 87/22/EEC concertation procedure. Thus, this includes obligatory applications made by companies for List A biotechnology products (see Chapter 15 for details). However, it also includes List B high technology products, where in the first place the company chooses to apply voluntarily and to justify the application under one of the headings in List B, and the EC Member State chosen as rapporteur then has to accept this case (or not). The main effect, in terms of second applicant protection for high technology products, is to increase the term of protection from six to ten years in Denmark, Ireland and Luxembourg.

6.3.3 Harmonisation of the rules for products which are copies of established medicinal products

The objective of stipulating the cases (for copy products) in which the results of the preclinical (animal toxicology and pharmacology) and clinical studies do not have to provided was to prevent unnecessary testing on humans and animals. The new section of Article 4(8)(a) (introduced in the Directive 87/21/EEC amendment) defines the circumstances where it is not necessary to provide the systematic results of animal toxicology and clinical studies. These are:

4(8)(a)(i): either that the new product is essentially similar to the original product authorised in the country concerned with the application and that the person responsible for marketing of the product has consented to the pharmacological, toxicological, or clinical references contained in the file on the original proprietary medicinal product being used for the purpose of examining the new application;

4(8)(a)(ii): or, that by detailed references to published scientific literature presented in accordance with the second paragraph of Article 1 of Directive 75/318/EEC that the constituent or constituents of the proprietary medicinal product have a well established medicinal use, with recognised efficacy and an acceptable level of safety;

4(8)(a)(iii): or, that the new product is essentially similar to a product which has been authorised within the Community, in accordance with Community provisions in force, for not less than six years, and is marketed in the Member State for which the application is made; this period shall be extended to ten years in the case of high technology products within the meaning of Part A in the Annex to Directive 87/22/EEC or of a medicinal product within the meaning of Part B in the Annex to that Directive has been followed; furthermore, a Member State may also extend this period to ten years by a single Decision covering all the products marketed on its territory where it considers this is necessary in the interests of public health. Member States are at liberty not to apply the abovementioned six-year period beyond the date of expiry of a patent protecting the original product.

However, where the proprietary medicinal product is intended for different therapeutic use from that of the other proprietary medicinal products marketed or is to be administered by different routes or in different doses, the results of appropriate pharmacological and toxicological tests and/or clinical trials must be provided.

6.3.4 Harmonisation of the rules for combination products

Article 4(8)(b) of Directive 65/65/EEC now deals with the question of combination products. It states that in the case of new products containing known constituents not hitherto used in combination, the results of pharmacological and toxicological tests and of clinical trials relating to that combination must be provided, but that it is not necessary to provide references relating to each individual constituent.

6.4 REQUIREMENTS FOR INFORMATION ON SECOND APPLICANT PRODUCTS

Volume II of *The rules governing medicinal products in the European Community* is entitled 'The Notice to Applicants ...'. The 1989 (second) edition indicates where the information about the section of the Directives under which an abridged application is made need to appear. Information is requested in the following sections:

- Part 1A (Administrative data), Section 2a asks in the case of a product claimed to be an 'essentially similar' product under Article 4(8)(a)(iii), for the following information:
  - □ the date and reference of the first authorisation in the EC (with appropriate verification), and
  - □ confirmation that the original product is on the market of the Member State to which application is made.
- Part 1C (Expert Reports, the Product Profile) asks under (a) 'Type of application' for a statement as to whether the product is:
  - □ a product essentially similar to one already on the market, or
  - □ a new active substance, or
  - □ a new combination of previously known active ingredients, or
  - □ a new pharmaceutical form, or
  - □ a new strength, or
  - □ an extension of indications.

6.5 EVIDENCE OF THE TEN YEAR AUTHORISATION AND MARKETING

Although, the 'Notice to Applicants...' asks for evidence of the date of the first authorisation in the EC, what is really needed is to show that a product has been approved for more than ten years in the EC, and that a product is still marketed in the

Member State(s) in which it is now proposed to market the new product. Evidence is needed to support the assertion of approval for more than ten years.

Evidence of current marketing of a product could be given by citing one of the commercial lists produced in the EC countries (such as the UK Monthly Index of Medical Specialities (MIMS) or the Chemist and Druggist Price List).

Evidence of marketing for more than ten years could be given by referring to an old edition of one of these commercial lists. Evidence can also be provided by reference to one of the official publications which are used to give details of marketing authorisations granted for medicinal products in each country (such as the *Moniteur Belge* in Belgium, the *Statstidende* in Denmark, the *Nederlandse Staatscourant* in the Netherlands, etc.). It is acknowledged, however, that some of the older information given in these publications may be misleading or incomplete in some respects. For example, in the UK, in the past, the date of marketing has been gazetted and not the date of authorisation. In Denmark the date gazetted in the past has been the date at which the company was offered a licence on condition that they supplied further satisfactory data. In other countries (such as the Netherlands and Italy) the information published in the past was incomplete. In these countries the authorities have agreed to provide information, on request, to applicants — where it cannot readily be found by other means.

6.6 ESSENTIAL SIMILARITY

For abridged applications under Article 4(8)(a)(iii) of Directive 65/65/EEC as amended, the question of demonstrating the essential similarity of their second (or subsequent) applicant product to an originator product arises.

6.6.1 The Smith Kline and French judicial review

On 2 October 1987, Smith Kline and French Laboratories (SKF) instituted judicial review proceedings against the UK Licensing Authority, seeking to restrain it in its use of their (the originator's) confidential data for cimetidine tablets (Tagamet) in the assessment of any second applicant's abridged application. On 23 February 1988, Mr Justice Henry declared that reference to such confidential data could not be made 'except with the express consent of the appellants'.

On 29 June 1988, the UK Court of Appeal set aside the Henry judgement. On 9 February 1989, the final appeal court in the UK (the House of Lords) dismissed SKF's appeal.

The House of Lords confirmed the right of the Licensing Authority in the UK to refer to the originator's confidential data, stating: 'It is for the Licensing Authority, comparing the information received from the second applicant and taking into account all other information available to the Licensing Authority, from whatever source and whether confidential or not confidential, to decide in the case of a particular application whether it shall be declined or granted'.

6.6.2 Essential similarity and the active ingredient

One of the arguments raised by SKF in their case was that the UK Licensing Authority had to require the generic product manufacturers (the second applicants) to provide data to show that their cimetidine drug substance was essentially similar to that of the originator (SKF).

It is this consideration of essential similarity of the active ingredient which has given rise to considerable difficulties for the second applicants (the generic product manufacturers). Different sources of an active ingredient may be made by different synthetic routes or variants of the same route. Such differences will inevitably give rise to differences in the impurity profile of the active ingredient. The words 'essential similarity' in the Directive do not mean absolute identicality of impurity profile, but what do they mean? The House of Lords did not specifically address this issue to give a legal definition, although it was mentioned in argument. One widely accepted view is that a second applicant's source of active ingredient can be regarded as 'essentially similar' if the physical form of the active ingredient and its attendant impurities make it similar in its biological properties to the patient. Thus, a new pattern of impurities in the second applicant's source of active ingredient should not then cause any difference to the safety or efficacy of the product in which it is used. The presence of (say) a new impurity which was known to be immunogenic in the second applicant's source of active ingredient might cause allergic reactions in some patients taking the product, and the product could not then be regarded as essentially similar.

The above highlights the need to have detailed information on the impurity profiles of the active ingredient used by the second applicant. The major impurities should be identified and their levels known in typical production batches. The levels of other minor impurities should also be known, approximately. The Pharmaceutical Expert Report should consider the impurities and cross refer to a detailed consideration of what is known about their toxicology in the Pharmacotoxicological Expert Report. The impurity limits need to be justified in relation to the toxicology of the impurity, the pharmacology and toxicology of the active ingredient itself, the route of administration, the daily dose, the duration of therapy, and the proposed indications for the product.

The essential steps in considering essential similarity are as follows:

- First, for the applicant to identify the impurity profile of his source of active ingredient and to comment on the potential toxicology problems as part of the justification for the proposed impurity limits in the active ingredient specification.
- Second, for the pharmaceutical assessor in the national authority to compare the impurity profile of the new source of active ingredient with that of the originator's active ingredient and to identify any major differences between them.
- Third, for the toxicological and clinical assessors in the national authority to consider the potential hazard to patients exposed to the different impurities or different levels of impurities and to decide whether they feel that they are satisfactory or not. If they do not accept the proposed levels or feel that insufficient information had been presented to make an informed judgement, they would probably need to refer the application to the national committee (see Chapters 17 and 18) for advice and or possible refusal.

As detailed in Chapter 7 (Drug Master Files), the information on impurities could come from either the active ingredient manufacturer himself, or from the product marketing authorisation applicant. In this latter case, the active ingredient manufacturer must impart the relevant information on the impurities and their potential toxicology to the applicant for the marketing authorisation for the dosage form — since it is he who will be responsible (and legally liable) if there are adverse reactions to the product which he should have foreseen.

6.6.3 Essential similarity and the finished product
Article 4(8)(a)(iii) requires the product to be essentially similar. The 'Notice to Applicants....' quotes the definition agreed in the Expert Working Group of the Council of Health Ministers:

> 'For the purposes of this provision, a proprietary medicinal product will be regarded as essentially similar to another product if it has the same qualitative and quantitative composition in terms of active principles, and the pharmaceutical form is the same and where necessary, bioequivalence with the first product has been demonstrated by appropriate bioavailability studies... .'

There are clearly many questions which arise from the above, and the CPMP will in due course revise and extend its guidance on the definition of essential similarity.

6.6.4 Essential similarity and the clinical indications
The second applicant has to demonstrate that an originator's product has been marketed for at least ten years, with the precise indications which are now being sought in one Member State, and is also currently marketed in the Member State in which the application is made. If the originator product added new indications or a new dose regimen within the ten year period, the second applicant can either cite published clinical and other data to provide the evidence, or provide evidence from new toxicology tests (where needed) and clinical trials to show that the new indications or dose are justified.

6.7 SECOND APPLICANT PRODUCTS BY DETAILED REFERENCE TO THE PUBLISHED SCIENTIFIC LITERATURE — ARTICLE 4(8)(a)(ii) OF 65/65/EEC

These are the so-called 'public domain' applications. As pointed out by Jefferys (1989) this heading can only be used in a small minority of cases. Its main area of use will probably be for very well-known active ingredients, where for one reason or another there is not an appropriate originator product with which the second product can be essentially similar. In such a case reference can be made to the published literature to establish the toxicology of the active ingredient and the clinical experience. It is also likely that patients will have been exposed to several sources of the active ingredient.

'Public domain' applications are sometimes attempted within the ten year period of second applicant protection — particularly where the main patent for the active ingredient has expired. However, Article 4(8)(a)(ii) requires 'detailed references' to the literature presented in accord with Article 1 of 75/318/EEC. This means that all of the headings in 75/318/EEC have to be considered — single dose toxicity, repeated dose toxicity, foetal toxicity, reproductive toxicity, mutagenicity, carcinogenicity, pharmacodynamics, pharmacokinetics, and clinical trials.

For an application within the ten year period, the quality of the active ingredient used in the various studies would also need to be documented (particularly the impurity profile of the active ingredient batches used in the toxicology studies). It is very rare indeed for such information to be presented in the published literature.

For an Article 4(8)(a)(ii) application, copies of all of the published papers (translated where necessary) should be included in the application.

6.8 CHEMISTRY AND PHARMACY OF ABRIDGED APPLICATIONS

The major requirements for all applications have been covered in Chapter 3 (New chemical active substance products: quality requirements). The purpose of this section is to summarise some of the main points of difference, and to highlight some of the principal issues which arise.

6.8.1 Composition/container/development pharmaceutics

The composition should be stated in the dossier with an indication of the function of each excipient, and a reference to the analytical standard for each ingredient.

A starting material (active or excipient) must comply with the requirements of the *European Pharmacopoeia* (Ph. Eur.) if there is a monograph. If a material has no Ph. Eur monograph but is included in an EC Member States' national pharmacopoeia (*British Pharmacopoeia, Deutsches Arzneibuch, Pharmacopeé Français*, etc), it must comply with that national monograph. It is only if a monograph is not included in any of these, that reference may be made to the monograph of a third country (outside the EC) pharmacopoeia — such as the *United States Pharmacopeia* (USP) or the *Japanese Pharmacopoeia*. There is considerable confusion about what an applicant must do if he wishes to routinely test excipients (or active ingredients) to specifications other than those in the *European Pharmacopoeia*. The routine tests he intends to carry out on each batch of material must be stated in the marketing authorisation application. If these tests are not the same as those stated in the Ph. Eur. monograph, then evidence must be supplied that batches of the material would meet the official Ph. Eur. monograph requirements.

The details of the container should be briefly stated (container materials, composition of container, closure materials, method of closure, method of opening, dosage measurement if special devices are used, etc.).

The CPMP guideline on Development Pharmaceutics is given in Volume III of *The rules governing medicinal products in the European Community*. According to this, the dossier should include reports to show how the dosage form was selected; that the formulation proposed is acceptable for the purpose specified in the marketing authorisation (MA) application; and that those formulation and processing aspects that are crucial for batch reproducibility have been identified and will be monitored routinely.

For a well-known active ingredient the formulator must be completely familiar with its properties — stability, degradation pathway, and its physical properties (such as whether the particle size distribution affects bioavailability or suspension properties).

Some examples of the areas of development which may be needed for an oral liquid product might include pH (effect of the specified range, including the effect on antimicrobial preservative efficacy); ease of redispersion of a suspension; particle size of suspended solids; crystal shape and form of suspended solids; rheological properties of the product; preservation of the fresh and aged product, using a suitable test (e.g. the *British Pharmacopoeia* antimicrobial efficacy test); and the effect of dissolved air on the product stability (to justify the presence and proposed level of an antioxidant).

For a solid oral dose-form (tablet or capsule), areas to be investigated and reported might include homogeneity of the active in a low-dose product (containing less than 2 per cent of the total uncoated tablet core mass or capsule plug mass); *in vitro* dissolution, using a suitable method and apparatus (e.g. the Ph. Eur. rotating paddle or basket, or the new proposed *Ph. Eur.* flow-cell method for very sparingly soluble active ingredients which would otherwise have to be tested under non-sink conditions or using nonphysiological pH conditions or solvent mixtures).

6.8.2 Method of preparation
The manufacturing formula must be stated with the batch size details. The process of manufacture has to be stated, with an indication of the type of equipment which will be used in the various manufacturing sites which are proposed.

Process validation data may be needed for critical products, such as sterile products with a nonstandard sterilisation cycle or sustained release products.

6.8.3 Control of starting materials
This has already been referred to in sections 6.6.2 and 6.8.1 in relation to active ingredients and excipients and monograph specifications.

For packaging materials, data must be included in the dossier on the specification and routine tests; the development studies on the various candidate packaging materials; batch analyses; and analytical results.

6.8.4 Control tests on intermediate products
The dossier needs to include relevant details on the tests, test methods, and method validation. An example of tests on an intermediate product are tests on a tablet core (e.g. core mass), which may not be repeated on the coated tablet.

6.8.5 Control tests on the finished product
The specification and routine tests must be stated in the dossier together with the analytical development and validation data to support them. Finished product tests might include active ingredient identification tests; assay of active constituent(s) (or for plant constituents, quantitative determination of constituents with known therapeutic activity); purity tests (that is, tests for degradation products of the active ingredient, solvent residues, microbial contamination); identification and assay of

antimicrobial agents or antioxidants; pharmaceutical tests (e.g. those laid down in the general monograph for the type of dose-form in the *European Pharmacopoeia*); and identification of approved colouring matters.

A new guideline is under development on Control Tests on the Finished Product (to be issued for consultation in 1990 and probably adopted in 1991). It is likely to call for more detailed information to be provided on the development of the final specification and on the justification for the choice of the tests which it is proposed to carry out routinely. It will certainly call for a more detailed comparison and justification of the manufacturing (release) and shelf life specifications.

6.8.6 Stability of the active ingredient and the finished product

Stability data may not be needed on a well-known active ingredient if the relevant information is in the public domain and there is no known problem with stability variation with material from different manufacturing sources.

Stability data on the finished product are needed, normally on at least three batches in the actual marketing pack, stored at a variety of stress test conditions, but certainly including 25°C as the EC kinetic mean test storage temperature.

6.9 PHARMACOTOXICOLOGICAL DATA

As mentioned in sections 6.6 and 6.7 of this chapter, an application for a new source of active ingredient (with a different impurity profile) needs to be supported by information on the toxicology of the impurities. An application under Article 4(8)(a)(ii) needs to be supported by a full survey of the toxicological literature under all of the relevant headings in Directive 75/318/EEC. The 'Notice to Applicants ...' in fact calls for the information to be tabulated, using the standard formats given in the section on the pharmacotoxicological Expert Report. This would certainly help to highlight any deficiencies in the data.

6.10 CLINICAL DATA

The clinical section of any abridged application needs to justify and provide evidence to support any claims that have not been previously authorised for essentially similar products (see the earlier comments under section 6.6.4 of this chapter).

The clinical Expert may also need to consider the question of new impurities in an existing active ingredient. The pharmacologist/toxicologist will have already considered the available animal data, and the clinician will need to consider any human epidemiological experience (including evidence from exposure to reagents/intermediates/materials in industrial workers handling them), and to try to draw conclusions that extrapolate from the preclinical data to the likely effects in patients.

Many abridged applications merely seek to extend the range of the company's products, for example by adding a paediatric dosage-form. In such a case, the clinical experience needs to be stated in respect of the additional dosage-form. However, if the company has already submitted voluminous data on another strength, with a complete package of preclinical and clinical data, this can be cross-referred to — it does not have to be repeated with the new product.

In the UK, a mechanism has been devised to allow companies to add a new major indication to existing licences. It is possible to do this by a change (variation) to the first authorisation, but the refusal of such an authorisation does not carry any rights of appeal. However, the company can apply for an authorisation for a product with the new indication, cross-referring to their own data for all other information. When granted, the new licence is administratively merged ('rolled back') into their existing authorisation. This device is known as the 'medically targeted' abridged application.

6.11 BIOAVAILABILITY AND BIOEQUIVALENCE DATA

Bioavailability studies will normally be needed where one or more of the following situations apply:

(1) where the physicochemical properties of the substance (e.g. its solubility) indicate that a change in formulation may affect bioavailability;
(2) where the substance is structurally related to one with known bioavailability problems;
(3) where absorption data obtained in animals or humans demonstrate a high degree of variability (possibly caused by effects of formulation or manufacturing variables on the bioavailability);
(4) where the dose-response curve is steep, the therapeutic range is narrow, or the pharmacokinetics are nonlinear (in the normal clinical range seen in man);
(5) where there are special claims made for the release characteristics (including modified release, enteric coating); and
(6) where the product contains more than one active ingredient and there is reason to suppose that one of these may affect the bioavailability of the other.

The design of bioequivalence studies should be such that the treatment effect (that is, the effect of the formulation on the bioavailability) can be separated from other effects. Normally, a crossover design is used, with randomised allocation to each leg of the study. Single dose studies are usually sufficient, but there are cases where steady state studies may be more appropriate (such as where the inter-individual variation in absorption is very large, or for sustained release products). Healthy volunteers (aged 20 to 40 years) are normally used, but there are some cases where only patients can be studied. Meals, other medication, and fluid intake need to be standardised.

Bioequivalence studies are usually carried out by measuring the plasma concentration versus time curve or the cumulative renal excretion and excretion rate.

The choice of any reference product needs to be made with care. It may be the 'innovator' product of the originator in the Member State concerned, or if this is not suitable, it may be useful to also include a solution or suspension of the active ingredient. If a multistate application is envisaged in several EC Member States, the choice of reference product(s) needs to be carefully justified so that the authorities in each country can be given the requisite assurance that there will be no untoward effect if prescribers in their country switch from their national brand leader product to the new product. It would be a mistake to assume that the composition of major products produced by multinational companies is the same in all European markets — the experience of the national authorities in assessing parallel import applications reveals that this is often not the case.

A 'decision rule' accepted by many of the regulatory authorities in the assessment of bioequivalence data is to determine if the 95% confidence interval for the ratio of the test variable (area under plasma curve or C_{max} — the maximum plasma concentration) and the reference variable lies entirely within the bioequivalence range of 0.8 to 1.2. For active ingredients with a narrow therapeutic ratio, a narrower range (e.g. 0.9 to 1.1) may be more appropriate. Simple null-hypothesis testing using a test such as the Student t test or similar (an approach used by many applicants) is not normally acceptable.

6.11.1 Verifiability of bioavailability and bioequivalence studies

In 1990, the CPMP reviewed its requirements for the verifiability of bioavailability and bioequivalence data, particularly in the light of evidence of fraud and misconduct found by the Food and Drug Administration in 1989/90 in studies in support of abbreviated new drug applications (ANDAs) for generic products. The CPMP issued a special clarification of their requirements and asked that all studies submitted after 1 September 1990 include this full verification. The verification steps now required are that the application should contain the following information — the name and address of the laboratory carrying out the study; the name of the investigator in the laboratory responsible for the study; the name of the laboratory study coordinator who administered the trial; the name and address of the laboratory/manufacturing site used for the manufacture of the experimental batches used in the studies; copies of the certificates of analysis for all batches, with batch reference numbers of experimental products (complete analysis) and reference products (active ingredient content and *in vitro* dissolution profile); copies of the batch manufacturing records of the batches of experimental product used in the studies; and results of *in vitro* dissolution studies using appropriate methodology on all batches of experimental and reference solid dose-form products used in the studies.

The application is required to contain a statement by both the pharmaceutical and clinical Experts in the Expert Report, as what steps they have taken to verify on behalf of the company (as the sponsor for the study) its authenticity. A statement certifying the authenticity of the study needs to be included.

The applicant or his testing laboratory must also keep sufficient retention samples of the test and reference products so that they are available for any laboratory examination (for example by a national control laboratory) if required.

The regulatory authorities have also stated that they reserve the right to request access to inspect the facilities and archives of testing laboratories (test protocol, documentation, analytical information, certificates of audit, etc.) or to request data and documents to be made available to them.

REFERENCES

Armstrong, S. M. L. (1989). Legal aspects of abridged licence applications. *BIRA Journal* **8** (3), Supplement, 18–20.

Cartwright, A. C. (1989). Procedural aspects of abridged product licence applications. *BIRA Journal* **8** (3), Supplement, 7–9.

Jefferys, D. B. (1989). Medical issues in the assessment of abridged applications. *BIRA Journal* **8** (3), Supplement, 10–11.

7

Drug master files

7.1 INTRODUCTION

Under the present terms of the European Community (EC) pharmaceutical Directives it is the responsibility of the applicant for or holder of a marketing authorisation to ensure that all relevant information and data are supplied. This includes the information relating to the active ingredient and any excipient.

In many cases the ingredients used in a pharmaceutical product are purchased from third parties. With some materials there are pharmacopoeial monographs on which the purchaser can rely when agreeing a purchasing specification with the vendor of the material. In some cases the pharmacopoeial monograph may not be adequate. Examples include where the route of administration is different from that for which the pharmacopoeial specification was developed or where the monograph does not contain sufficiently specific impurity controls to ensure adequate limitation of potentially toxic impurities arising from a modified or different synthetic route. In other cases there will be no pharmacopoeial monograph at all.

Suppliers of chemicals are sometimes unwilling, for reasons of confidentiality, to supply full details of their syntheses and quality control to the pharmaceutical company using their materials. In such cases some regulatory authorities permit the submission of information direct to the authorities from the ingredient suppliers or their agents with agreed confidentiality. Such submissions are often referred to as 'drug master files' (DMFs).

In this chapter the provision of DMFs is discussed with particular reference to the EC, using the current procedures in the United Kingdom (UK) as an example.

7.2 WHAT IS A DRUG MASTER FILE AND WHEN MAY ONE BE USED?

7.2.1 In the United Kingdom

In the UK a DMF is a set of documents submitted voluntarily to the Medicines Control Agency by the manufacturer of an active ingredient, excipient, or container component or by his agent. The information is submitted on a commercially confidential basis and access to it is authorised by the person or company originally supplying the information.

DMFs may be submitted at any time but are not assessed until a marketing authorisation or a clinical trial certificate application is submitted which cross refers to it, and for which a letter of authorisation of access has been received from the DMF provider. Reference to a DMF is not usually permissible in connection with a clinical trial exemption application, and 'approval' in such cases would in any case be of limited value in the light of the negative vetting procedures applied to this type of application.

'Approval' relates to an application for a specific product and not to the DMF itself. It should not be considered that approval for use in one product means that the DMF is automatically approved in connection with another — for example, a material approved for use in a tablet may not be considered suitable for inclusion in an injection solution.

DMFs may be submitted or required in the UK in connection with substances having a pharmacopoeial monograph which does not adequately characterise the substance for its intended use.

As of April 1990, 1225 DMFs had been submitted to the Medicines Control Agency/UK Licensing Authority. A summary of their distribution is given in Table 7.1, and those substances for which ten or more DMFs have been submitted are listed in Table 7.2.

7.2.2 In the European Community

DMFs are accepted in Denmark, France, Greece, Ireland, and the Netherlands, as well as the UK. They are probably acceptable in Spain and Portugal. The German authorities are not prepared to accept DMFs — this is of course in line with a strict interpretation of the EC pharmaceutical Directives as presently worded.

7.2.3 Comparison with United States Food and Drug Administration DMFs

There are a number of similarities between the handling of DMFs in the EC and in the United States. For example, DMFs are not normally assessed until an application is made which cross-refers to them, and it is the product and not the DMF that is subject to approval. European DMFs are usually equivalent to FDA DMFs for drug substances, excipients, and occasionally containers. Those relating to good manufacturing practice aspects are not generally required, but some of the information is included in other types of DMF.

Information in accord with the FDA guidelines and the Code of Federal Regulations may or may not be adequate for EC purposes, depending on the specific case. Due account is necessary of local requirements (e.g. national or *European Pharmacopoeia* requirements).

Table 7.1 — Frequency distribution of drug master file (DMF) submissions in the United Kingdom

Number of DMFs	Number of substances
1	344
2	98
3	47
4	24
5	21
6	15
7	5
8	4
9	5
10	6
11	3
12	1
13	1
14	1
15	1
16	1

Table 7.2 — Substances for which ten or more drug master files (DMFs) have been submitted in the United Kingdom

Substances
Allopurinol
Amoxycillin trihydrate
Ampicillin trihydrate
Atenolol
Erythromycin
Frusemide (furosemide)
Heparin sodium
Ibuprofen
Methyldopa
Nifedipine
Propranolol hydrochloride
Tamoxifen citrate
Trimethoprim
Verapamil hydrochloride

The FDA inspects manufacturers named in DMFs. There is no inspection of such manufacturers by most EC regulatory authorities at present.

7.3 ASSESSMENT PROCEDURES FOR DMFs IN THE UNITED KINGDOM

7.3.1 Introduction

It has been indicated that a DMF may be submitted at any time, but it is not assessed until an application for a product licence or for a clinical trial certificate is received which cross-refers to it. The assessment is not begun unless a letter of authorisation from the supplier of the drug substance, etc., has been submitted. Approval is granted in appropriate cases, but is for the product and not for the DMF. DMFs by themselves are not approved.

DMFs are required to be submitted in English, or a translation of the whole of the information provided. The data requirements are in line with those for a new active substance or for a known substance or for an excipient, as appropriate, as outlined in Chapters 3 and 6. The most significant sources of data requirements are Directives 65/65/EEC, 75/318/EEC, and 75/319/EEC. Due account is also to be taken of the Committee for Proprietary Medicinal Products (CPMP) guidelines and Notice to

Applicants. The requirements are not relaxed because the data are included in a DMF rather than the main applicant dossier.

The assessment procedure followed is the same as for normal applications, except that the DMF is not examined for completeness at the time of receipt. If it is subsequently found that it is deficient at the time of assessment — for example if no Expert Report has been submitted — the DMF provider is approached to make good any deficiencies before assessment starts. If further deficiencies are found during assessment, additional information may be requested informally (for example, by a telephone call) or formally (in a letter sent under section 44 of the Medicines Act 1968). If the information is grossly deficient it may form part of the basis for a recommendation being put to an advisory committee to refuse the grant of a licence or certificate, and, if this is agreed, a letter raised under section 21 of the Medicines Act. If confidentiality restrictions applied by the DMF provider require it, the grounds of concern are sent in a separate letter addressed to the DMF provider and not to the applicant for a product licence. More information on the assessment procedure and appeal procedures is included in Chapter 17.

7.3.2 Data requirements

The following notes are a brief outline of the data requirements. More information is included in Chapters 3 and 6.

The nomenclature of the material is stated, using International Nonproprietary Names (INNs), *European Pharmacopoeia* monograph titles, other EC Member State monograph titles, EC Member State approved names, United States Adopted Names, or the systematic scientific names, laboratory codes, or proprietary names.

A description is provided, modelled on those of the *European Pharmacopoeia*. This includes information on the physical form, structural and molecular formulae, relative molecular mass of the whole molecule and the active part of it as necessary, and stereochemistry, using standard notation.

The synthetic route is described in sufficient detail. Information is included on starting materials, reagents, solvents, catalysts, critical reaction conditions, and yields at key stages. Isolated intermediates are described and any control tests given. Particular attention is paid to the final purification stages. Justification is provided for alternative reaction routes or reagents, and the equivalence of the product obtained when using the various options shown. The name and address of the manufacturer(s) are stated. Any changes from the originator's synthetic route are discussed if appropriate, especially with reference to the nature of any different impurities that may result. Sufficient batch analysis data are presented relating to material prepared by the proposed synthetic route at full manufacturing scale.

Adequate specifications are given for key starting materials and intermediates. The criteria used to establish any primary or secondary working standards are stated.

For new compounds and new synthetic routes adequate proof of structure is provided. In the case of known materials comparative spectral evidence may suffice. In other cases full information is required on structure, conformation, configuration, potential isomerism, and stereochemistry.

The chemical and physicochemical properties of the material are discussed, especially with respect to any characteristics that may affect bioavailability or bioequivalence. Potential and actual impurities are discussed, taking into account the requirement for 'essential similarity' required for materials used in products which are the subject of applications submitted under Article 4 (8) (a) of Directive 65/65/EEC. This is discussed in Chapter 6. Validation data on analytical methods are submitted. Toxicity of unusual impurities is discussed, and, where necessary, results from toxicology studies are provided.

The proposed specification for the material is included in the dossier and should include a statement of characteristics, identity tests, purity tests, physical characteristic controls, and potency controls.

Stability data on known materials are provided if the synthetic route has been changed from that previously submitted to the regulatory authorities. Such data are required for all new chemical entities.

Expert Reports are required for DMFs. The report on the quality of the ingredient should be prepared by an appropriately qualified pharmaceutical Expert. Where the DMF provider wishes to use a non-pharmacist as the author of the pharmaceutical Expert Report, this has to be justified. Certain aspects of the application as a whole will need to be discussed by the DMF Expert Report author and the authors of the Expert Reports on the main dossier. In particular, the pharmaceutical and toxicopharmacological Experts need to discuss the toxicology of the active ingredients, the toxicology of impurities, the daily dose of the material, the target population, the indications proposed, and the duration of therapy.

7.3.3 Experience with DMFs in the United Kingdom

The quality of DMFs seen by the Medicines Control Agency varies from excellent to almost useless. Common areas of deficiency include inadequate information on the synthetic route, illegible spectra or chromatographic traces, poor interpretation of spectra, and inadequate analytical validation data.

Other deficiencies are found in the batch analyses presented — especially the omission of recent, sequential analyses. The discussion of potential and actual impurity profiles is often poor. Too often the DMF provider puts forward a pharmacopoeial specification without any consideration as to whether the monograph offers adequate controls on impurities likely to arise specifically from a modified synthetic process.

Frequently, the stability studies are inadequately designed and/or reported. Another common fault is the failure to update old data, for example to reflect changes to the route of synthesis, modified specifications, etc. Expert Reports are also often of poor quality, failing to include accurate data summaries or critical overviews or both.

7.4 THE EUROPEAN DRUG MASTER FILE PROCEDURE

7.4.1 Introduction

The Committee for Proprietary Medicinal Products (CPMP) has recently been considering the introduction of a European drug master file procedure for active ingredients in connection with the EC pharmaceutical Directives. This is to rationalise the existing arrangements. A document has been approved on which a new procedure is to be based. A modification will be needed to the pharmaceutical Directives to allow the full introduction of the scheme, to allow some information to be provided by a party other than the applicant.

7.4.2 The European drug master file procedure

The European drug master file procedure (EuroDMF) is to be available to any active ingredient manufacturer (AIM) who is not the applicant for a marketing authorisation. It is intended to be an alternative option to the inclusion of all data within the marketing authorisation application. The EuroDMF documentation is to include sufficient information to establish the quality of the active ingredient and to show that the material is adequately controlled by the specification proposed by the marketing authorisation applicant. The shared responsibility of the AIM and the marketing authorisation applicant in providing all necessary information is emphasised.

To maintain confidentiality the AIM is to give a letter of access to the regulatory authority for each marketing authorisation application with which the data may be used. This is to indicate the name and address of the marketing authorisation applicant, the name of the product and date of the application (if possible), the name and address of the AIM, the name and address of the importer of the active ingredient (if appropriate), and the name and address of the distributor, agent, or broker as applicable. It is also to be stated that there is a formal agreement between the AIM and the applicant ensuring that any significant changes to the manufacturing methods or the specification of the active ingredient will be notified to the applicant and to the regulatory authorities.

The applicant for the marketing authorisation retains the responsibility for inclusion in the Expert Reports of the necessary critical evaluation of the dossier. For those parts of the data to which the applicant does not have access a critical appraisal is to be included in the restricted part of the EuroDMF. In particular this is expected to address how the manufacturing method guarantees consistent material of the desired quality, to discuss the batch analysis data and whether consistency of manufacture has been demonstrated by them, and to demonstrate how the proposed specification and routine tests in the applicants part can be justified by data in the restricted part of the dossier.

It is intended that the EuroDMF procedure apply to new active ingredients covered by a patent and not described in the European or Member States' pharmacopoeias, non-patented active ingredients not covered by a pharmacopoeial monograph, and for active ingredients described in a pharmacopoeia but prepared by a method liable to produce impurities not adequately controlled by the monograph.

Data requirements are as for any other case covered by the relevant pharmaceutical Directives, the EC Notice to Applicants, and the EC guidance notes.

To maintain the necessary commercial confidentiality two parts are proposed for a EuroDMF — one part to be provided to the marketing authorisation applicant (the 'applicant's part') which is confidential and not to be released to third parties without the permission of the AIM, and a second part confidential to the AIM and the regulatory authority (the 'restricted part').

The applicant's part of a EuroDMF is to include sufficient information for the applicant to take responsibility for an evaluation of the active material in terms of its suitability for the intended use. This includes a brief summary of the synthetic route, information on potential impurities, and where necessary on the toxicity of named impurities. The AIM is expected to provide available information on the toxicology of potential impurities, using references to the published literature, or by presenting data to justify the proposed limits. If the information is incomplete, additional information is to be provided by the marketing authorisation applicant.

The restricted part of the EuroDMF contains detailed information on the manufacturing method and the quality control applied during manufacture.

A possible distribution of information is indicated in Table 7.3.

Table 7.3 — Possible distribution of information in a European Drug Master File Procedure document

Information	Restricted part	Applicant's part
Name(s)/site(s) of manufacturer(s)	+	+
Specification/routine tests		+
Nomenclature		+
Description		+
Manufacturing method — brief outline (for example flow chart)		+
Manufacturing method — details	+	
Quality control during manufacture	+	
Process validation/data evaluation	+	
Development chemistry		
— evidence of structure†		+
— potential isomerism		+
— physicochemical characterisation		+
— analytical validation		+
Impurities		+
Batch analyses (including impurities)		+
Stability†		+

Note: † if necessary.

7.4.3 Related matters

Arising from the introduction of the EuroDMF procedure, consideration will need to be given to the need for inspection of active ingredient manufacturing sites. At the moment this is not undertaken by most regulatory agencies in the EC (unlike in the

United States, where such manufacturers are subject to FDA inspection). It seems likely that the chemical industry's trade associations will not object to the concept of inspection.

The identification of impurities not adequately controlled by *European Pharmacopoeia* monographs or those in the pharmacopoeias of the Member States will also draw attention to the need for regulatory authorities to advise the pharmacopoeia authorities of such problems. This requirement is already built in to the pharmaceutical Directives, but difficulties have arisen in its implementation because of confidentiality restrictions on data submitted in connection with marketing authorisation applications and drug master files. Suitable mechanisms will be needed to provide the necessary information to the European Pharmacopoeia Commission and national pharmacopoeial authorities.

REFERENCES

Helboe, P. (1990) Drug master files, *BIRA Journal* **9**(3), 3–5.

Matthews, E. R. (1990) The drug master file, Pharmaceutical Manufacturing International, 115–118, ISSN 0951–9696, Sterling Publications International Ltd, London.

8

Radiopharmaceutical products

8.1 INTRODUCTION

The market for radiopharmaceuticals is specialised, being estimated at about £300m per annum worldwide. There are a relatively few manufacturing companies — not more than six major companies service the European Community (EC) market.

The products themselves are unusual in that they are generally supplied only to specialised radiopharmacies or to health physicists, or direct to specialised and specially licensed medical practitioners. Most are used for diagnostic purposes on one or a small number of occasions in a given patient, and the amount of chemical administered is usually very small. The effects of the radiation administered with the products is, of course, unavoidable. It is an unavoidable side effect of the use of diagnostic agents, and is the wanted effect of therapeutic products.

The current regulation of radiopharmaceutical products is not consistent between Member States of the EC. These products are regulated in Belgium, Denmark, Ireland, France, Germany, Luxembourg, and the United Kingdom (UK), but not in Italy, Greece, the Netherlands, Spain, and Greece. In countries where there are no formal regulations in place at a national level the provisions of the *European Pharmacopoeia* still apply — for example in Greece and in Italy.

The regulation of radiopharmaceuticals is to change in the near future as a result of the adoption of Council Directive 89/343/1989 on 3 May 1989. This has the effect of adding radiopharmaceuticals to the range of products controlled under Directive 65/65/EEC. The radiopharmaceuticals extension Directive is due to take effect for new products not later than 1 January 1992 (unless necessary amendments to Directive 75/318/EEC are not adopted by that date, in which case the implementation date is to be deferred until the date those amendments are adopted). For products already on the market the Directive requires that its requirements be progressively extended so that all products are covered by 31 December 1992. This date does not seem to be movable.

In this chapter the present controls applying to radiopharmaceutical products in the UK are discussed, and the future controls that may be applied under Directive 89/343/EEC will be speculated on.

8.2 RADIOPHARMACEUTICAL AND RELATED DEFINITIONS

8.2.1 UK definitions
8.2.1.1 The Medicines Act 1968

Section 130 of the Medicines Act defines what is meant by the term 'medicinal product': any substance or article (not being an instrument, apparatus, or appliance) which is manufactured, sold, supplied, imported, or exported for use wholly or mainly in either or both of the following ways — by being administered to one or more human beings or animals for a medicinal purpose; or for use as an ingredient in the preparation of a substance or article which is to be administered to one or more human beings or animals for a medicinal purpose.

'Medicinal purpose' is defined in terms of the following: treating or preventing disease; diagnosing disease or ascertaining the existence, degree, or extent of a physiological condition; contraception; inducing anaesthesia; or otherwise preventing or interfering with the normal operation of a physiological function, whether permanently or temporarily, and whether by way of terminating, reducing or postponing, or increasing or accelerating, the operation of that function or in any other way.

8.2.1.2 The Medicines (Radioactive Substances) Order 1978

This is an Order made under section 104 of the Medicines Act (which enables the Health Ministers to bring under the Medicines Act articles or substances which are not medicinal products but which are manufactured, sold, supplied, imported, or exported for use wholly or partly for a medicinal purpose). It includes the following definition of a radioactive substance: any substance that contains one or more radionuclides of which the activity or the concentration cannot be disregarded as far as radiation protection is concerned.

The Order covers four categories of product. The first of these is interstitial and intracavitary appliances (other than nuclear powered pacemakers) which contain or are to contain a radioactive substance sealed in a container (otherwise than solely for the purpose of storage, transport, or disposal) or bonded solely within material and including the immediate container or bonding that are designed to be inserted into the human body or body cavities.

The second category is surface applicators (plates, plaques, and ophthalmic applicators) which contain or are to contain a radioactive substance sealed in a container or bonded solely within material designed to be brought into contact with the human body.

The third category is any apparatus capable of administering neutrons to human beings in order to generate a radioactive substance in the person to whom they are administered for the purpose of diagnosis or research.

The fourth category is other substances or articles (not being an instrument, apparatus, or appliance) which consist of or contain or generate a radioactive substance which consist of or contain or generate that substance in order, when administered, to utilise the radiation emitted therefrom, and are manufactured, sold, or supplied for use wholly or mainly by being administered to one or more human beings solely by way of a test for ascertaining what effects it has when so administered.

8.2.2 Relevant *European Pharmacopoeia* definitions

Radiopharmaceutical preparations are defined as preparations containing one or more radionuclides. Radionuclides are nuclides which are radioactive and which transform spontaneously into other nuclides by a mechanism which may involve the emission of charged particles (α or β^+ or β^-), electron capture, or isomeric transition. Gamma- or X-ray emissions may accompany certain types of transitions.

Radioactive source is defined as a radioactive material used to provide ionising radiation. A sealed source is a radioactive source intended to be used in such a manner that the radioactive material does not come into immediate contact with the environment. It consists of radioactive material firmly incorporated in solid material or sealed in a resistant container which will not result in contamination during normal use.

A non-sealed source is one which allows the radioactive material to come into immediate contact with the environment. The radioactive material is directly accessible for physical or chemical manipulation. Radiopharmaceutical preparations belong to this category.

Radionuclidic purity is the ratio of a particular radionuclide's radioactivity to the total radioactivity expressed as a percentage. Alternative terms with the same meaning are radioactive purity and radioisotopic purity.

Radiochemical purity is the ratio of the radioactivity from a given radionuclide in a stated chemical form to the total radioactivity from that radionuclide in the material, expressed as a percentage.

A carrier is a non-radioactive isotope of the same element as the radioisotope present in the same chemical form as the radionuclide.

Specific [radio]activity is the radioactivity of the nuclide per unit mass of the element or the chemical form concerned. Radioactive concentration is the radioactivity of a nuclide per unit volume of the solution in which it is present.

8.2.3 Definitions from Directive 89/343/EEC

A radiopharmaceutical is any medicinal product which, when ready for use, contains one or more radionuclides (radioactive isotopes) included for a medicinal purpose.

A generator is any system incorporating a fixed parent radionuclide from which is produced a daughter radionuclide which is removed by elution or by any other method and used in a radiopharmaceutical.

'Kit' means any preparation to be reconstituted or combined with radionuclides in the final radiopharmaceutical, usually prior to its administration.

'Precursors' or precursor radiopharmaceuticals are any other radionuclides produced for the radiolabelling of another substance prior to administration.

8.2.4 Definitions from Directive 65/65/EEC

A medicinal product is any substance or combination of substances presented for treating or preventing disease in human beings or animals, or any substance or combination of substances which may be administered to human beings or animals with a view to making a medical diagnosis or to restoring, correcting, or modifying physiological functions.

In this context a 'substance' is any matter irrespective of origin, which may be human, animal, vegetable, or chemical.

8.3 UK CONTROL OF RADIOPHARMACEUTICALS

8.3.1 Introduction

Radiopharmaceuticals are presently controlled under the Medicines Act 1968. Products are subject to the licensing provisions of the Act. Manufacturers within the UK are also licensed, and those outside the UK are subject to inspection by the UK Medicines Inspectorate or by local inspectors under reciprocal arrangements such as the Pharmaceutical Inspection Convention. The application of good pharmaceutical manufacturing practices is expected, such as those described in the current *Guide to good pharmaceutical manufacturing practice*.

The licensing of radiopharmaceuticals under the Medicines Act is carried out by the Medicines Control Agency, with reference of applications for product licences to the Committee on Safety of Medicines if necessary. However, a number of aspects of radiopharmaceuticals control are exercised under the aegis of the EURATOM Directives 76/579/EURATOM, 80/836/EURATOM, and 84/467/EURATOM concerned with radiation safety, and these are dealt with by other agencies in the United Kingdom. (In other EC Member States these aspects may be dealt with by the same authorities.)

Under certain circumstances a radiopharmaceutical product licence application can become the subject of compulsory or voluntary EC procedures. For example, a radiolabelled monoclonal antibody is covered by the compulsory List A concertation procedure. A novel radiopharmaceutical may be included in the 'high technology' List B concertation procedure; and a radiopharmaceutical may become the subject of a multistate application following approval in one Member State and then the subject of applications to two or more other Member States.

8.3.2 Basis of data expectations

Although covered by national legislation in the UK radiopharmaceuticals are treated as if they were medicinal products under Directive 65/65/EEC in terms of the data requirements and the format of the applications. During assessment due account is taken of the special nature of the products, and any special considerations necessary are applied. These include the infrequent administration likely for diagnostic products (depending on the indications claimed), the small amounts of materials administered, and the inherent properties of the radiation unavoidably associated with the use of the products.

A guideline on certain chemistry and pharmacy and 'special particulars' aspects of the application is included as an Annexe to the UK *Guidance notes on applications for product licences (MAL 2)*.

8.3.3 Expert Reports
Expert Reports are required with all applications for product licences for radiopharmaceutical products, as for any other product.

8.3.4 Pharmaceutical data requirements
The UK national legislation covers radiopharmaceuticals of all categories as defined in Directive 89/343/EEC—'radiopharmaceuticals', generators, precursors, and kits. The data requirements are generally as per the pharmaceutical Directives, guidance notes, and Notice to Applicants, for either new substances or for abridged applications as appropriate, and taking into account the UK guideline. The general requirements are discussed fully in Chapters 3, 4, 5 and 6 (for chemical substances).

In the following sections attention is drawn to those areas of data requirements which differ from other types of product.

8.3.4.1 Composition
In the case of generators, information is required on both the mother and daughter radionuclides, the generator column material, the elution medium, and components of the elution pathway.

For products containing radionuclides information is required on the concentration of the radioactive component expressed in MBq (or GBq, etc.), although additional units of measurement are not excluded. This concentration is expressed in terms of the amount of radioactivity per millilitre or per dosage form or per container at a stated reference date and time. The time should include a reference to GMT or BST or other time zone as appropriate. Adequate information is also required on the composition of any diluent or other material supplied for use with the radiopharmaceutical.

In the case of non-radioactive kits, normal requirements apply.

8.3.4.2 Development pharmaceutics
For generators, information on factors affecting the suitability of recommended elution media is required.

Normal requirements apply to radioactive radiopharmaceuticals.

For radiopharmaceutical kits, data are provided to justify the ranges of reconstitution volumes and amounts of radioactivity recommended for use in the radiolabelling procedure, together with data to validate and justify any manipulation required to effect satisfactory radiolabelling. A full discussion on factors affecting radiochemical purity is included. It is sometimes necessary to provide data to show that the eluate from a number of typical generators or precursors from different manufacturers are suitable for use with the kit (e.g. where the amount of a reducing agent is particularly low in a kit to be used with $^{99}Tc^m$-pertechnetate eluate, or where particular purity criteria are applied to precursor radiopharmaceuticals for use with the product as with ^{111}In-indium chloride solutions for labelling monoclonal antibodies). The excipients and the amounts of each included are justified, especially for materials such as reducing agents or other materials playing a major role in the radiolabelling process of formation of the radiolabelled species. Compatibility of the product and the container system is discussed.

In all cases the animal and human biodistribution of the product is discussed. Animal studies are often described in the development pharmaceutics section to demonstrate that biodistribution of the product is not variable from batch to batch and is not affected by variations in the reconstitution/radiolabelling procedure. References are included to the appropriate parts of the preclinical and clinical parts of the dossier as well as to the pharmaceutical data.

8.3.4.3 Manufacture

A full description of the manufacturing process is required for all products.

In the case of radioactive materials, information is required on the manufacture and separation of the radionuclides. Factors affecting radiochemical or radionuclidic purity are discussed.

In the case of generators, full information is included regarding the assembly of the parts of the generator, and attention is paid to those aspects which may affect eluate quality.

8.3.4.4 Impurities

Particular attention is paid to the presence of potential or actual impurities which could affect the human biodistribution or dosimetry. Adequate validation data for tests for radiochemical purity are provided. In the case of generators, particular consideration is given to the presence of mother nuclide, elution column derived material, or other impurities.

8.3.4.5 Other constituents

Information is included on all ingredients in the formulated product. Any recommended reconstituting or diluting media or materials used in the manufacturing process are described. If licensed medicinal products are used — e.g. sodium chloride intravenous infusion bought from a licensed source — little additional information is required. If an unlicensed source is used, then full supporting data are required.

Pharmacopoeial specifications are not invariably acceptable for materials used in radiopharmaceuticals: demonstration of suitability of material of the appropriate specification for use in the product is sometimes required.

8.3.4.6 Control tests on the finished product

Compliance with relevant pharmacopoeial requirements is expected. Monographs in the *European Pharmacopoeia* should be given priority for specifications, followed by monographs in the Member States' pharmacopoeias. The use of other pharmacopoeial specifications has to be justified.

Several parts are sometimes necessary to the control specifications on the finished product. One part of the specification relates to the product as supplied to the user. Release and shelf life (or check) specifications are often appropriate for this.

A second specification relates to the product after any manipulation, radiolabelling, and other processes required prior to administration of the product to the patient. This specification often includes two parts: one applying at the end of any incubation period necessary after radiolabelling and one at the end of a defined storage period, for example. The latter is supported by data to show that material of this age is consistently within specification if the recommended storage conditions are used.

In the case of a product with a very short radioactive half life, it may not be possible to carry out the full range of finished product tests before the release of the product for sale. The tests should nonetheless be carried out, and the results recorded. A defined procedure should be in operation so that it is clear at what stage the product is released by the Qualified Person and on the basis of what data.

A user test for radiochemical purity is usually required, and, wherever possible, this should be the same as the test applied by the manufacturer so as to allow comparison of results obtained by the user and the manufacturer in cases of dispute.

8.3.4.7 Stability data

In many cases the shelf life claimed for a radioactive material is limited by the physical half life of the radionuclide rather than by chemical stability. In the case of radiolabelled materials it is necessary to undertake stability trials to establish the shelf life of the product supplied to users.

Where a product is reconstituted or otherwise manipulated it is necessary to provide stability data to establish the shelf life and storage conditions for the processed material. Biodistribution studies in animals are often provided as a useful part of this data. In practice the storage life may be limited by factors other than the chemical or radiochemical stability — e.g. the lack of a antimicrobial preservative in a multi-dose container may restrict the in-use shelf life of the product.

8.3.5 Preclinical data requirements

In the case of a product containing a new non-radioactive material it is necessary to provide data from a mutagenicity package. The need for further data will depend on the results in the mutagenicity studies, the intended uses of the product, the probable frequency of use, and the intended target population. For such products, data are also required on repeat dose toxicity of appropriate duration and on biodistribution studies in animals (which are compared with the results in man presented in the clinical studies).

8.3.6 Clinical data requirements

Safety and efficacy are demonstrated in all claimed indications. Recommended dosages are in accord with the recommendations of the Administration of Radioactive Substances Advisory Committee (ARSAC), or any deviation fully justified.

Sec. 8.4] EC involvement in the regulation of radiopharmaceutical products

These recommendations are published in the *Notes for guidance on the administration of radioactive substances to persons for the purposes of diagnosis, treatment or research*.

8.4 EC INVOLVEMENT IN THE REGULATION OF RADIOPHARMACEUTICAL PRODUCTS

8.4.1 Introduction

The EC is involved in the control of radiopharmaceutical products in two ways. The first of these is the EURATOM Directives which are concerned with the production, supply, transport, and use of radioactive materials. (ARSAC's remit owes its origins to these Directives.) The second is the specific control of radiopharmaceuticals introduced with Directive 89/343/EEC.

The effect of the adoption of Directive 89/343/EEC is to bring radiopharmaceuticals under the aegis of the pharmaceutical Directives 65/65/EEC *et seq*. The Directive has effect throughout the EC, so that all radiopharmaceuticals will become the subject of national laws in each Member State, implementing the Directive by the effective dates.

The data requirements in the original pharmaceutical Directives, particularly 75/318/EEC, do not take into account the special nature of many radiopharmaceutical products. Certain modifications are required to take account of these.

Directive 89/343/EEC itself introduces two new areas of data requirement. Article 3 requires for generators a general description of the system together with a detailed description of the components of the system which may affect the composition or quality of the daughter nuclide preparation. Article 4 requires for radiopharmaceuticals full details of internal radiation dosimetry and additional detailed instructions for extemporaneous preparation and quality control of such preparations, and, where appropriate, maximum storage time during which any intermediate preparation such as an eluate or the ready-to-use pharmaceutical conforms to its specifications. Since these are included in the Directive itself they have mandatory effect.

There is at the time of writing no guideline on data requirements for radiopharmaceuticals, nor does the Notice to Applicants apply. (In fact there is a specific statement in the Notice to Applicants that it does not apply to radiopharmaceuticals!) A new supplement is also needed for the recently published EC *Guide to Good Pharmaceutical Manufacturing Practice* to cover the special aspects of radiopharmaceuticals manufacture.

At the time of writing (August 1990) four draft documents are at various stages of circulation for comment by interested parties. These are a draft amendment to the Annex to Directive 75/318/EEC (which relates to the technical data requirements for applications for marketing authorisation); draft guidance notes for radiopharmaceuticals and for radiopharmaceuticals based on monoclonal antibodies; and a draft supplement to the good manufacturing guide. A draft revision for the Notice to Applicant is in hand but is not yet out for consultation. The following sections are, therefore, based on what might happen: the final outcome depends on the account taken of comments submitted by the interested parties following the consultation process, and may differ in some or many respects from what is discussed below.

8.4.2 Predicted data requirements for radiopharmaceuticals under EC Directives

8.4.2.1 Introduction

The following notes are intended to identify only those areas of difference from the normal requirements applying to all products under the pharmaceutical Directives, the guidance notes, and the Notice to Applicants.

8.4.2.2 Pharmaceutical, chemical, biological, and microbiological data requirements

(a) Qualitative particulars

In the case of ready-made radiopharmaceuticals and precursors the name of the radionuclide is stated. For generators the name of the mother and the daughter radionuclides are stated. The nature of any added material present, especially in kits, which is essential for the radiolabelling process is stated.

(b) Quantitative particulars

For radioactive materials the amount of radioactivity is stated in terms of MBq (etc.) at a stated time and date, with the time zone used being specified. A statement of the specific activity of the radioactive material and an indication of whether it is present in carrier-free or carrier-added condition is useful. The normal requirement to declare the content of active ingredient by weight normally does not apply.

(c) Development particulars

The chemical and radiochemical purity and the biodistribution of the material are discussed. The maximum and minimum volumes and radioactivity recommended for the preparation of the radiolabelled material are justified. If special purity requirements are necessary for radiolabelling media, these are established in this section. In the case of radiopharmaceutical kits, the development of a suitable test by which the user is able to ascertain the suitability of the radiolabelled product for use in patients is described in this section.

(d) Method of preparation

For radioactive materials, information is required on the nuclear reactions used to prepare the radionuclide as well as the separation processes applied. For sterile products, particular attention is paid to the maintenance of sterility, possibly in the presence of radioactivity, and the validation of the process of manufacture since the manipulation concerned are often complex.

For radiopharmaceutical kits a description is also included in this section of the radiolabelling process which is used to obtain the finished radiopharmaceutical. Particular attention is paid to any special manipulations necessary. For radioactive compounds, information is supplied on the specificity of the radiolabelling process and of the specific activity of the product.

Sec. 8.4] EC involvement in the regulation of radiopharmaceutical products 123

(e) Control of starting materials

For radioactive materials the controls extend to any irradiation target material. Chemical purity and isotopic abundance are discussed. The significance of any permitted impurities is discussed in terms of the nuclear reactions that may result under the conditions of irradiation employed.

Where a *European Pharmacopoeia* monograph is available for the material it is expected to apply. In certain circumstances additional purity standards are required, for example where the manufacturing method produces impurities not controlled by the pharmacopoeial specification. In the absence of a *European Pharmacopoeia* monograph one from the pharmacopoeia of a Member State may be used (subject to the same proviso). The proposed use of other pharmacopoeial specifications needs to be justified.

If ingredients are not the subject of acceptable pharmacopoeial monographs it is necessary to provide adequate information to justify a proposed specification. For a radioactive material this includes tests for identity, radionuclidic and radiochemical purity, specific activity, and a validated and properly calibrated assay procedure.

(f) Control tests on the finished product

In the case of kits, some form of radiolabelling efficiency test is expected to form part of the release and check specifications.

The assay limits for radioactive components may be within ± 10 per cent of the nominal amount, since the normal limits of ± 5 percent expected for therapeutically active ingredients involves operatives in unnecessary exposure to radioactivity.

Radionuclidic purity and specific activity of radioactive material are controlled.

For radiopharmaceutical kits that do not contain radioactive material, therapeutically active ingredients are expected to comply with the normal nominal ± 5 per cent requirement. Deviation from this is justified in specific applications. Control tests for radiochemical purity of radiolabelled material are included in the release and shelf life specifications.

With generators, information is included on testing for both the mother and the daughter radionuclides and consideration is given to the inclusion of adequate controls on the elution of the mother radionuclide or any other unwanted material.

Identity tests for radioactive materials include methods for characterisation of emission types and energy levels.

Impurity controls reflect any potential effects on radiochemical purity and biodistribution, based on potential effects on human patients.

Excipients essential for radiolabelling are assayed and identified.

In the case of radiopharmaceuticals containing a short-lived radionuclide it is recognised that it may be necessary to release the product for sale before all the necessary quality control tests have been completed. In such cases the stage at which the decision is taken to release the product for sale is stated. The full release testing programme should be undertaken in all cases as a monitor for the production process. The finished product specification should differentiate between those tests undertaken on a routine basis and those undertaken on an occasional basis (with a statement on the frequency with which the tests will be applied). For certain terminally sterilised products it is possible that acceptable justification can be advanced for parametric release. This depends on the adequacy of the facility, staff, and quality system concerned. It is not usual for the requirement for a product to comply with a sterility test if tested to be deleted from the finished product specification, however. In the case of aseptically prepared products a sterility test is likely to be required on a routine basis.

(g) Dosage form-related points
It is unlikely that the weight of radioactive material needs to be stated for solid dosage forms. Dosage expressions in terms of the amount of radioactivity (in MBq, etc.) are more usual.

In the case of parenteral products it is likely that a rabbit pyrogens test or a limulus amoebocyte lysate test for endotoxins will be permitted, provided that the latter is validated. However, once a choice is made between the two tests, the other will not be permitted as an alternate release criterion. Products intended for the intrathecal route normally are expected to be tested by using a validated limulus amoebocytelysate endotoxin test.

(h) Stability testing
Data are required for all products. With products containing radionuclides it is sometimes necessary to investigate the effects of radioactive decay on the overall stability of the product.

In the case of radiopharmaceutical kits it is necessary to report on the stability of both the kit and the reconstituted/radiolabelled product. Particular attention is paid to the radiochemical purity and the biodistribution of the product as prepared for clinical use. For a product presented in a multi-dose vial, data are submitted on the effects of removal of a number of doses from the vial, as is likely to be done in the clinic, on the stability of the remaining product.

8.4.2.3 *Toxicological and pharmacological data requirements*
(a) General
It is recognised that the radiation associated with radiopharmaceutical products is inevitably associated with toxicity: this is unavoidable in the case of diagnostic products and is the wanted effect in the case of therapeutic agents. The toxicity of the chemicals, etc., included in radiopharmaceuticals and the radiation toxicity are therefore considered separately.

Toxicology studies are, as far as possible, carried out by using non-radioactive product either without using a radioactive material at all or allowing the radioactive component to decay before carrying out the tests in those cases where the radiolabelling process modifies the ligand. Distribution and elimination studies are carried out using radiolabelled material since the low concentrations of material used would otherwise not be easily detectable. Where radioactive material is used it is prepared by the radiolabelling procedure described for the clinic.

No-carrier-added radionuclides or simple salts are unlikely to require additional toxicity studies where the toxicity of the non-radioactive equivalent material is known and is available for submission.

Sec. 8.4] EC involvement in the regulation of radiopharmaceutical products 125

(b) Subacute toxicity studies
The normal recommendations are followed, the duration of the necessary studies being dependent on the number of doses to be given to humans and the period over which they will be given.

(c) Mutagenic potential
All new chemicals are evaluated for mutagenic potential be using studies designed to identify gene and chromosome mutations. Both radiolabelled and unlabelled materials are investigated.

(d) Carcinogenic potential
The evaluation of the carcinogenic potential is presented. In many cases this is a paper exercise based on the absence of demonstrable genotoxicity in the mutagenicity studies. If no specific studies have been undertaken, this is stated in the summary of product characteristics.

(e) Reproductive studies
The claims for use of the product determine whether such studies are required. If the product is likely to be given to the same patient repeatedly, studies may be required. If studies are reported, the chemical and radiation aspects are discussed separately.

(f) Pharmacodynamics
In most cases it is not expected that radiopharmaceutical products will have measurable pharmacodynamic effects. However, this is not a reason for not looking for such effects in the various studies.

(g) Pharmacokinetics
Animal biodistribution studies are reported for diagnostic radiopharmaceuticals to assess the *in vivo* stability of the radiolabelled complex.

(h) Radiation dosimetry
Data are provided to identify the target organs and to establish the systemic tolerance. Calculated absorbed radiation dose estimates and effective dose equivalents are reported.

8.4.2.4 Clinical data requirements
Controlled clinical trials are reported wherever possible. Controlled and uncontrolled trials are summarised separately. Adverse events encountered in the trials are reported together with a summary of the investigations undertaken to find them. In the case of some radiopharmaceuticals it is more relevant to compare the radiopharmaceutical product with products or techniques of proven value. The use of healthy volunteers is avoided wherever possible.

Diagnostic or therapeutic efficacy is established for each claimed indication.

An adequate discussion is included on the possibility of interaction between the radiopharmaceutical product and other radiopharmaceuticals or other products likely to be in use in the target population group(s).

The radiation dose recommended is established from the results of the clinical trials, due account being taken of any accepted guidelines on the amount of radioactive material to be administered for particular procedures.

8.4.3 Labelling and instruction leaflets
8.4.3.1 *Introduction*
Directive 89/343/EEC requires that radiopharmaceuticals labels are in accordance with the requirements of the regulations for the safe transport of radioactive materials laid down by the International Atomic Energy Agency.

8.4.3.2 *Directive 89/343/EEC specific requirements*
The Directive requires the following information to appear:

(a) On the label on the shielding
   — The name of the product (brand name, common name accompanied by a trade mark or the name of the manufacturer, or a scientific name accompanied by a trade mark or the name of the manufacturer).
   — Where the product contains only one active ingredient, the International Nonproprietary Name (INN) or the usual common name of that ingredient if the main title is a brand name.
   — A qualitative and quantitative statement of the active ingredients using INNs or usual common names.
   — The manufacturer's batch number.
   — The marketing authorisation number.
   — The name/corporate name and address of the person placing the product on the market, and where applicable the manufacturer.
   — The method of administration.
   — The expiry date in plain language.
   — Any special storage conditions.
   — The pharmaceutical form and contents (volume, weight, number of unit dosage forms).
   — An explanation of the codings used on the vial and the amount of radioactivity per dose/vial/number of capsules/number of millilitres in the container.
(b) On the label on the vial
   — The name or code of the product, including the name or chemical symbol of the radionuclide.
   — The batch identification and expiry date.
   — The international symbol for radioactivity.
   — The name of the manufacturer.
   — The amount of radioactivity (as above).

However, a draft revision to the labelling requirements included in Directive 65/65/EEC is presently under development. It is not clear whether this will affect the labelling required for radiopharmaceuticals.

8.4.3.3 European Pharmacopoeia *requirements*
The general monograph on radiopharmaceutical preparations in the *European Pharmacopoeia* includes the following labelling requirements:

(a) On the container
- The name of the preparation.
- The name of the manufacturer.
- An identification number.
- For liquid preparations, the total radioactivity in the container or the radioactive concentration per millilitre at a stated date and, if necessary, time, and the volume of liquid in the container.
- For solid preparations, the total radioactivity at a stated date and, if necessary, time.
- For capsules, the radioactivity of each capsule at a stated date and, if necessary, hour, and the number of capsules in the container.

(b) On the package:
- That the preparation is intended for medical use.
- The route of administration.
- The expiry date (or period of validity).
- The name and concentration of any added antimicrobial preservative.
- Any special storage requirements.

8.4.3.4 *Instruction leaflet*

Directive 89/343/EEC requires that Member States ensure that a detailed instruction leaflet is enclosed with the packaging of radiopharmaceuticals, generators, kits, or precursor radiopharmaceuticals. The information to be included is as in Article 6 of Directive 75/319/EEC. This includes the following requirements:

- The leaflet applies only to the product concerned.
- The information is in accordance with the information submitted under Article 4 of Directive 65/65/EEC (which lists the documents and particulars accompanying an application for a marketing authorisation) and approved by the regulatory authorities.
- At least the following information:
  - The name and address/corporate name and address or registered place of business of the person responsible for placing the product on the market, and, where necessary, the manufacturer.
  - The name and quantitative particulars of the product in terms of the active ingredient, using the INN where available.
  - In the absence of a decision to the contrary by the regulatory authorities, the therapeutic indications, contraindications, side effects, and special precautions for use, taking into account the results from clinical trials and pharmacological tests as required by Directive 65/65/EEC and of experience gained in use after marketing.
  - Directions for use of the product, including method of administration, duration of treatment if this is limited, and usual dosage.
  - Any special storage requirements.

Any other information provided is clearly separated from that described above.
Article 6 of Directive 89/343/EEC also requires information to be included on the precautions to be taken by the user and the patient during the preparation and

administration of the product, and special precautions for the disposal of the container and its unused contents.

Leaflets may be in more than one language provided that the information is identical in all languages.

A proposed revision of the leaflet requirements is presently under consideration, but the effect of this on the requirements for radiopharmaceutical product leaflets is unclear.

9

Medicated devices

9.1 INTRODUCTION

This chapter includes a discussion of the control of medicated devices in the Member States of the European Community (EC). In 1987 this would have involved a listing of the different controls applied in each Member State, and indeed a short part of the present chapter does this for some of the countries concerned. However, in 1987 the Commission of the European Communities† (CEC) was convinced by the European medical device trade associations that the state of affairs existing at that time, and proposals for changes to the systems of control within Member States, amounted to a technical barrier to trade. It was agreed that Directives would be developed to harmonise the controls on medical devices. Furthermore, it was agreed that the Directives would be developed under the so-called 'new approach' (which will be further discussed and explained in section 9.4).

The CEC invited the trade associations to submit proposals on which it could base a series of medical device Directives. The original plan was for four Directives — one for powered implantable electromedical devices (such as heart pacemakers), one for other powered electromedical devices (such as X-ray machines), one for *in vitro* diagnostic products, and one for all other medical devices.

This chapter includes sections discussing the development of the medical device Directives and their implications, as well as information on the controls at present applied to medical devices in some Member States of the EC. The provisions applying to contact lens care products and intrauterine contraceptive devices in the United Kingdom (UK) are discussed in more detail in Chapter 10.

9.2 THE DEVELOPMENT OF THE MEDICAL DEVICE DIRECTIVES

9.2.1 Introduction

In this section the development of the medical device Directives is described.

9.2.2 The present EC market for medical devices

The European market for medical devices at present demonstrates a wide range of

† European Economic Community, Iron and Steel Community, European, Atomic Energy Commission.

different approaches to controls on how those products are placed on the market and are subsequently marketed.

The range of products covered by the term 'medical device' is enormous, and includes implants, drug delivery systems, apparatus, appliances, and *in vitro* diagnostics. It is possible to consider medical devices according to their function — for example diagnostic, therapeutic, surgical, monitoring. The mode of use of the products may also be of relevance — for example use outside the body (such as *in vitro* diagnostics or wheelchairs); use on the body by an expert (for example X-ray equipment); or left in contact with the body (for example heart valves, pacemakers, sutures, or contact lenses).

The medical device industry, in 1987 or earlier, viewed with some concern the variety of controls applied to these products in different Member States of the EC (and indeed beyond the EC). This was not only because of the effects of those different controls as a technical barrier to trade and the costs of working to the various different systems, but also because of the potential for Member States to introduce different or additional controls, which could make the situation more complicated (and potentially increase costs).

Another factor was the increasing complexity of the borderline between products that could be considered *bona fide* medical devices and those that could be considered as pharmaceutical products. The medical device industry was not enthusiastic about the potential for the application of the types of controls applied to pharmaceuticals to what they saw as legitimate medical devices.

It was widely recognised that some unified system of control was needed for medical devices on an EC-wide basis, and that the controls applied should be proportional to the risks associated with the devices (rather than to the risks associated directly with their uses). Following a meeting organised by the European Confederation of Medical Suppliers Associations (EUCOMED) in Brussels in 1987 (which followed discussions between the CEC and the trade associations) the CEC was convinced of the need for harmonised controls for medical devices.

The CEC invited the trade associations to put forward proposals for the development of 'new approach' Directives for medical devices. Given the vast range of products, more than one directive was considered likely to be needed, and several European trade associations were invited to participate in the preparation of proposals.

The first proposals submitted to the CEC related to 'active implantable electromedical devices' — products such as pacemakers ('active' implies powered by means other than those derived from the human body or gravity). These were submitted by the International Association of Medical Prosthetics Manufacturers (IAPM). The proposals were used as the basis for the first of the proposed Directives, and, after considerable effort and frantic consultative stages, the proposals were submitted to the Council of Ministers for initial approval as a common position paper in January 1990. The final version of the Directive was adopted by the Council of Ministers on 20 June 1990.

Meanwhile, other sets of proposals were submitted from EUCOMED (for non-active medical devices — a category covering a vast range of products) and from the Coordination Committee of Radiological and Electromedical Equipment (COCIR)

Sec. 9.2]   **The development of the medical device Directives**   131

(for active medical devices). A further set of proposals developed by the European Diagnostic Manufacturers Association (EDMA) to cover *in vitro* diagnostics was submitted to the CEC in 1988.

Work on the development of directives for non-active medical devices and active medical devices is under way at the time of writing (August 1990), although the latest draft document combines the two types of product into a single draft directive. Work on the development of the fourth (*in vitro* diagnostics) directive has yet to commence at the Community level.

9.2.3 Control of medical devices in the Member States of the EC

The most stringent controls on medical devices in the World are those applied in Japan and the United States. Many other markets — including those of the EC Member States — have some form of control over the marketing of at least some medical devices. There is, however, considerable variety in the form and extent of controls in force.

At the EC level there is a specific Directive (84/539/EEC) on electromedical equipment; this was developed under the 'old approach'.

In the UK there are two types of control in operation. That with the narrowest application is for those products (such as contact lens care products, intrauterine contraceptive devices, and dental root filling materials) which are considered to be covered by the provisions of the Medicines Act and its Regulations and Orders. The level of scrutiny in this pre-market approval system is the same as that applying to pharmaceuticals, including inspection of manufacturers and the need for evidence of clinical safety and efficacy as well as quality. Clinical trial certificate and exemption schemes apply to such products.

The second scheme is a voluntary registration scheme operated by the Procurement Directorate of the Department of Health (now the Medical Devices Directorate). In this case there is no compulsion to register, although failure to appear on the approved manufacturers' list may result in difficulties when products are to be supplied to National Health Service hospitals. However, the scheme involves no detailed consideration of the design or clinical performance of the products concerned. It involves confirmation that the manufacturer's manufacturing facility and quality systems are satisfactory. (Compliance with appropriate good manufacturing practices guidelines is the basis for the scheme.)

The provisions of the *European Pharmacopoeia* and of national pharmacopoeias apply to materials that are the subject of monographs — for example some surgical sutures and surgical dressings.

The Committee on Dental and Surgical Materials and the Medicines Commission (bodies appointed under the UK Medicines Act) have expressed concern at the lack of adequate control of certain categories of devices including heart valves and other products whose failure could be catastrophic.

There is no comprehensive list of products available on the UK market.

In 1987 there were plans for the introduction of comprehensive controls on medical devices in West Germany, Denmark, Italy and possibly Belgium.

In West Germany in 1987 power-driven equipment and apparatus were covered by a 1985 Regulation on medical technical equipment (implementing the EC Directive 84/359), and certain products were controlled under the drugs law (including materials temporarily or permanently implanted in the body; dressings and surgical sutures; and *in vitro* diagnostics). Further categories of product were to be controlled under the drug law in 1988 (including sterilised disposable medical, dental and surgical instruments). It was proposed that all devices would be transferred to a planned medical devices law when enacted. In all cases quality assurance aspects were fundamental. In the proposed new device law it was intended to cover production, packaging, storage, marketing, quality assurance and inspection, and sterility assurance as well as safety and efficacy.

The National Board of Health in Denmark introduced a voluntary registration scheme in 1971, mainly for sterile products. Purchasers were encouraged to use registered products. This scheme was stopped in 1985 owing to inadequate resource and poor take-up. It was later proposed that compulsory registration be introduced, with controls being introduced progressively for different categories of product — infusion, injection, blood transfusion, and collection equipment to be controlled in 1988; catheters etc. in 1989; sterile products for wounds in 1990; implants in 1991; and other devices in 1992. The proposed system was also to cover sampling, with the possibility that faulty products would have to be modified in design, manufacture, labelling, etc.

Italian regulations have existed since 1927 and were extended in 1941 to cover a wide range of products (disinfectants, insecticides, contact lens fluids, oral hygiene products containing fluoride, vermin poisons; vaginal pessaries, irrigators, and apparatus, and intrauterine contraceptive devices; syringes, blood and infusion fluid containers, etc; cardiac catheters, vascular prostheses, cardiac valves, and pacemakers; and other products such as trusses, hearing aids, orthopaedic shoes and surgical sutures). These provisions were replaced in 1986 by a new device law recognising three groups of product — chemical aids (for environmental use), medical devices, and *in vitro* diagnostics for laboratory and for home use. The implementation of the new law relied on the publication of several Ministerial decrees to specify the information required; the technical standards required; inspection, analytical and clinical tests; labelling, etc. Standards exist for hearing aids, pacemakers, and cardiac leads, lasers, transcutaneous stimulators, bone cements, and contact lenses. In practice, the device law has been applied only patchily.

In Belgium surgical sutures, sterile bandages, sterile materials used for therapeutic or diagnostic intervention, and materials inserted into the body for long periods are controlled. Contraceptives are controlled under the drugs laws. Clinical thermometers are controlled by the Ministry of Economic Affairs metrology division. Approval requires satisfaction on manufacturing facilities, sterilisation procedures, labelling, and notification of product particulars. It was proposed that new regulations be introduced to control more closely all sterile products and implanted materials and products, with attention to good manufacturing practices, and clinical data assessment for critical products. Some products were to be subjected to post-marketing surveillance, with compulsory adverse event reporting and labelling regulation.

Limited controls are applied in the Netherlands under a 1982 law which had, in 1987, been applied only to sterile products.

There are five categories of controlled device in France. The first category is the subject of a homologation procedure (based on a 1950 procedure renewed in 1983) with testing against manufacturing and some physical standards. Only products approved by this process may be purchased by public hospitals. Some 200 AFNOR (French Standardisation Committee) standards apply to medical devices. Clinical evaluation is in accredited hospitals prior to approval. The process may be applied only to imaging systems; electrosurgical equipment; anaesthetic, infusion, and intensive care equipment; artificial organs, prostheses, and extracorporeal circuits; and equipment for monitoring and processing data from physiological systems.

There is a certification system for sterile products such as surgical implants, extracorporeal systems, surgical instruments, packaging for sterilisation, antiseptics and disinfectants, anaesthetic gases and medical gases, dental materials and equipment, injection and infusion equipment, intrauterine contraceptives, and gloves.

Other devices are classed as sterile products processed as pharmaceuticals, devices for disabled persons, and 'others'. Local control systems may be applied.

There were no effective control mechanisms in Spain or Portugal in 1987.

9.3 IDEAL CHARACTERISTICS FOR A NEW SYSTEM OF CONTROLS FOR MEDICAL DEVICES

In the opinion of the author any new system should possess as many as possible of the following characteristics.

It should be simple to operate, practical, and resource sparing.

Every device on a particular market should be known to the responsible competent authority. Some form of adverse event reporting scheme should be introduced to enable defective or unsafe devices to be identified quickly. This should require all serious events to be reported, and the competent authorities should then investigate as necessary to establish whether further action is required.

Relevant good manufacturing practices should be enforced or policed by adequate inspection of manufacturers' facilities, using a previously submitted and approved statement of what is done (and how it is done) as the basis for the inspection.

Where available, relevant published standards should be applied by manufacturers. If such standards are not used, alternatives should be allowed, but the specifications etc. should then be the subject of review by the relevant authorities prior to marketing. If a particular standard is found to be unsatisfactory a suitable mechanism should be available for competent authorities to refuse to accept it, with the deficiencies being drawn to the attention of the CEC and the standards body which generated the specification.

Critical devices (those that could result in foreseeable catastrophic failure with death or serious injury as a result) should be the subject of premarket approval, and the approval process should include an assessment of clinical 'usefulness' ('efficacy' being the term used in pharmaceutical contexts) and safety, and a suitable system should be available to identify such critical products.

Product literature and labelling should be suitably monitored, with adequate guidance on what should be included in it.

Removal of unsafe or otherwise unsatisfactory products from the market should not be unduly restricted, provided that there are appropriate appeal procedures to protect the interests of both the national authorities and the manufacturers. All products marketed in the EC should carry a CE mark to indicate that the manufacturer claims compliance with the appropriate essential requirements. The conditions for application of the CE mark to a device should be clearly stated.

Any system should build in levels of control proportional to the risks associated with the product (not with the procedure with which they are intended to be used).

9.4 'OLD APPROACH' AND 'NEW APPROACH' DIRECTIVES

Reference has been made to 'old approach' and 'new approach' directives. 'Old approach' directives are developed by a procedure which requires unanimity in the voting for their acceptance by the Member States. They contain detailed and mandatory technical specifications which lead to a risk of the specification (and therefore the Directive) becoming obsolete owing to technical developments. They are difficult to modify quickly once adopted. Some 300 to 400 'old approach' Directives have been adopted.

If the Single Market is to be achieved in a reasonable time it is obvious that an alternative is required to the cumbersome process of the 'old approach'. The answer to this was the introduction of the 'new approach'.

A Council Decision on 7 May 1985 introduced this procedure, with a modified process for the generation of Directives based on adoption by qualified majority voting (the number of votes available to each Member State being determined by the size of its population).

The Directives adopted by this procedure are of broad scope and contain essential requirements to be met by the products covered by the Directive, but do not include technical detail such as test methods or requirements. Another key aspect to these Directives is that once a product had been approved by the appropriate notified body in one Member State it can be marketed in any or all of the others without further approval. There is also an obligation on Member States to prevent the marketing of products which do not comply with the essential requirements. The fundamental basis for approval is a manufacturer's declaration of conformity with the essential requirements, together with monitoring procedures for the production processes and quality systems.

Documents of relevance in this context are Directive 83/189/EEC; Directive 88/182/EEC; and the Council Decision of 7 May 1985 (published in the Official Journal 85/C 136/01).

9.4.1 The role of CEN and CENELEC
As indicated above, the Directives contain essential requirements but not any technical detail. The recognised source of published standards under the 'new

approach' is the European Standardisation Committee (CEN) or the European Electrotechnical Standardisation Committee (CENELEC). These two standards-making bodies usually start with available International Standards from the International Standards Organization (ISO) or the International Electrotechnical Commission (IEC). Where possible these are adopted unchanged. If necessary, they may be modified (but the modification is based closely on the international document). If the international standard is totally unsuitable, then a European standard is developed, based on available national standards of the member organisations of CEN and CENELEC. It should be noted that the membership of these two bodies is not restricted to members states of the EC — the EFTA countries' national standards organisations belong, too.

CEN and CENELEC standards are not intended to be obligatory on individual manufacturers with respect to specific products. Compliance with an appropriate CEN or CENELEC standard is, however, taken as confirmatory evidence for compliance with relevant essential requirements.

European Standards (ENs) must replace any conflicting national standards. Because of this there is a complicated voting system for the adoption of an EN. The voting rights are shown in Table 9.1. In the case of a Harmonisation Document

Table 9.1 — Voting rights on the adoption of CEN and CENELEC standards

Country	Votes	Country	Votes
Austria	3	Italy	10
Belgium	5	Luxembourg	2
Denmark	3	Netherlands	5
Finland	3	Norway	3
France	10	Portugal	5
Germany	10	Spain	8
Greece	5	Sweden	5
Iceland	1	Switzerland	5
Ireland	3	United Kingdom	10

(HD), national variations are permitted where particular regulations or technical requirements make them necessary for a specified transitional period.

In order to be adopted, four criteria must be met when a draft standard or harmonisation document is voted on. Excluding abstentions, the number of votes cast in favour of the adoption of the proposal must be greater than the number against. At least 25 of the weighted votes must be in favour of adoption. There must be not more than 22 weighted votes against adoption. Not more than three members may vote against if adoption is to succeed. If these conditions are not met, the votes of those members which are in the EC are counted separately. The proposal is adopted if the conditions are met on the basis of those votes alone.

CEN and CENELEC work through an extensive system of Committees and Working Groups. CEN has more than 250 technical committees split into working groups or subcommittees. CENELEC has more than 50. Membership of the Committees is through national standards organisations, although other interested parties may observe at meetings. Individual national experts and observers attend Working Party Group meetings.

Observer status has been granted to a number of trade associations, including COCIR, EUCOMED, EDMA, IAPM, the Association of International Industrial Irradiation (AIII), the Commission on World Standards of the World Association of Societies of Pathology (COWS of WASP), the Disposable Hypodermic and Allied Equipment Manufacturers' Association of Europe (DHAEMAE), European Association of Surgical Suture Industry (EASSI), European Federation of Pharmaceutical Industry Associations (EFPIA), the European Federation of National Associations of Contact Lens Manufacturers (Euromcontact), the European Federation of Precision Mechanical and Optical Industries (Eurom VI), the Federation of European Dental Industry (FIDE), the International Committee for Standardisation in Haematology (ICSH), and the International Federation of Clinical Chemistry.

In addition, the International Association of Surgical Blade Manufacturers (IASBM) and the Regulatory Affairs Professionals Society (RAPS) have an informal status.

The working practices are such that experts attend and participate in the work of the Working Groups. National delegations at the Committee meetings are of restricted size. The secretariat of each of the various Committees and Working Groups is provided by one of the national standards organisations. The development of ENs and harmonisation documents is by a process of consensus.

In the case of medical devices there is a small group of products whose published standards have traditionally been included in pharmacopoeias — both national and, since 1971, the *European Pharmacopoeia*. The initial non-acceptance of these published standards for the purposes of the medical device directives was the cause of some debate. The *European Pharmacopoeia* is binding on those countries who have become party to the Convention for its elaboration (which includes all those countries listed in Table 9.1 and, in addition, Cyprus), and the CEC has recently signed the Convention, and as a full member (that is after ratification by all 19 Member States) will be similarly bound to recognise its supremacy. For pharmaceuticals this is built into the Pharmaceuticals Directives — 65/65/EEC *et seq*. The status of some (unspecified) *European Pharmacopoeia* monographs is recognised in the latest draft of the medical device Directive.

9.4.2 The consultative processes in the EC in the development of a Directive

When the need for a new Directive has been identified — for example where there are technical barriers to free movement of goods within the EC — Community-level interest groups such as European trade associations or consumer interests may approach the CEC or be approached by the CEC for preliminary consultations. National authorities can contribute usefully to this process. Proposals may be generated by or put to the CEC Services, who then study them. The Economic and

Social Committee and European Parliament committees are consulted. The CEC then prepares a proposal which is referred to the Council of Ministers.

When the proposals are submitted to the Council of Ministers the formal consideration and bargaining begin. Study groups of national authority Experts are formed. Other interested parties may take part in the deliberations by the national authorities if time permits, for example representatives of trade associations, interested professional groups, etc. National authorities and national parliaments are also involved. The European Parliament is consulted again. All relevant information is funnelled into the Committee of Permanent Representatives of the Member States, and the consideration and bargaining process is continued.

After completion of the earlier stages, the proposal is submitted as a Common Position to the Council of Ministers and is adopted, using a weighted majority voting procedure. A further consultation with the European Parliament leads to the CEC considering any points made before final submission to the Council of Ministers. The Directive is then adopted.

As indicated above, the European Parliament is consulted several times during the development of a Directive. The initial CEC proposal is submitted to the Council of Ministers and to the European Parliament for an opinion, which the CEC takes into account. After the consultative and bargaining process and the adoption of the Common Position by a qualified majority, the matter is referred back to the European Parliament under the Co-operation Procedure.

Within three months of reference to the Parliament, the Parliament may approve the Council position or take no position (in which case the Council will adopt the Directive); or reject the Council Common Position by an absolute majority (in which case the Council may adopt the Directive only if there is a unanimous vote for adoption). The Council Common Position may be amended by an absolute majority of the members of the Parliament (in which case the CEC reviews the Parliament's amendments within one month and may revise its proposals, following which the Council will within a period of three months adopt the CEC proposal by a qualified majority. If the CEC should fail to act, Parliament may agree to a one-month extension, failing which the CEC proposal lapses. The Council may adopt the Parliamentary amendments not approved by the CEC by a unanimous vote; or otherwise amend the CEC proposal by unanimous vote.

After the adoption of the Directive and its publication in the *Official Journal* in the national languages of the Member States, a timetable is set for the introduction of national laws to give it effect. The time required for this is taken into account in setting deadlines for various stages of the implementation schedule specified in the text of the Directive.

9.4.3 Constituent parts of a 'new approach' Directive
The main constituents of a 'new approach' Directive are:

- the definitions of the class of products to be covered, other necessary definitions, and the field of application of the Directive (including any exclusions);

- the essential requirements worded with sufficient precision to create legally binding obligations which can be enforced, and a statement recognising the status of harmonised standards;
- provision for the marketing of the product throughout the Communities once the CE mark has been applied in conformity with the provisions of the Directive;
- provision for the appointment of Notified Bodies;
- details of the accreditation and certification procedures and conformity assessment procedures;
- requirement for the application of the CE mark to products in compliance with the essential requirements and provisions for the removal from the market of non-complying products (and products found to be unsafe in use);
- the establishment of Standing Committee(s) and the definition of its (their) role.

9.5 CONTENTS OF THE ACTIVE IMPLANTABLE MEDICAL DEVICE DIRECTIVE (90/385/EEC)

9.5.1 Article 1: Application, definitions, provision re: medicinal products, reference to Directive 89/336/EEC

The Directive applies to active implantable medical devices.

A medical device is defined as follows:

'Medical device' means any instrument, apparatus, appliance, material, or other article, whether used alone or in combination, together with any accessories or software for its proper functioning, intended by the manufacturer to be used for human beings in the:

- diagnosis, prevention, monitoring, treatment, or alleviation of disease or injury,
- investigation, replacement, or modification of the anatomy or of a physiological process,
- control of conception,

and which does not achieve its principal intended action by pharmacological, chemical, immunological, or metabolic means, but which may be assisted in its function by such means.

An active medical device is defined as:

'any medical device relying for its functioning a source of electrical energy or any source of power other than that directly generated by the human body or gravity'.

An active implantable medical device is defined as:

'Any active medical device which is intended to be totally or partially introduced, surgically or medically, into the human body or by medical intervention into a natural orifice, and which is intended to remain after the procedure'.

A custom-made device is an active implantable medical device specifically made in accordance with a medical specialist's written prescription which gives, under his responsibility, specific design characteristics and is intended to be used only for an individual named patient.

A device intended for clinical investigation is any active implantable medical device intended for use by a specialist doctor when conducting investigations in an adequate human clinical environment.

'Intended purpose' means the use for which the medical device is intended and for which it is suited according to the data supplied by the manufacturer in the instructions.

'Putting into service' is defined as:

making available to the medical profession for implantation.

In the case of medicinal products administered by use of a medical device the Directive differentiates two cases. The first is where an active implantable medical device is intended to administer a substance which is a medicinal product as defined in Directive 65/65/EEC: that substance is subject to the system of marketing authorisation provided for in Directive 65/65/EEC.

The second case is where the active implantable medical device incorporates as an integral part a substance which, if used separately, might be considered to be a medicinal product within the definition of Directive 65/65/EEC, in which case the device is evaluated and authorised in accordance with the requirements of Directive 90/385/EEC.

Directive 90/385/EEC is a specific Directive within the meaning of Article 2 (2) of Directive 89/336/EEC relating to electromagnetic compatibility.

9.5.2 Article 2: Marketing of custom-made and investigational devices
This article places on the Member States an obligation to allow onto the market and to be put into service only those active implantable medical devices and custom-made devices which do not compromise the safety and health of patients, users, and in appropriate cases other persons, provided that they are properly implanted, maintained, and used in accordance with the intended purposes.

9.5.3 Article 3: Compliance with essential requirements
It is a requirement that active implantable medical devices, custom-made devices, and devices intended for clinical investigation (collectively termed 'devices') comply with the essential requirements defined in Annex 1 to the Directive.

9.5.4 Article 4: Member States' obligations and rights
Member States are required not to impede the placing on the market or putting into service devices bearing the CE mark nor to create any obstacles to devices intended for clinical investigation being made available to specialist doctors for that purpose, provided that they satisfy the conditions laid down in Article 10 and Annex 6. Custom-made devices are also to be allowed to be placed on the market and put into service, provided that they satisfy the conditions laid down in Annex 6 and are accompanied by the statements referred to in that Annex. Neither of these two types of device are allowed to carry the CE mark.

Provision is made for the display of non-conforming devices at trade fairs, exhibitions, demonstrations, etc., provided that a visible sign clearly indicated that the devices do not conform to the Directive requirements and that they cannot be put into service until they have been made to conform.

National language(s) labelling requirements are permitted for information included in sections 14 to 15 of Annex 1.

9.5.5   Article 5: Role of harmonised standards
Member States are required to presume compliance with the essential requirements for devices which comply with the requirements of relevant national standards adopted pursuant to the harmonised standards, reference to which have been published in the *Official Journal of the European Communities*. References to such national standards are to be published by the Member States.

9.5.6   Article 6: Unsatisfactory harmonised standards; implementation and practical application of the Directive — the role of the Standing Committees
If a harmonised standard referred to in Article 5 is considered by a Member State or the CEC not to meet entirely the essential requirements the matter is to be brought to the attention of the Standing Committee set up under Directive 83/189/EEC, giving the reasons. The Committee is required to deliver an Opinion without delay, and the CEC is required to inform the Member States of the measures to be taken with regard to the standards and the publications referred to in Article 5

Any matters relating to the implementation of and practical application of this Directive is to be referred to another Standing Committee composed of representatives of the Member States and chaired by a representative, of the CEC, who is also to submit a draft of the measures to be taken. The Opinion of the Committee on the matter before it is recorded by the CEC representative, and any Member State also can have its position recorded. The CEC is required to take the utmost account of the Opinion delivered by the Committee, and is to inform the Committee of the manner in which its Opinion has been taken into account.

9.5.7   Article 7: Removal of products from the market
Provision is included here for products to be removed from the market or prevented from being marketed on grounds of compromise to the health and/or safety of patients, users or other persons. There is an obligation to report to the CEC, the grounds for this action. In particular this should identify whether non-compliance with the requirements of the Directive is due to failure to meet the essential requirements where the product does not fully comply with the harmonised standards; or due to the incorrect application of those standards; or due to shortcomings in the standards.

The consultative procedure to be followed in such cases is laid down. These involve the Member states concerned, the CEC, and the manufacturers concerned. If the measures are justified, all Member States are advised of the problem and, where necessary, the Standing Committee referred to above is advised too. If the measures are considered to be unjustified, the Member State concerned and the manufacturer or his representative are informed.

Sec. 9.5]   Contents of the active implantable medical device Directive   141

The removal from the market of a product not complying with the requirements of the Directive but bearing the CE mark is allowed. Appropriate action is to be taken against the person applying the mark. The CEC and the Member States are to be informed of that action. The CEC is to keep Member States informed of progress and outcome of actions under this procedure.

9.5.8   Article 8: Records of adverse events and withdrawals from the market
Member States are required to keep centralised records of cases of the deterioration of product characteristics or performance, or inaccuracies in instruction leaflets, which result in death or deterioration of health of a patient, or any technical or medical reason for a manufacturer's withdrawing a device from the market. All such cases are to be reported to the CEC and the Member States with details of the measures taken or contemplated.

9.5.9   Article 9: Conformity assessment options
This states the various options for conformity assessment. For the majority of devices the choices (to be made by the manufacturer) are for an EC declaration of conformity; or for an EC type-examination procedure involving either EC verification or EC declaration of conformity. For custom-made devices the procedure in Annex 6 is to be followed, including the provision of the declaration described there.

9.5.10   Article 10: Clinical investigation provisions
Proposed clinical investigations are to be advised to the competent authority of relevant Member States at least sixty days before the commencement of the investigations. The statement referred to in Annex 6 is to be submitted. The investigation may commence at the end of the period of sixty days unless the competent authority has advised the manufacturer of a decision to the contrary. Such adverse decisions are based on considerations of public health or public order.

9.5.11   Article 11: Appointment and withdrawal of notified bodies
This Article requires the Member States to advise the CEC and the other Member States of the appointment of 'notified bodies'. The CEC is to publish a list of such bodies. The minimum criteria to be taken into account in designating the notified bodies are set out in Annex 8. If the nomination of a notified body is withdrawn for any reason this is to be advised to the other Member States and the CEC. Notified bodies and manufacturers are to agree time limits for the completion of the verification operations.

9.5.12   Article 12: Application of the CE mark and the notified body's logo to products
All devices other than those for clinical investigation or those which are custom made are to bear the CE mark if they are considered by the manufacturer etc. to meet the essential requirements. The form in which this appears is required to be visible, legible, and indelible. It must be accompanied by the logo of the notified body responsible for its approval.

9.5.13 Article 13: Inappropriate application of the CE mark

It is the responsibility of the notified body to advise the competent authority in the Member State of cases where the CE mark has been inappropriately applied. This applies to cases where the device does not conform to the relevant standards referred to in Article 5; or does not conform to an approved type; or where the device conforms to an approved type but does not meet the relevant essential requirements; or where the manufacturer has failed to fulfil his obligations under the EC declaration of conformity.

9.5.14 Article 14: Refused or restricted marketing provisions

If the manufacturer is refused an authorisation to market a device, or if restrictions are placed on the marketing of the product or its being put into service, the exact grounds for the decision are advised, and the manufacturer is also advised of the remedies available under the law in force in the Member State concerned.

9.5.15 Article 15: Confidentiality

All parties concerned in the application are bound to observe confidentiality with regard to information obtained in the performance of their duties. This does not affect the obligations of Member States and notified bodies with respect to the dissemination of warnings and mutual information as required under this Directive.

9.5.16 Article 16: Effective dates

Member States are required to adopt and publish laws and other provisions giving effect to this Directive before 1 July 1992, and inform the CEC of their publication. These provisions are to be applied from 1 January 1993. Up to 31 December 1993 products may be placed on the market and put into service if they comply with the national laws in force on 31 December 1992.

9.5.17 Article 17: Addressees

This states that the Directive is addressed to the Member States.

9.5.18 Annex 1: Essential requirements

9.5.18.1 *Introduction*

The essential requirements are subdivided into general requirements and requirements regarding design and construction. Confirmation that the device meets the requirements regarding characteristics and performance in normal conditions of use and the evaluation of side effects or undesirable effects must be based on clinical data established in accordance with Annex 7.

9.5.18.2 *General requirements*

The essential requirements are that (1) the product, when properly used in accordance with the manufacturer's recommendations, does not compromise the clinical condition or the safety of the patient, persons implanting the product, or other persons; (2) the product meets the manufacturer's intended performance requirements; (3) the characteristics and performance of the device do not compromise the clinical condition and safety of patients or other persons during the lifetime of the

Sec. 9.5] **Contents of the active implantable medical device Directive** 143

product under normal conditions of stress; (4) the design, manufacture, and packaging ensure that the characteristics and performance of the device are not adversely affected during normal transportation and storage; (5) side effects and other undesirable effects constitute an acceptable risk when weighed against the performance intended.

9.5.18.3 *Requirements regarding design and construction*
The device is designed and constructed according to the latest acknowledged state of the art with respect to safety.

The product is sterile when placed on the market and remains so until the packaging is removed and the product implanted.

Design and manufacture of the products minimises the following risks: (1) physical injury arising from physical features of the product; (2) those associated with the use of the energy sources (and in the case of electricity especially with insulation, leakage currents, and overheating); (3) those associated with foreseeable environmental conditions such as magnetic fields, electrostatic discharge, pressure, and acceleration; (4) those associated with medical treatment — for example defibrillators, high-frequency surgical equipment; (5) those associated with the ionising radiation from any radioactive material included in the device (in accordance with EURATOM Directive requirements); (6) those associated with situations where maintenance and calibration are impossible, such as an excessive increase in leakage currents, the effects of ageing on the materials used, or decreased accuracy of any measuring or control mechanisms.

In designing and constructing devices to comply with the general requirements, particular attention is paid to the toxicity of chosen material, biocompatibility with particular reference to the anticipated use of the device, compatibility of the device with any substance that it is intended to administer, connectors (especially with regard to their safety), the reliability of the energy source, that the device is leakproof if necessary, and the proper functioning of the programming and control systems (including any software).

Where the device incorporates substance(s) which, if used separately, are likely to be considered to be medicinal products under Directive 65/65/EEC which is (are) likely to be bioavailable, then the safety, quality, and usefulness of the substance (taking into account the uses of the device) must be verified by analogy with the relevant requirements of Directive 75/318/EEC. No definition of 'bioavailability' is included. (A possible definition for this term was under discussion in one of the CEN Technical Committees at the time of writing.)

There are a number of requirements which relate to labelling and information provision. These include:

- that the device or component parts are identified to allow appropriate measures to be taken if a potential risk is identified associated with them;
- a code by which the type of device and year of manufacture can be identified without the need for a surgical operation;
- if a visual system of instructions for operation or adjustment is used, then the information is intelligible to the user and to the patient if necessary;

- the following information is to appear on the sterile pack (using generally recognised symbols if possible): method of sterilisation; information for the identification of the product; the name and address of the manufacturer; the device description; 'exclusively for medical investigation' or 'custom-made device' if appropriate; a declaration that the product is sterile; the month and year of manufacture; an indication of the time limit for implantation of the device.
- the sales packaging is to include the following information: the name and address of the manufacturer; the device description; the purpose of the device; relevant characteristics; 'exclusively for clinical investigation' or 'custom-made device' if appropriate; a declaration that the product is sterile; the month and year of manufacture; an indication of the time limit for implantation of the device; storage and transportation instructions.
- instructions for use are to be provided, including the following: the year of authorisation to apply the CE mark; the information required for the labelling except for the manufacturing date and the latest date for implantation; design performance information and undesirable side effects; information to allow the clinician to select a suitable device and the appropriate accessories and software; information for the clinician and patient for the correct use of the device and its accessories and software together with information on the nature, scope, and times for the operation of controls and trials and maintenance measures; information to allow the avoidance of risks associated with the implantation of the device; information on effects on the device caused by instruments present at the time of investigation (or vice versa); instructions on what is to be done if the packaging is damaged and methods of resterilisation (if appropriate); an indication that reuse of the device requires reconditioning by the manufacturer to comply with the essential requirements, if appropriate.
- information is required for use by the doctor in briefing the patient, particularly with respect to contraindications and precautions to be taken, such as how to determine the life of the energy source; what action or precautions should be taken if the performance of the device changes; warnings about exposure to magnetic fields etc; adequate information about medicinal products which the device is intended to administer.

9.5.19 Annex 2: Declaration of conformity (full quality system)

The manufacturer applies an approved quality system to the design and manufacture and final inspection of the product, and is subject to EC surveillance. Having drawn up a written declaration of conformity the manufacturer applies the CE mark and the identifying logo of the notified body responsible. Details are given with respect to the quality system, the examination of the design of the product, and surveillance for this type of declaration of conformity.

The manufacturer has to apply for approval of his quality system. The application includes information on the categories of product manufactured, quality system documentation, and an undertaking to maintain the approved quality system in an adequate and efficacious condition and to fulfil the obligations arising from the approved system. An undertaking is also required regarding the introduction and maintenance of a post-marketing surveillance system. The competent authorities are

Sec. 9.5]   **Contents of the active implantable medical device Directive**   145

to be advised of cases where deterioration of characteristics or performance of a device or inaccuracies in the instruction leaflet for a device might lead or has led to the death of or deterioration in the clinical condition of a patient, or any technical or medical reason resulting in the withdrawal of a device from the market by the manufacturer.

The quality system applies to all stages of the product from design to finished product controls. Every relevant aspect is the subject of written procedures, etc. This includes the manufacturer's quality objectives; the organisation of the business; monitoring and verification procedures for the device(s); quality assurance and control techniques; and the tests and trials undertaken before, during, and after production and the frequency with which they are carried out.

Conformity with the requirements is assumed for quality systems which correspond to the corresponding horizontal harmonised standards. The evaluation procedure on the part of the notified body includes a site inspection. Any changes planned to the quality system are reported to the notified body concerned by the manufacturer.

In the case of the original request and any changes requested, the notified body advises the manufacturer of the conclusions it arrives at and provides a reasoned evaluation.

A design dossier is submitted to the notified body for approval. This includes the design specifications and standards applied, and proof of their appropriateness (especially if the harmonised standards have not been applied in full); a statement of the inclusion as an integral part (or not) of a substance which might be considered to be a medicinal product and which may be bioavailable; and data from relevant trials, clinical data, and a draft instruction leaflet. Notified bodies may require additional data to demonstrate compliance with the Directive requirements. A compliance certificate issued by a notified body includes conclusions on the examination, the conditions of its validity, data needed for the identification of the approved design, and a description of the intended use of the product where appropriate.

Any modifications to the approved design which may affect conformity with the essential requirements of the Directive or the prescribed conditions of use of the product are subject to approval by the notified body which issued the original certificate of approval for the product. Supplementary approvals are given as addenda to the EC design examination certificate.

Notified bodies are to notify each other of the approval, refusal, and withdrawal of approvals.

9.5.20   Annex 3: EC type-examination procedure

This describes the EC type-examination procedure in which the notified body observes and certifies that a representative sample of the production satisfies the relevant provisions of the Directive.

The manufacturer or his representative in the EC makes an application to a notified body which includes the name and address of the manufacturer or representative, a declaration that no other application has been made to another notified body; and appropriate documentation to allow the evaluation to be made of the conformity with the Directive requirements of a representative sample of the product, otherwise referred to as a 'type'. A type is made available to the notified body.

The necessary documentation includes information on the design, manufacture, and performance of the product. This includes a description of the product with design drawings and diagrams of parts, subassemblies, and circuits together with descriptions and explanations; methods of manufacture, especially sterilisation; a list of the harmonised standards applied in full or in part; and a description of how the essential requirements have been met where harmonised standards have not been applied. The results of design calculations, investigations, and tests are supplied. The applicant also furnishes a statement as to whether or not a substance otherwise likely to be considered a medicinal product is incorporated as an integral part of the device which may become bioavailable together with data from relevant trials. Clinical data and draft instruction leaflets are also provided.

The notified body is required to examine and evaluate the written evidence and to verify that the type has been manufactured in accordance with the documentation. Those items based on harmonised standards and those not so based are recorded. Necessary inspections and tests are undertaken to verify that the product complies with the essential requirements where harmonised standards have not been applied. Where standards are said to be applied it is necessary to carry out appropriate inspections to ensure that those standards have actually been applied.

Where a type meets the requirements of the Directive an EC type-examination certificate is issued to the applicant by the notified body. This includes the name and address of the manufacturer and other information such as the conclusions of the examination of the information provided, the conditions under which the certificate is valid, and information necessary for the identification of the type concerned. Significant parts of the documentation are attached by the notified body, which keeps a copy.

Any modifications to the approved product are advised by the manufacturer to the notified body. These must be approved by the notified body which issued the original certificate of type-examination where the modifications may affect the conformity of the product with the essential requirements. Any new approval is issued as an addendum to the initial EC type-examination certificate.

Notified bodies are to advise each other of approvals, refusals, and withdrawals of products. Copies of the EC type-examination certificates and any supplements may be supplied to any notified body. The annexes to those certificates and supplements may be obtained if the notified body that wants them makes a reasoned application and advises the manufacturer.

9.5.21 Annex 4: EC verification procedures

These are the procedures by which a notified body verifies and certifies that the type described in an EC type-examination certificate conforms to and meets the relevant requirements of the Directive.

Prior to manufacture the manufacturer prepares documents defining the manufacturing procedure and all routine operations necessary to ensure homogeneity of production and conformity of the products with type used to establish the EC type-examination certificate and with the requirements of the Directive. A post-marketing surveillance system is also set up by the manufacturer to identify faults.

The notified body is required to apply a statistical verification procedure. The product is presented in homogeneous batches, and random samples are taken from each batch. These samples are examined individually for conformity with the type used to establish the EC type-examination certificate. The sampling system is required to be such as to achieve a level of quality corresponding to a probability of acceptance of 95 per cent with a non-conformity of between 0.29 and 1.0 per cent, and a limit quality corresponding to a probability of acceptance of 5 per cent with a non-conformity of between 3 and 7 per cent.

A written certificate of conformity is provided for accepted batches. All of that batch may be marketed with the exception of those samples tested and found not to comply. Rejection of a batch requires that the notified body takes measures to ensure that the batch is prevented from being marketed.

The CE mark and the identifying logo of the notified body responsible for the statistical verification may be applied during manufacture if this is justified on practical grounds.

9.5.22 Annex 5: Assurance of production quality in connection with the EC declaration of conformity to type

Manufacturers are required to apply for quality system approval for the manufacture of the device and to conduct the final product inspection according to an agreed programme. The fulfilment of the manufacturers' obligation is ensured by EC surveillance.

The declaration of conformity is a written statement made by manufacturers satisfying the quality system obligations and guarantees that the product(s) concerned conform to the type described in the EC type-examination certificate and meet the relevant requirements of the Directive.

The CE symbol and the identifying logo of the relevant notified body are affixed to the device.

In the application for quality system approval the manufacturer includes appropriate information on the products to be made and quality system documentation, and undertakings to fulfil obligations arising from the quality system as approved. It is also necessary to undertake to maintain the quality system in an adequate and efficacious form.

Technical information relating to the EC approved type and the type-examination certificate are submitted. The usual requirement for post-marketing surveillance and reporting applies.

Quality system documentation is to be systematic and orderly and include procedures and policies, allowing a uniform interpretation of quality programmes, plans, manuals, and records as appropriate. The quality system is audited by the notified body. Conformity with the Directive requirements is presumed if the quality system conforms to the appropriate horizontal harmonised standards requirements. At least one member of the evaluation team from the notified body is required to have experience of the evaluation of the technologies concerned.

Any proposed plans to modify an approved quality system are advised to the notified body. Such changes are evaluated to determine whether the modified quality system is still acceptable. Decisions on initial applications for approval and those for changes are notified to the manufacturer, together with a reasoned evaluation.

Notified bodies are required to undertake surveillance of manufacturers by means of periodic inspections and evaluations to ensure that the approved quality system is being applied. Evaluation reports are to be provided following inspections etc. The visits to the manufacturing facility may be announced or unannounced.

Notified bodies are required to advise each other of approvals, refusals, or withdrawals in connection with quality systems.

9.5.23 Annex 6: Custom-made devices and devices intended for clinical investigations

Custom-made devices are to carry statements with the following information: (1) data allowing the device to be identified; (2) a statement that the product is for use in connection with a particular (named) patient; (3) the name of the doctor who drew up the prescription and the name of the clinic concerned if necessary; (4) the features of the device's prescription; (5) a statement that the device complies with the essential requirements of the Directive and, if necessary, indicating which essential requirements have been wholly met. Documentation is kept available on the design, manufacture and performances of the product so as to allow an assessment to be made of compliance with the Directive. Manufacturers are to ensure that the product meets the requirements of this documentation.

Statements for devices intended for clinical investigation carry the following information : (1) data to identify the device; (2) an investigational plan including the purpose, scope, and number of devices concerned; (3) the name of the responsible doctor and institution; (4) the place, date of commencement, and scheduled duration of the investigations; (5) a statement regarding the essential requirements being complied with except for those aspects being investigated, and that with regard to those aspects every precaution has been taken to protect the patient.

The manufacturer maintains documentation to allow the notified body to assess compliance with the Directive. This includes a general description of the product and design drawings, diagrams of parts, subassemblies, and circuits, etc., and the methods of manufacture. A list of the harmonised standards complied with in full or in part and a description of any alternative ways of meeting the essential requirements are included as necessary. Results from design calculations and checks and technical tests are kept, too.

The manufacturer takes all necessary steps to ensure conformity with the documentation.

9.5.24 Annex 7: Clinical evaluation

The adequacy of the data submitted is to be assessed against the background of harmonised standards and the current scientific literature covering the intended use of the device, with a critical assessment report on the summary of this information, or results from clinical investigations.

Data are to remain confidential unless it is considered essential to divulge them.

Clinical investigations are to verify under normal conditions of use that the product performs in such a way that it is suitable for the intended functions, and also to determine any undesirable side effects under those conditions and the acceptability of the risks with regard to the performance of the product. Conformity with the provisions of the Helsinki Convention is required with respect to the protection of human subjects.

The Annex also discusses the design of clinical trials in general terms.

9.5.25 Annex 8: Minimum criteria for inspection bodies to be notified

The notified body shall have no direct interest in the products being evaluated and verified. The staff of the notified body shall operate with the highest degree of professional integrity, impartiality, and technical competence, free from improper pressures and inducements. Professional secrecy is to be observed with regard to all information obtained except for the provision of necessary information to the competent authorities in the country concerned.

Notified bodies may undertake tasks themselves or have them carried out under their responsibility. Necessary staff, equipment, and facilities are to be available to allow them to undertake the tasks associated with the relevant types of evaluation and verification.

Staff for control operations are to be adequately trained for all the evaluations required of the notified body, have a satisfactory knowledge and experience of the controls being applied, and possess the ability to draw up certificates records and reports to demonstrate how the controls have been applied.

Unless liability is assumed by the government of the country concerned, the notified body is required to be adequately covered by third-party insurance.

9.5.26 Annex 9: CE mark

The CE mark of conformity is described in this Annexe.

9.6 THE DRAFT DIRECTIVE ON MEDICAL DEVICES

9.6.1 Introduction

It is indicated above that the original intention was for a series of four directives covering the medical device field. The first of these, on active implantable medical devices, has now been adopted and has been discussed in section 9.5. The development of separate directives for active medical devices and for non-active medical devices was being pursued up to mid-1990. The latest draft available at the time of writing (dated 15 July 1990) is for a Directive covering both active and non-active medical devices. It is emphasised that this is not the final draft of the document, and that it might be considerably modified before the final version of the Directive is published. The following sections are therefore not definitive, but may be of use to readers in following the development of the thinking behind the Directives.

9.6.2 Definitions

The definitions for medical device and related terms have been amended in this draft. The latest (but not finalised) definitions are included below:

'Medical device': Any instrument, apparatus, appliance, material, or other article, whether used alone or in combination, intended by the manufacturer to be used for human beings wholly or mainly for the purpose of:
- diagnosis, prevention, monitoring, treatment, or alleviation of disease, injury, or disability
- investigation, replacement, or modification of the anatomy or of a physiological process
- control of conception,

and which does not achieve its principal intended action in or on the human body by pharmacological, chemical, immunological, or metabolic means, but which may be assisted in its function by such means.

Accessories are treated as medical devices for the purpose of this Directive.

'Accessory': An article which contributes to the functioning of a medical device while not being a medical device in itself within the meaning of the definition of a medical device.

'Active medical device': Any medical device directly connected to or equipped with a power source necessary for its functioning regardless of whether it is of electrical energy or of any source of power other than that directly generated by the human body or gravity.

'*In vitro* diagnostic medical device': Any medical device which is a reagent, reagent product, kit, instrument, apparatus, or system, whether used alone or in combination, intended by the manufacturer wholly or mainly to be used *in vitro* for the examination of substances derived from the human body for the purpose of providing information relevant to the detection, diagnosis, monitoring, or treatment of physiological states, states of health or disease, or congenital abnormality.

'Custom-made device': Any medical device specifically made in accordance with an appropriately qualified practitioner's written prescription (or any other person who is authorised to establish the prescription in question on the grounds of professional qualifications) which gives, under his or her responsibility, specific design characteristics and is intended to be used only for an individual identified patient.

'Device intended for clinical investigations': Any (medical device) intended for use by an appropriately qualified practitioner (or other appropriately-qualified person) when conducting investigations in an adequate human clinical environment.

'Implantable device': Any medical device which is intended to be totally or partially introduced into the human body or a natural orifice; or to replace an epithelial surface or the surface of the eye by medical or surgical intervention, and which is intended to remain after the procedure for at least thirty days and which can only be removed by medical or surgical intervention.

'Manufacturer': The person or organisation with overall responsibility for the design, manufacture, and packaging of a medical device with a view to its being placed on the market, regardless of whether these operations are carried out by that person or organisation themselves or by a third party or organisation. The person or organisation which on its own account assembles, packages, processes, and/or labels one or more ready-made products and/or assigns to them their intended purpose as a medical device with a view to their being placed on the market is deemed to be a manufacturer. (The latter does not apply to persons or organisations not 'manufacturers' as defined above but who assemble or adapt within their intended purpose for an individual user medical devices which already exist on the market.)

'Intended purpose': The use for which the medical device is intended and for which it is suited according to the data supplied by the manufacturer in the labelling instructions and/or the promotional materials.

'Placing on the market': The first disposal against payment or free of charge of a medical device other than that which is intended for clinical investigation for distribution and/or use on the Community market.

'Putting into service': The first use in the Community market of a medical device in accordance with its intended purpose.

The Directive will not apply to *in vitro* diagnostic devices, nor to active implantable medical devices except where the requirements are complementary.

9.6.3 Products containing medicinal substances

Similar provisions to those included in the active implantable medical device Directive apply to medical devices with regard to substances which might be otherwise considered medicinal products (within the terms of Directive 65/65/EEC) which are to be administered by the device (when the substance is subject to the system of marketing authorisation described in 65/65/EEC); and with regard to such substances which are incorporated in devices as an integral part (which are authorised under the medical device Directive).

9.6.4 Classification of medical devices

The medical device Directive draft includes different classifications for different types of product: active medical devices may be included in classes I and IIb; other medical devices may be included in classes I, IIa, and III. The rules for the classification are included in an Annex in the draft document, together with special rules and definitions and decision trees. (These are discussed in section 9.6.10.)

Where there is a doubt about the classification of a particular device the competent authority can be asked to decide by the manufacturer or his representative. If there is a dispute between a notified body and a manufacturer concerning the classification of a product the competent authorities are to decide. If it is considered that the rules in Annex 9 may be applied differently by different notified bodies, then a competent authority may refer the matter to the CEC and ask that it be referred to the Standing Committee set up under the active implantable medical device Directive to deal with matters arising from the implementation of the device Directives.

9.6.5 Provisions which differ from the active implantable medical devices Directive

In addition to the reference to harmonised standards produced by CEN and CENELEC, this draft Directive also refers to conformity with monographs of the *European Pharmacopoeia* (where the references have been published in the *Official Journal*) as being a method of presumed compliance with the relevant essential requirements. These *European Pharmacopoeia* monographs are specifically stated to be considered to be equivalent to harmonised standards.

Member States are required to take steps to ensure that incidents of the following types are recorded and evaluated in a 'centralised manner': any deterioration in the characteristics or performance of a device, inaccuracies in labelling or in instruction leaflets which might have resulted in the death or serious and irreversible deterioration of the state of health of a patient, or any technical or medical reason for the withdrawal of a device. However, this extends only to class IIa, IIb, or III devices.

Conformity asessment procedures are included, as follows:

- For class III devices, other than those which are custom-made or for clinical investigation, either EC declaration of conformity (complete quality assurance system); or EC type-examination and EC verification or EC declaration of conformity (assurance of production quality); the requirements for the design examination apply.
- For class IIa devices, other than those which are custom-made or for clinical investigation, EC declaration of conformity (complete quality system) or EC verification procedure and EC verification procedure or EC declaration of conformity (assurance of production quality); the requirements for design examination do not apply.
- For class IIb devices, other than those which are custom-made devices or for clinical investigation, EC declaration of conformity (full quality system); or EC type-examination and EC verification or EC declaration of conformity (assurance of production quality); the requirements for design examination do not apply.
- For class I devices, other than for clinical investigation, only a manufacturer's declaration of conformity is required.

For class IIa, IIb, and III devices that are custom-made an appropriate declaration is also required.

Notified bodies' decisions have a maximum period of validity of five years and may be renewed for further periods of five years.

An appeal process by which Member States may request reclassification of a device or a class of devices is described.

Manufacturers of class I devices (or their representatives or persons marketing devices made outside the EC) are required to notify the competent authorities concerned of the offices or manufacturing sites in the Member State and the nature of the devices concerned. If requested other Member States and the CEC may be given this information.

Class I devices do not have to carry the CE mark, but those not intended for clinical investigation or which are custom-made may carry it. Class IIa, IIb, and III devices are required to carry the CE mark unless they are custom-made or for clinical investigation (when it cannot be applied). Where the CE mark is applied, the logo of the authorising notified body is also carried. Where the intended use of the device is changed, approval of the change is to be gained before the CE mark is affixed.

Ethics committees are required to be set up within the Member States to consider relevant points concerning proposed clinical investigations.

9.6.6 Provisions in common with the active implantable medical devices Directive

One common requirement is that only medical devices which do not compromise the safety and health of patients, users, and other persons when properly installed, maintained, and used in accordance with their intended purpose are to be allowed access to the market.

Compliance with the essential requirements is required, although the detail of those requirements differs (see section 9.6.7).

Products bearing the CE mark are to be allowed free access to the EC market.

Devices for clinical investigation and custom-made devices are to be made available subject to the relevant conditions being met. Such devices are not to carry the CE mark.

Provisions with regard to exhibitions, trade fairs, demonstrations, and the like, are common to the two documents.

National language requirements for certain information are permitted.

The two Standing Committees referred to in the active implantable medical devices Directive are also referred to in the latest draft for the medical device Directive. The safeguard clause concerning withdrawal from the market of unsafe devices and the appropriate appeal procedures is also included in both documents.

Clinical investigation provisions are included. Notification of such investigations to competent authorities is required for class III devices and implantable devices in class IIa 45 (rather than 60) days before the commencement of the trials. The trial can continue after that time unless the competent authority objects. Objections are not expected where a proposed trial has received a favourable opinion from an ethics committee. These provisions do not apply fully to investigations on devices which can carry the CE mark.

Procedures for the appointment and withdrawal of notification of notified bodies are described. The manufacturers and the notified bodies agree timetables for the evaluation and verification procedures.

Where the CE mark has been wrongly affixed, notified bodies are required to take the appropriate action.

Decisions to restrict or refuse the placing of a device on the market or the undertaking of clinical trials are communicated to the companies concerned with a statement of the grounds on which the decision was based.

Normal confidentiality restrictions apply.

9.6.7 Essential requirements

9.6.7.1 *General requirements*

There are certain changes to the content and wording of the general requirements.

Devices are required to be designed and manufactured to ensure that under normal conditions of use they are not to compromise the clinical condition or safety of the patient. Taking into account all the essential requirements they do not present unacceptable risks to the person using them or other persons.

Design and construction taken up by the manufacturer are to be in line with the generally acknowledged state of the art.

The intended characteristics and performances are to be achieved. Normal use stresses are not to result in compromised safety for the patient or other persons during the expected lifetime of the device. The characteristics and performances are not affected adversely by normal conditions of storage and transport, and the design, manufacture, and packaging of the device are to take this into account.

Any side effects or undesirable conditions arising from the use of the device are to be acceptable in the light of the intended performance.

9.6.7.2 *Design and construction*

Similar considerations apply to the design and manufacture of medical devices as to active implantable medical devices. The toxicity of materials, mutual compatibility, and related topics are to be taken into account. Risks of contamination are to be minimised, as are risks associated with leaching of substances from the device during use. The device is to be safe for use with other products with which it is intended to come into contact during normal use.

Where a device incorporates as an integral part a substance likely to be considered to be a medicinal product under Directive 65/65/EEC and if that substance becomes bioavailable, then the quality, safety, and usefulness of that substance are to be verified by analogy with the appropriate methods specified in Directive 75/318/EEC.

Risks of infection of the patient are to be minimised. The risks of cross-infection from devices incorporating human or animal tissue are to be minimised by appropriate tissue selection, collection, and testing. Sterile devices are to remain sterile until the sterility barrier is breached. Devices claimed to be sterile are to have been subjected to a validated sterilisation process.

Where products are not intended to be sterile they are packed in such a way as to maintain the product without deterioration. Products to be sterilised before use are packed to minimise the risk of microbial contamination. If a product is marketed in both sterile and non-sterile forms the packaging is to differentiate between the two states.

Connections between medical devices and/or other equipment used together are to be safe and are not to adversely affect the performance of the device. Limitations for use are to be stated in labels or instructions.

Devices are to be designed and manufactured to minimise or remove risks of physical injury associated with their physical features and mechanical hazards of the device, risks associated with foreseeable environmental factors (for example electromagnetic effects), risks associated with medical investigation and treatment, and risks arising from inability to maintain or calibrate the device (for example an implant). Risks associated with use of a device with flammable materials or materials that promote combustion are to be minimised by appropriate design and construction. Vibration and noise levels are maintained within acceptable limits. Connections for hydraulic, pneumatic, or electrical supplies (etc.) minimise potential hazard. The temperature of accessible parts of the device is not to constitute a hazard.

Measuring functions are to be undertaken with adequate stability and accuracy, taking into account the intended use of the device. Appropriate units of measurement are to be used.

Radiation emissions are to be within the appropriate dose limits to the user indicated in EURATOM Directives. Precise information on the characteristics of radiation-emitting devices and on appropriate protection for patient and users are to be included in the instructions for use of such devices. Unintended radiation exposure of patients and users is to be minimised by adequate design and construction. Visual and/or audio warning systems are to indicate when radiation is being emitted from such devices.

Hazards arising from errors in the software of software-controlled devices are to be minimised by adequate design.

Where the safety of the patient is dependent on an internal power source the user is to be able to determine the state of the power source. If dependent on an external power source a suitable power failure alarm is to be provided.

Powered devices are to be designed to minimise the risks related to electromagnetic field production which could affect other devices or equipment functioning correctly in the vicinity. The risk of electric shock for correctly installed devices in normal use and single-fault conditions is to be minimised as far as possible.

Devices intended to deliver energy or substances to the patient are to be designed and constructed to allow output from the device to be set and maintained with an adequate level of accuracy. Hazardous conditions and settings are to be prevented or indicated by using interlocks and/or warning devices.

Information provided by the manufacturer is to include the identity of the manufacturer and that information necessary for the safe use of the product. Wherever possible such information is to appear on the device itself and/or the pack. Leaflets may also be used. Symbols and colour identification used are to be in accordance with harmonised standards.

Labels are to include the following information: the name/trade name and address of the manufacturer; information to identify the device or pack contents; 'STERILE', if appropriate; a batch reference; a time limit for the use of the device if necessary; an indication if the product is for use on a single occasion; for class IIa, IIb, and III devices the statement 'custom-made device' or 'exclusively for clinical investigation' if appropriate; relevant storage and handling conditions; instructions for use as relevant; warnings and precautions as relevant. The intended purpose of the device is to be stated unless this is self-evident. Devices and detachable components are to be identified to allow necessary action to be taken in the event of a potential risk being discovered.

Instructions for use are to include the following information: for class III devices, the year of authorisation for the application of the CE mark; the information to appear on the label with the exception of the batch number and expiry date; performance and undesirable effects; adequate information on the products with which the device is intended to be used (to allow the use of safe combinations); information on checks for correct installation, proper functioning, and routine maintenance; information allowing certain risks associated with the implantation of the device to be avoided; risks of reciprocal interference; instructions about damaged packs of sterile products and instruction on resterilisation if appropriate; information on the processing necessary for reusable devices (including cleaning, repackaging, resterilising, etc.), and information on any limitation on the number of reprocessing operations that may be undertaken, if appropriate; information relating to any additional processing required before a device can be used.

In addition the instruction leaflet is to include information to allow medical staff to brief the patient on the contraindications and precautions to be taken, particularly relating to changes in the performance of the device, exposure to foreseeable environmental conditions, medicinal products which the device is intended to administer, and precautions to be taken against any specific unusual risks associated with the disposal of the device.

9.6.8 Conformity assessment procedures

Annexes 2 to 7 of the draft document relate to the conformity assessment procedures. The various options are:

- EC declaration of conformity (complete quality assurance system);
- EC type-examination;
- EC verification;
- EC declaration of conformity (assurance of production quality);
- EC declaration of conformity (product quality assurance);
- EC declaration of conformity.

Many of the characteristics of these options have been discussed under the section (9.5) on active implantable medical devices, and will not be expanded on further here. Suffice to say that the conformity assessment procedures are derived from a proposal for a Council Directive concerning the modules for the various phases of the conformity assessment procedures which are intended to be used in the technical harmonisation directives, under reference COM(89) 209 final — SYN 208 (89/C 231/03) (published in the *Official Journal of the European Communities* No C231/3 of 8 September 1989).

9.6.9 Statement concerning devices intended for special purposes

The provisions included in this Annex are closely similar to those applied to the active implantable medical device Directive. They apply only to class IIa, IIb, and III devices.

9.6.10 Classification decision criteria

The medical devices Directive draft includes classification decision rules for devices other than active medical devices and for active medical devices. Decision trees are also included, although they are to have no mandatory legal effect in the final Directive.

For the purpose of the Directive it is proposed that the term 'transient' is defined as normally less than 15 minutes (of use); 'short-term' is up to 30 days; and 'long-term' is more than 30 days.

Invasive devices are those penetrating wholly or mainly through body surfaces or into a natural orifice (itself defined as a natural opening in the skin, including the exterior surface of the eyeball and a surgically created opening such as a stoma). A surgically invasive device is one which penetrates body surfaces during surgical intervention. A surgical instrument is one intended for use in several different surgical procedures for action such as cutting, drilling, sawing, scraping, retracting, or clamping.

Devices are classified according to their most critical intended use. Where more than one classification can be allocated it is proposed that the highest applies.

The classification rules are listed according to categories of product. These are summarised in the order in which they appear in the draft Directive.

9.6.10.1 *Non-active medical devices*

(a) Non-invasive devices coming into contact with intact skin

Rule 1

Products are class I if they do not come into contact with blood or other body liquids which will be infused into the body; liquids or gases which will be infused or delivered into the body; or breached or compromised external body surfaces. The exception is products which are placed on limbs for the purpose of compression in order to prevent thromboembolism (class IIa).

Rule 2

Products which are non-invasive and intended for channelling or short-term storage of blood, other body liquids, liquids, or gases for eventual infusion or delivery into the body are class I. However, if they are used in connection with active medical devices they become class IIa devices.

Rule 3

Non-invasive devices intended to modify biological or chemical composition of blood, other body liquids, or liquids which will be infused into the body are class III unless the treatment consists of filtration, centrifugation, exchange of gas, heat, or solute (when they are class IIa). (This proposed rule in particular includes a number of points still under discussion.)

(b) Non-invasive devices coming into contact with breached skin

Rule 4

Devices intended to be used as mechanical barriers for compression or for absorption of exudates are class I.

Devices intended to replace any of the functions of the skin (other than those of mechanical barrier or for exudation) are class IIa.

Devices intended to be used on third degree burns are class III.

(c)   Invasive devices with respect to natural body orifices

Rule 5

Invasive (but not surgically invasive) devices are class I if intended for transient use other than those intended for use in the urethra which are class IIa.

Products intended for short-term use are class IIa (other than those placed in the oral cavity as far as the pharynx, anterior nostril, or the anterior ear canal as far as the ear drum, or reusable instruments, which are class I).

Products intended for long-term use are class IIa.

(d)   Surgically invasive devices

Rule 6

Surgically invasive devices not intended for diagnosis, monitoring, or correcting a defect in the cardiovascular system by manipulation and/or progression inside this system are class IIa; devices for those purposes are class III. The exception is reusable instruments, which are class I.

Rule 7

Surgically invasive devices intended for short-term use are class IIa with the following exceptions: devices intended to diagnose, monitor, or correct a defect in the cardiovascular system or manipulation and/or progression inside this system, or used in direct contact with the central nervous system (class III).

(e)   Implantable devices and long-term surgically invasive devices

Rule 8

Devices intended for use in direct contact with the cardiovascular or central nervous systems are class III; other products are class IIa.

Rule 9

Devices intended to undergo chemical change in the body, have biological activity, be absorbed, or deliver energy or medicinal products are class III, unless placed in the teeth (class IIa).

(f)   Special rules

Rule 10

Devices incorporating as an integral part a substance otherwise considered to be a medicinal product under Directive 65/65/EEC and which may result in the bioavailability of that substance are class III.

Rule 11

Devices intended to prevent conception or the transmission of viral diseases by sexual contact are class III devices.

9.6.10.2 *Active medical devices*

All active medical devices are class IIb unless they cannot be used in direct connection with another active device, and/or they are not intended to deliver or exchange energy or substances to the human body, in which case they are class I devices.

9.6.11 Clinical evaluation

The provisions are similar to those applying to active implantable medical devices (Annex 7), but they apply only to class III devices.

9.6.12 Criteria to be met when designating inspection bodies to be notified

These are in line with the requirements laid down in Annex 8 of the active implantable medical device Directive.

9.6.13 CE mark of conformity

This is the same as that described in Annex 9 of the active implantable medical devices Directive.

9.7 COMMENTS ON THE MEDICAL DEVICE DIRECTIVES

The similarity in the wording of the definition of medical device and that for medicinal product is noteworthy. In Directive 65/65/EEC a medicinal product is defined as:

> Any substance or combination of substances presented for treating or preventing disease in human beings or animals.

> Any substance or combination of substances which may be administered to human beings or animals with a view to making a medical diagnosis or to restoring, correcting, or modifying physiological functions in human beings or animals is likewise considered a medicinal product.

The same Directive defines a 'substance' in the following terms:

> Any substance irrespective of origin which may be human (for example human blood and human blood products), animal (for example microorganisms, whole animals, parts of organs, animal secretions, toxins, extracts, blood products, etc.), vegetable (for example microorganisms, plants, parts of plants, vegetable excretions, extracts, etc.), chemical (for example elements, naturally occurring chemical materials, and chemical products obtained by chemical change or synthesis).

There is therefore a potential area of overlap between the two sets of Directives. This has to some extent been recognised by the provision in the device Directives that in the case of devices intended to administer a medicinal product, that substance is to be the subject of controls under the pharmaceutical Directive 65/65/EEC as amended last by Directive 87/21/EEC.

Where a medicinal product is incorporated as an integral part of the device, then the device is evaluated and controlled under the device Directive that is appropriate. In the essential requirements it is indicated that where the medicinal product is bioavailable, the safety, quality, and 'usefulness' of that substance are evaluated by analogy with the appropriate methods specified in Directive 75/318/EEC as last amended by Directive 89/341/EEC. Products containing such bioavailable medicinal products are classified as class III devices where a classification system applies. Unfortunately, the term 'bioavailable' has not been defined in the draft Directive.

The reference to specific amendment dates for the pharmaceutical Directives will presumably require amendment to take account of future amendments and developments.

It is likely that some disputes will arise as to whether a particular product is a medical device or a medicinal product in certain cases. In addition, disputes will undoubtedly arise from the classification system and its application. It is to be admitted that the US system of classification has shortcomings, but it may be that the main way of avoiding classification disputes will be the published lists of classifications applied to products (thus setting precedents for the notified bodies and competent authorities to take into account).

It has also been suggested that the way of overcoming the potential difficulties of the pharmaceutical–device borderline is to modify the definition of a medicinal product in Directive 65/65/EEC.

The necessity for appropriate arrangements for verification and certification to be made by all competent authorities may result in difficulties once the initial problem of dealing with the huge number of existing products on the market has been dealt with. Since it is for the manufacturer to select which notified body to submit his product to for verification and certification (if necessary), it is possible that some of the notified bodies will be lightly loaded with at least some types of work in the foreseeable future. In addition, the provision of national systems of approval (and the possible need to indicate the notified body's logo along with the CE mark) is seen by some as an opportunity for the introduction of new barriers to trade where some purchasers might give preference to products approved in their own countries.

Another possible problem of this system is that there may be differences in practices between the various notified bodies. All of these problems might have been overcome had the approval process been centralised in the first place. This would also have helped minimise the problems likely to arise from the limited numbers of professional staff qualified to undertake the verification and certification procedures.

The application of the CE mark may be seen as a useful assurance of the satisfactory nature of the product. It is therefore surprising that it has been considered optional for class I medical devices to carry the symbol. This would appear to undermine the whole application of the concepts behind the 'new approach' to medical devices, since the user will not be able to buy only CE mark-carrying devices when some class I devices may not be available which carry the mark. It is not clear how the user is to know which class I devices comply with the essential requirements.

The suggested omission of class I products completely from the requirement for manufacturers to report incidents related to death or deterioration of the clinical condition of patients and of medical or technical reasons for the withdrawal of the product from the market, is also surprising. It is noteworthy that the wording of the relevant Article from the active implantable medical device Directive ('might lead or might have led to the death of a patient or to a deterioration in his state of health') has been amended in the latest draft of the medical device Directive (to 'might lead to or might have led to the death of a patient or to a serious and irreversible deterioration in his state of health').

The proposed acknowledgement of the status of certain *European Pharmacopoeia* monographs is welcome to some if not all manufacturers. However, it is noted that only those monographs to which reference is made in the *Official Journal of the European Communities* are to be so recognised. The basis of selection of the monographs to be recognised could be usefully expanded.

With respect to the necessity that an adequate number of CEN and CENELEC standards be available to support the essential requirements for as many devices as possible, it might be considered that the standards-generating bodies have been set an impossible task. Priority is being given to the development of horizontal standards (for example sterilisation, good manufacturing practice, connector compatibility, biocompatibility, symbols and labelling, etc.), and this appears to be reasonable.

However, in due time vertical standards (that is those applying to individual products or small groups of closely related products) will also be needed, and the amount of time and effort that will be required to generate standards which are adequate and acceptable is enormous. Particular difficulties may arise where products have formerly been considered to be pharmaceuticals, where the authorisation authorities' approach relies on the flexible application of guidelines rather than full compliance with published standards and the tailoring of requirements to particular situations. It might be difficult to build such flexibility into a standard whilst still ensuring that the essential requirements are met. (A standard normally requires a method to be defined — usually after considerable collaborative trial work to ensure that it is robust enough to be applied successfully by a number of laboratories — together with a stated performance which is to be achieved.)

With regard to the provisions for the advance notification of a manufacturer's intention to carry out a clinical investigation it is noted that the period of time in advance of the commencement of the trial which is required has been amended from 60 days in the active implantable medical device Directive to 45 days in the draft Directive on medical devices. This is in line with an amendment to the former approved by the European Parliament but not incorporated into the final Directive. However, it does not seem to take into account the practicalities of the necessary assessment work required by the notified bodies. If an unreasonably short deadline is set, then extra resource will be needed by the notified bodies: this must increase costs without necessarily offering a significant improvement in performance. (The clinical trial exemption scheme operated by the UK Medicines Control Agency for pharmaceuticals requires 35 days' notice but this can be extended by a further 28 days if necessary. Such a two-tier system might be useful for the clinical trial approvals for medical devices. Similarly, it might have been useful to have a clinicians exemption scheme for medical devices similar to that operated by the Medicines Control Agency for pharmaceuticals.)

10

Contact lens products and intrauterine contraceptive devices

10.1 INTRODUCTION

Chapter 9 discusses the controls on medical devices under present and proposed future scheme in general. This chapter discussed the application of controls to two types of medical device — contact lenses and lens care products, and intrauterine contraceptive devices. The United Kingdom procedures for the control of these products will be used as the basis for the chapter.

The choice of these two types of device is not entirely random. Both were brought under the UK Medicines Act in the same Order made under section 104 of that Act. A further explanation of the UK's system of controls and the role of section 104 Orders is included in Chapter 17.

The Order bringing contact lenses and their associated care products under the Medicines Act was the Medicines (Specified Articles and Substances) Order 1976 (No. 968). This covers contact lenses, the blanks used in their manufacture, and products (solutions and others) used for cleaning, disinfecting, irrigating, lubricating, wetting, storing, and soaking the lenses, or used as a barrier between the contact lens and the eyeball, or any other substance used in connection with lens care. In practice, only those parts of the Order relating to contact lens care products used by lens wearers or practitioners have been activated.

The same Order also brought under control of the Medicines Act intrauterine and intracervical contraceptive devices.

In addition to the 1976 Order a number of other Orders and Regulations were introduced to give effect to various aspects of the control of these products. These may be found in the listing of Statutory Instruments in Chapter 17.

10.2 CONTACT LENS CARE PRODUCTS

10.2.1 Contact lenses and contact lens care products in the UK

In the UK all contact lenses and lens care products were brought under the Medicines Act by Statutory Instrument 1976: No. 968. The provisions relating to contact lenses have not been activated.

10.2.2 Controls in the EC

The controls applied to contact lenses and contact lens products in the European Community (EC) are summarised in Table 10.1. This gives an example of how individual national controls can vary between Member States. This was one of the reasons for the medical device industry trying to get medical devices covered by harmonised, mutual recognition Directives as discussed in Chapter 9. A Working Group of the European Standardisation Committee (CEN) (TC 170 WG 5) is developing harmonised standards to support the control of these products under the medical device Directives.

10.2.3 Requirements in the UK

Table 10.1 — Controls applied to contact lenses and contact lens care products in the EC

Country	Lens controls	Care products
Belgium	None	None
Denmark	None	None
France	None	All controlled
Greece	None	All controlled
Ireland	None	In-eye products
Italy	Suspended	All controlled
Luxembourg	None	None
Netherlands	None	Labelling
Portugal	None	None
Spain	None	All controlled
Germany	Anomalous drug	In-eye products

At one time a separate Medicines Act leaflet was available giving advice on the data requirements for contact lens products (MAL 53), but this has now been incorporated in the Guidance Notes on Applications for Product Licences (MAL 2) (MCA, 1989) as Annexe VII.

10.2.3.1 General requirements

The application should be in the EC-suggested format, as if the pharmaceutical Directives applied fully. MAL 201 application forms should be used. Expert Reports are always needed for the chemistry and pharmacy parts of the application and might be required for the experimental and biological and the clinical sections, especially in the case of products containing a novel ingredient or an ingredient used in a particular way for the first time.

Contact lens care products have no legal status. The subject of legal status is discussed more fully in Chapter 17. However, the relevant advisory Committee in the UK, the Committee on Dental and Surgical Materials, has indicated that it considers that all contact lens care products should be supplied only through professional outlets (pharmacies, dispensing opticians and optometrists, as well as hospital clinics). This limitation is usually written into product licence applications forms.

10.2.3.2 *Chemical and pharmaceutical documentation*
The normal data requirements of MAL 2 and the EC requirements apply, with the following amendments or modified emphasis.

(a) Microbiological studies
Details should be included in the application of the results obtained for antimicrobial preservative efficacy testing by an appropriate method (details of which should be included) and suitable organisms. The test method should be validated, including details of results from recovery experiments using low levels of inocula. In particular the inactivation of preservatives present in the product should be discussed if relevant.

The level of antimicrobial activity expected is related to the intended use of the product — thus, in-eye products and cold disinfection products are expected to show a higher level of activity than, say, a cleaner that is used prior to a rinsing/disinfection cycle.

Kill curve data should be provided on at least two batches of product over a suitable period (which should be related to the recommended method of use). The level of inoculum used should be sufficient to allow 3 or 4 log orders of reduction in viable count to be followed. Fresh and aged product should be examined. The organisms used should include those recommended in the *British Pharmacopoeia* antimicrobial preservative efficacy test, although additional organisms may be included. In some cases it might be appropriate to include *Acanthamoeba* species or other clinically significant organisms. Adequate data may be required to demonstrate activity of cold disinfectant products against cystic forms of *Acanthamoeba* species.

(b) Compatibility studies
Product/container compatibility studies are required for all products. In addition, data are required to demonstrate compatibility of the product with representative examples of the types of lenses with which the product is to be used. Factors such as preservative uptake and release and the physical parameters and properties of the lenses following the normal recommended use procedures for the product should be reported. In the case of physical parameter studies a range of lens prescriptions should be used including high + and high − power lenses. Depending on the claims for use, the product/lens compatibility studies may need to incorporate polymethylmethacrylate (PMMA) lenses, representative types of rigid gas permeable (GP) lenses, and representative high and low water content (i.e <55 per cent and >55 per cent water content) ionic and non-ionic hydrogel lenses, for example.

The compatibility studies should use methods that mimic the recommended usage of the product, or represent a greater challenge.

(c) Container sizes

Products intended for use on more than one occasion should contain sufficient product for use for not more than 28 days unless the container is pressurised or satisfactory additional data to justify a longer use period are supplied. In the case of single-use products the container should not hold an excessive overage and should not be resealable. All containers should have tamper-evident closures. A suitable labelling statement regarding sterility of the product until the seal is broken is often included for products intended to be used on more than one occasion.

10.2.3.3 Experimental and biological studies

For all products coming into contact with the eye, adequate local toxicity data are expected, including sensitisation and ocular irritation tests. Tests should be undertaken on the product to be marketed. The period of testing should be justified but should not be less than four weeks, although longer studies may be appropriate in the case of products containing novel ingredients or novel combinations of ingredients. The studies should mimic as far as possible recommended clinical usage. Full justification should be provided for the omission of such studies.

Mutagenicity data should be submitted as suggested in the usual guidelines. Provided that the results of these do not indicate mutagenic potential, and provided that the systemic exposure to components in the product is low, it may not be necessary to undertake carcinogenicity studies.

Non-animal test systems may be used where they have been validated and shown to be reliable. Where it is necessary to undertake animal tests, dosage should be over seven days per week, with lenses worn for at least six hours per day in appropriate cases. Where lenses are worn the control eye should be fitted with a lens of the same design and of the same material. Lenses should be examined for changes. Daily examinations should be undertaken, with frequent slit-lamp examinations of the eyes. Terminal histological preparations should be made of the eyes and eye lids. Corneal thickness and the status of the corneal endothelium might be of particular interest. Animals' organs may need to be preserved in case any clinical findings indicate a need to examine them.

10.2.3.4 Studies in humans

Statistically valid evidence of safety and efficacy in all the claimed indications is required. Protocols should reflect the recommended usage of the product. Randomised comparative trials should be used, although it may be possible to present arguments against the need for comparative efficacy data for certain products − e.g. some disinfectants − where satisfactory *in vitro* data are available. Unsubstantiated testimonials are not acceptable in the place of clinical trial data. Clinical trial reports should include reference to the condition of lenses at appropriate test intervals and the end of the study. All adverse clinical findings should be reported, and a summary of all adverse reaction reports (worldwide) should be included in the data package.

10.2.3.5 Product literature

The product literature should include adequate instruction on the hygiene necessary in the care of lenses, lens cases, or other auxiliary equipment, including advice on the frequency and nature of cleaning. In particular, appropriate mention should be included in the product literature of the use of daily surfactant and weekly protein cleaners, as appropriate. If it is claimed that such products are not required, then supporting data will be required in the application.

10.3 INTRAUTERINE CONTRACEPTIVE DEVICES

10.3.1 Introduction
SI 1976 No 968 specifically brought under the Medicines Act intrauterine and intracervical contraceptive devices. A Medicines Act leaflet covers the data requirements for these products — *Guidance notes on applications for product licences and clinical trial certificates for intrauterine contraceptive devices* (MAL 61) (MCA, 1977) — and parts of MAL 2 (*Guidance notes on applications for product licences*) (MCA, 1989) and MAL 4 (*Guidance notes on applications for clinical trial certificates and clinical trial exemptions*) (MCA, 1985, 1986) are also relevant. Normal administrative data are required.

10.3.2 Data requirements in the UK
10.3.2.1 Chemical and pharmaceutical documentation
Information is required on the components used in the device and their manufacture and composition. In addition to description it is helpful to include drawings and samples of the product. The product development sections of the application should include the derivation of the design characteristics, the choice of materials for the device, and factors affecting the choice of sterilisation method. The packaging system choice should be discussed too.

The manufacturing process should be described and discussed and information provided on the routine bioburden of the product, and the validation of the sterilisation method discussed as appropriate especially where ethylene oxide sterilisation or radiation doses of less than 25 kGy or parametric release are requested.

Quality assurance arrangements should be stated, especially those relating to the physical characterisation of the device and its components including tensile strength, extension to break, modulus, melt flow index, glass transition temperature, and molecular weight distribution. The specification of any metallic component — for example copper wire — should be stated. In-process controls should be stated.

The finished product specification should include tests for physical properties including dimensions, identity tests for essential components, sterility requirements, etc.

Stability data should establish that the product maintains its physical attributes as well as showing that the packaging does not deteriorate to such an extent that sterility of the product is threatened.

10.3.2.2 Experimental and biological studies
Provided that the materials used in the intrauterine or intracervical contraceptive device have been widely and safely used in similar products for some time, few toxicity studies will normally be required.

The need for pharmacodynamic or pharmacokinetic data will depend on whether there is a constituent which will be released from the device that has not been used widely before: extraction studies may be of some significance here, and the polymer or material chemistry will be taken into account. If studies are required (for example where the composition or production method is changed significantly, or in the case of materials that do not have a history of safe clinical use) the material used for those studies should have been exposed to the normal production and sterilisation procedures as far as possible.

Implantation tests in two mammalian species may need to be included, using one non-rodent species. Six-month studies using the subcutaneous, intramuscular, and intraperitoneal routes as well as intrauterine or intracervical routes should be used where necessary, with frequent histological examination of the implantation sites as well as terminal histology. The initial ratio of surface area of device to surface area of animal should be similar to that experienced with women. An increase in this ratio may be required in the case of evidence of extractable materials being found.

If carcinogenicity studies are required these should be carried out in two species, but using a single dose level comparable to the human exposure. Subcutaneous, intramuscular, and intraperitoneal routes should be used.

Reproductive studies are not required.

10.3.2.3 Studies in humans

Clinical studies should be carried out in women of child-bearing age who are regularly exposed to the risk of pregnancy. Initial studies should provide about 100 women-years of data with not more than five percent loss to follow-up.

For main studies some 600 women should be followed up for a year, with a minimum of fifty per investigator. The loss to follow-up should not exceed ten per cent.

Guidance is included in the guidance note MAL 61 on the inclusion of women who had previously taken oral contraceptives or had been previously fitted with an IUCD.

The clinical data should be statistically analysed by stated and appropriate methods. Information should be included on the incidence of pregnancy, device expulsion, removal (analysed separately according to reason for removal), loss to follow-up, release from follow-up, and any difficulties found in fitting or removing the devices. Any foetal abnormalities or defects in children born to women wearing the device should be reported. Clinical examination results should be reported.

11

Experts and Expert Reports in marketing authorisation applications

11.1 INTRODUCTION

The requirement for Expert Reports was introduced in 1975 in Directive 75/319/EEC. This stated that the 'documents and particulars' for marketing authorisation applications must be drawn up by 'experts with the necessary technical and professional qualifications'. The Experts were supposed to provide a detailed report. However, this requirement had not been implemented systematically by the authorities in all of the EC Member States — in most it was honoured more in the breach than the observance.

The changes brought about by Directive 83/570/EEC made the authorities review this requirement for Expert Reports. This Directive had introduced the new requirement on the authorities to draw up an 'assessment report' which they needed to have available immediately on request for products containing a 'new active substance' (NAS). The concept of an NAS now replaced the more archaic term 'new chemical entity' (NCE) which was previously applied to all types of active whether synthetic, semi-synthetic, biosynthetic, a product of biotechnology, an endogenous compound extracted from human or animal tissue, or a novel active derived from a plant (vegetable) source. NASs can be divided into new chemical active substances (NCAS) and new biological active substances (NBAS).

The Committee for Proprietary Medicinal Products (CPMP) set up an *ad hoc* working party of representatives of the Member States to consider how best to implement this new requirement. They concluded that the new 'assessment report' should be firmly based on the framework which could be provided by the companies' own Expert Reports. The Working Party reviewed these legal requirements and their own practical needs and devised a guideline. This was the first (1986) edition of the *Notice to applicants for marketing authorizations for proprietary medicinal products in the European Community*. This guideline was adopted by the CPMP and published by the Commission of the European Communities (CEC).

The 'Notice to applicants'... underwent a very substantial revision before the second edition was published, and drew on the two to three years' experience of the authorities with Expert Reports. The second edition gives much more detailed guidance on the qualifications and experience necessary for the three types of Expert (the pharmaceutical Expert, the pharmacotoxicological Expert, and the clinical Expert). It defines the format and content of the Expert Report in much more detail than hitherto.

11.2 WHY ARE EXPERT REPORTS NEEDED?

The Expert Reports are needed for a variety of cogent legal, technical and administrative reasons, which are set out below.

11.2.1 To comply with the requirements of Articles 1 to 3 of Directive 75/319/EEC

Articles 1 and 2 require that the 'documents and particulars' are drawn up by Experts, who have to provide information according to Directive 75/318/EEC (the 'norms and protocols' Directive). The Expert is required to provide a detailed report.

The authorities are required, according to Article 3 of 75/319/EEC, to refuse the application if Expert Reports are not included. In many EC Member States the application is regarded as invalid and returned to the applicant without any detailed assessment if it does not contain the appropriate Expert Report.

11.2.2 To be used in the compilation of assessment reports (for multistate and concertation applications)

Article 9(1) of Directive 75/319/EEC requires the national authorities to take into 'due consideration' the marketing authorisation of another Member State. Some commentators have (mistakenly) implied that this should mean automatic mutual recognition of the first authorisation. However, what it really means is that a second authority can, by referring to the assessment report, see all the issues that were considered by the first authority, and all the issues it raised with the applicant before it granted the authorisation. As can be seen later, there are reasons why a second authority may (quite legitimately) take a different view of an application from the first, and grant different therapeutic indications, require different contraindications, different quality requirements, etc. In the future, these differences in approach will need to be harmonised, but at the moment they represent legitimate differences in prescribing and diagnostic practice in the Member States; differences in access to sophisticated specialist care in hospitals and clinics; different types of products authorised in the Member States; different indications and dosages for the same pharmacotherapeutic classes of active ingredients; etc. The assessment report enables a second authority to reconsider the major issues in the light of its own national practices.

An assessment report will be supplied for use in consideration of a second national application (on request). It will also be supplied by the 'rapporteur' Member State in the multistate and concertation procedures.

An assessment report will always be available for a NAS product. In the UK it may not, however, at the moment be available for an 'abridged' (second applicant product, copy product, new strength, new dosage form of existing active ingredient etc.) application. In many of the EC Member States it will also not be available for a reviewed product licence (old product licence brought up to date according to the current requirements according to the legal requirements of Article 39 of Directive 75/319/EEC). In some other EC Member States (such as France and the Netherlands) an assessment report may be specially written on request if needed for one of the EC procedures.

An assessment report usually consists of the following documents:

- the applicant's Expert Report (if suitable);
- the comments from the assessors (either the internal assessors or the outside independent Experts for a country which uses such a system);
- the official Committee advice/decision;
- the appeal data (formal or informal appeal);
- notes on the consideration of the appeal;
- the final approval (including a copy of the approved summary of product characteristics);
- notes on any major changes (variations) to the marketing authorisation;
- notes of the pharmacovigilance experience in the Member State (adverse drug reaction reports from the company itself or from health-care professionals — physicians, pharmacists, opticians, etc.);
- reports of any formal post-marketing surveillance studies (PMS).

11.2.3 To provide a summary and overview of the product for any subsequent action by the authorities on the authorisation

The original data are very voluminous for many marketing authorisation applications. The original data are often stored by the authorities separately from the (paper) working file. The Expert Report provides a convenient summary of the dossier which can be placed on the working file. This can then be referred to by the assessors in considering any proposals from the applicant to change the authorisation. Any adverse drug reaction (ADR) data and product defect reports can also be considered in the light of the original data as summarised in the Expert Report. The use of the Expert Report in this way enables an assessor to make an informed judgement on any proposed change more quickly. For example, a major new proposed indication can be reviewed not only in the light of the new clinical trial data submitted in support of the new claim, but also the previous clinical data on related claims and the earlier overall analysis of the product safety profile in patients.

11.2.4 To identify the major issues raised by the data in the dossier for its subsequent consideration nationally or in the Committee for Proprietary Medicinal Products (CPMP)

An assessment report is prepared in the following circumstances — for use by a national Committee (such as the Committee on Safety of Medicines in the UK, the Commission A in the Federal Republic of Germany, the Dutch College, etc.); and

Sec. 11.2] **Why are Expert Reports needed?** 171

for use in the CPMP for a multistate application or a concertation application (for a biotechnology or high technology product).

There are three parts to an Expert Report:
(1) the summarised tabulated information,
(2) the optional written summary (usually only included in the Clinical section of the Expert Report),
(3) the critical analysis of the information by the Experts.

It is this critical analysis section which provides a unique opportunity for the Experts to explain the development of the product and to try to identify the major issues raised by the application, and to explain and reassure the assessors and the national Committee/CPMP on these points. It could be argued that the most critical aspect of the role of the Expert is to try to identify any potential points which the national Committee or CPMP might wish to raise and to try to answer them in advance.

To carry out this role the Expert needs to be completely *au fait* with the EC legal technical requirements as set out in Directive 75/318/EEC and in the guidelines (which are the harmonised views of the authorities on many technical issues). In addition, the Expert needs to be familiar with precedent for similar products on a national market for a purely national application, or in a number of markets for a multistate application or concertation application. If major new therapeutic claims are made, are these justified by sufficient clinical data?

11.2.5 To ensure that all marketing authorisation applications have had critical review

Many applications received by the national authorities are incomplete. In many Member States in the EC, applications are subjected to a validation check — a check for the essential completeness of the application. In the UK, for example, about 15 to 25 per cent of applications submitted are invalid (the higher figure represents applications received in the periods before the change in licence fees). Some applications are held for a while, and further data are added to enable them to be accepted; others are returned to the applicant.

The need to write an Expert Report should mean that the data in the dossier are thoroughly reviewed in the light of the current European legal and technical requirements (as defined in the Directives, the Guidelines, and the 'Notice to Applicants'), and any deficiencies identified before the application is submitted.

11.2.6 To provide the core of the Evaluation Report in the Product Evaluation Report (PER) scheme

Chapter 16 reviews the need for companies to develop a regulatory strategy in the EC and European Free Trade Area (EFTA) countries. The PER scheme described in Chapter 16 includes some EC Member States as well as the EFTA countries.

In this scheme an evaluation report is provided on request for NAS products. In essence this is identical to the assessment report used in the EC countries. Thus, a well-written Expert Report will also provide the core of the PER report, and can considerably expedite the granting of authorisations in the PER countries (which now includes Canada and Australia).

11.2.7 To provide the core of the assessment/evaluation report in the future in a wider European or global application

In the coming months and years as the newly liberalised governments in Eastern Europe link more closely to the EC, it is likely that the use of PER or similar schemes will expand to enable them to have access to the evaluation reports of the EC Member States. Thus the Expert Report is likely to be a vital element in any future internationally harmonised marketing authorisation application (the so-called 'global application').

11.3 THE EXPERT — LEGAL DEFINITIONS AND PRACTICAL REQUIREMENTS (TRAINING, POSITION, AND EXPERIENCE)

11.3.1 Legal definitions (Directive 75/319/EEC)

The Directive merely defines the Experts as having 'the necessary technical and professional qualifications'. The three Experts are designated as the analyst, the pharmacologist/toxicologist, and the clinician.

11.3.1.1 The analyst
The duties of the analyst are stated to be to ensure that the product is consistent with the declared composition and to give substantiation of the control methods employed in the manufacture.

11.3.1.2 The pharmacologist/toxicologist
The pharmacologist/toxicologist is referred to as 'a pharmacologist or specialist with similar experimental competence', and his duties are to state the toxicity of the product and the pharmacological properties observed.

11.3.1.3 The clinician
The clinical Expert is described as a 'clinician', and his duties are to state whether he has been able to ascertain whether the effects of the product (actions and side effects) are as described, and whether the product is well-tolerated, what is the dosage regimen required, and what are the recommended indications and contraindications.

11.3.1.4 Legal requirements as to qualification of Experts
In the case of the clinician it is clearly implied that medical training is needed. For the pharmacologist/toxicologist, the Directive indicates the need for a pharmacologist or specialist with similar experimental competence.

No such clear guidance is given on the education and training requirements for the 'analyst' (the pharmaceutical Expert), and we therefore need to investigate these by considering what job he is asked to do.

Sec. 11.4]   **The three Experts: further exploration of their roles**   173

11.3.2 The practical requirements as defined in the 1989 edition of the 'Notice to Applicants'

The CPMP has given further guidance on the suitable qualifications and experience of the three Experts in the 1989 edition of the 'Notice to Applicants'.

Their general recommendations are as follows:

- It is recommended that the pharmaceutical Expert should have a formal qualification in pharmacy (or for biotechnology products, a qualification in another relevant discipline) and practical experience in research and development and/or the physicochemical, biological or microbiological control of medicinal products.
- It is suggested that the pharmacotoxicological Expert should have, a formal qualification in toxicology and/or pharmacology, or another relevant discipline, and have sufficient practical experience.
- It is necessary for the clinical Expert to have a formal qualification in medicine with relevant practical experience.

The 'Notice to Applicants' also makes it clear that the Expert does not necessarily have to have been personally involved in the performance of the tests whose results are reported in the dossier. He should, however, prepare a critical review of the relevant part of the dossier on behalf of the applicant. The 'Notice to Applicants' also recommends that the Expert must be conversant with the EC legislation (the Directives) and the relevant guidelines (both those cited in Volume III of the *Rules governing medicinal products in the European Community* and any guideline adopted by the CPMP subsequently).

11.4 THE THREE EXPERTS: FURTHER EXPLORATION OF THEIR ROLES

11.4.1 The pharmaceutical Expert

Article 2 of Directive 75/319/EEC refers to the role of the 'analyst' as 'substantiation of control methods'. Since 1975 the role of this Expert has considerably widened, and it now includes the responsibility for making a critical analysis of the data on development pharmaceutics, process validation, biopharmaceutics, analytical validation, active ingredient stability, and finished product stability. It is for this reason that the CPMP has now recommended that in general the suitable person is now the pharmacist, with his broad training which includes all these areas. Some companies are still using non-pharmacists (particularly in Italy and in the UK where there seems to have been a shortage of industrial pharmacists), but this may cause disadvantages later, particularly if an application is made in several Member States in the multistate procedure, or after 1992 using the 'decentralised' procedure (see Chapter 21).

11.4.2 The pharmaco-toxicological Expert

Article 2 of Directive 75/319/EEC refers to the role of the 'pharmacologist or the specialist with similar experimental competence' and defines his responsibilities as having to state 'the toxicity of the product and the pharmacological properties observed'. Since 1975 the role of this Expert has widened to include critical comments on the pharmacological/toxicological data in relation to potential problems in man and in relation to the statements of pharmacological particulars and clinical particulars in the proposed summary of product characteristics (SPC). In particular, the Expert needs to comment on the target-organ toxicity, the undesirable effects, and use during pregnancy and lactation.

It has been suggested that the pharmacotoxicological Expert's role is mainly confined to new active substance (NAS) applications. This is not so — an evaluation of the toxicological data/literature on impurities in a new source of an active substance forms an important part of his task in relation to a 'second applicant' abridged or copy product. There may be local or systemic toxicity associated with the (well-known) active ingredient used in a product, and the Expert would be expected to justify and comment on the proposed formulation in association with the pharmaceutical Expert. For example, if the active ingredient is known to be irritant to the oesophagus, is the formulation one that is likely to adhere to the mucous membrane in the oesophagus? Have tests been carried out in an animal model to provide reassurance? For a non-steroidal anti-inflammatory drug (NSAID) in a bolus sustained release dose-form (i.e. one that largely remains intact during the release of the active, unlike a pellet dose-form which is likely to disperse throught the gastrointestinal tract during its release), what is the effect if the dose-form is trapped in the intestine? Many elderly patients who are likely to be prescribed NSAIDs may suffer from intestinal fistulae etc.

Most Member States accept a combined pharmacotoxicological/clinical Expert Report — particularly for a well-known active ingredient used in the accepted indications. However, the application needs to make this clear, and to justify the use of such a combined Expert. It would be less acceptable to use such a combined Expert for an abridged application submitted without full pharmacological and toxicological data and clinical data under Article 4(8)(a)(ii) of Directive 65/65/EEC. An example of such a case would be an active ingredient licensed in the EC for less than ten years where the Expert would be expected to cite and summarise the published toxicology data from the literature under all of the relevant headings from Directive 75/318/EEC. This includes single dose toxicity, repeated dose toxicity, foetal toxicity, reproductive toxicity, mutagenic potential, carcinogenic potential, pharmacodynamics, and pharmacokinetics.

As the 1989 'Notice to Applicants' recommends, the Expert Report needs to include a summary of these published data, preferably using the formats in the 'Notice . . .', and commenting on whether the studies were carried out under good laboratory practice (GLP) or not. The fact that these data might have been scrutinised by another authority (e.g. the Food and Drug Administration (FDA)) who then referred to their review in a public document (e.g. the FDA Summary Basis of Approval document) is not regarded as sufficient in this context.

11.4.3 The clinical Expert

Article 2 of Directive 75/319/EEC requires the clinician to state whether he has been able to ascertain effects on persons treated with the product which correspond to the particulars given in Article 4 of Directive 65/65/EEC (the Summary of Product Characteristics); whether the patient tolerates the product well; and the posology (dosage regimen) advised; and any contraindications and side effects.

11.4.4 The three Experts: their role in defining the applicability of published references (for abridged applications)

According to Article 2(c) of Directive 75/319/EEC, all of the Experts have to state the grounds for using the published literature in relation to Article 4(8)(a) and (b) — particularly for abridged marketing authorisation applications for medicinal products containing established active ingredients. Thus, the Experts need to discuss the 'essential similarity' (according to Article 4(8)(a)(iii) of 65/65/EEC) of the product which is the subject of the new application (i.e. the 'copy' product) to the originator's product.

They will need to review the quality of the drug substance (polymorphic form, particle size, impurity profile — particularly the presence of impurities which may be toxic); the evidence of bioequivalence to the originator's product; and the evidence that it is the same type of pharmaceutical dose-form, given at the same dose, route of administration, etc.

In relation to Article 4(8)(a)(ii) of 65/65/EEC, the Experts will need to review all the published evidence on the pharmacology, toxicology, and clinical trials.

The requirements for abridged applications was discussed in more detail in Chapter 6. It should be noted that the CPMP has decided that it is not acceptable to merely refer to the fact that another authority has reviewed this information and has accepted it. Thus, citing the FDA Summary Basis of Approval document on the originator's product, does not meet the requirements of Article 4(8)(a)(ii) of Directive 65/65/EEC.

11.5 THE EXPERTS: WHO SHOULD THEY BE?

Although the wording of Articles 1 to 3 of 75/319/EEC defining the three Experts, and of the subsequent detailed interpretation in the 'Notice to Applicants' is very clear, there have been many enquiries from the pharmaceutical industry on the requirements for the Experts to see how their work can be integrated into the structure and procedures of the particular company concerned. The following section is an attempt to further define the type of person who might be used.

11.5.1 Single versus multiple Experts

One question often asked is whether there can be more than one Experts for a single Report. In fact some of the very early Expert Reports were signed by several Experts, each signing a section. It was quite common to find that the pharmaceutical Expert Report was signed by an organic chemist, an analyst, the research and development manager, a process validation chemist, etc. This use of a number of Experts to sign the Expert Report is no longer regarded as acceptable. Only one Expert should now sign the Report, although a number may have contributed to its preparation.

The practicalities of preparing an Expert Report in a large multinational company are that the summarised data on the formats are often drafted by the regulatory affairs department. The written 'bridging' summary (particularly used for a NAS clinical report) will either be written by the regulatory affairs staff or the

Expert. However, although the critical overview section of the Expert Report may be drafted by a number of hands, it is the Expert signatory himself alone who takes final responsibility — and if he is not satisfied with any of the individual elements suggested by his colleagues it is up to him to ask for further information or even require more work to be done to supplement the information in the (unsatisfactory or incomplete) dossier.

This use of a single Expert avoids the kind of difficulties which arise when there are divided responsibilities and no one person is responsible for the whole task. Thus, an organic chemist might ignore the fact that the active substance is very sparingly water soluble and lipophilic and will be used without further processing in a solid oral dose-form. If the particle size distribution/surface area of the batches of active substance used in the animal toxicology studies, the clinical trials, and the production batches are not defined, then the relevance of these studies to the proposed use in man may be unclear. They may not provide the supporting data on safety and efficacy which the applicant hopes they do.

The use of a single Expert is formalised in the 1989 edition of the 'Notice to Applicants' where it states that 'only one expert may assume responsibility for the report'.

11.5.2 The consultant Expert

If a company does not have the expertise itself, it may employ an outside Expert to give the necessary review of the data and to write the Expert Report. Where this happens, however, the Expert needs to have been brought in at sufficiently early a stage for him to be able to influence the content of the report — and where necessary to ask for further work to be done to complement that already available. It is preferable, if a consultant is used, for him to be used in the design of the studies generating the data, so that he can ensure that problems and deficiencies are identified at an early stage.

The independent consultant has an important role to play in some of the smaller companies, or even in larger companies where he can step back from the day to day pressures and provide a more objective analysis of the evidence. However, the reputation of the consultant will depend on how objectively he can perform the vital task of making a critical analysis and review of the data. It is his first task to carry out the review and to see whether the data even justify the submission of an application. If they do, then he can apply his expertise to the task.

11.5.3 The 'foreign' Expert versus national Expert

The Expert does not have to be based in the UK or indeed any of the EC Member States. For a foreign company with its research headquarters outside the EC, a foreign Expert will obviously be more readily available. However, it may be necessary for the Expert to take part in discussions with the authorities in the countries in which the application is to be made, and to be concerned with national or CPMP hearings/appeals etc. For these reasons the accessibility of the Expert and his language abilities may also need to be considered.

An Expert already used in one EC Member State for a marketing authorisation application will normally be acceptable in another EC Member State. In the EC there is no need to have an Italian Expert for an Italian application, a French Expert for a French application, or a British Expert for a British application. Even where a national application is made simultaneously in several different EC countries, one application and one single set of Experts can and should be used. This enables European companies to centralise and rationalise their regulatory affairs departments and to make considerable cost savings in the preparation of applications.

This position is formalised in the 1989 edition of the 'Notice to Applicants', where it states that 'authors of reports should be chosen on the basis of their qualifications and experience; their nationality is not relevant'.

11.6 THE FLOW OF INFORMATION — RAW DATA IN THE LABORATORY TO THE EXPERT REPORT AND THE PRODUCT PROFILE

The flow of information for the compilation of Expert Reports can be shown as follows:

- Raw data
- →Study reports
- →Documentation
- →Summary tabulations (using the Expert Report formats)
- →Expert Report.

It must be emphasised that in writing his critical Expert Report, the Expert must have access to at least all of the study reports and documentation. In cases of difficulty he may need to refer back to the raw data.

The Product Profile need not be compiled by any of the Experts. It is often written by the regulatory affairs staff. However, the information given in it must be wholly consistent with the Expert Report. It would be sensible for the three Experts to have seen and agreed the text. The Product Profile consists of a one to two page summary, and includes the following:

(a) Type of application (NAS, new combination, new indications).
(b) Chemical and pharmacokinetic properties (chemical structure of the active, physicochemical properties of the active, and characteristics of the dosage-form which could affect the pharmacokinetic properties and clinical efficacy).
(c) Indications (therapeutic indications, pharmacological and therapeutic classification of the active defining the mode of action).
(d) Precautions (precautions and warnings from the principal results of the preclinical studies.
(e) Marketing/post-marketing (a list of any PMS studies, a list of marketing authorisations issued in other countries).

11.7 LINKS BETWEEN THE THREE EXPERTS

The marketing authorisation application will ultimately be considered as a whole, so that issues raised in one section must be integrated in their answer in that section and others where that issue has relevance. Thus the Experts must not carry out their tasks in a compartmentalised way — and each must consider what is the relevance of particular aspects of their section to the reports of the other two Experts. Some particular issues where the links between Expert Reports may need to be emphasised are documented below.

If the active ingredient has been shown (in the pharmaceutical Expert Report) to be sparingly soluble and lipophilic, has the particle size of the batches of active used in the oral route animal toxicology studies and the clinical trials been controlled? If so, what is the bioavailability of the active in the animal species tested compared to man? If the proportion absorbed in the animals was much lower than in man, does this affect the calculation of the safety margin before target organ toxicity etc. will be seen?

Has the impurity profile of the active been fully defined? The pharmacotoxicological Expert Report will need to consider what is known of the toxicity of the impurities and justify the proposed limits. The pharmaceutical Expert Report will include a complementary discussion of the proposed impurity specification for the drug and the product.

Is the active a NAS where the route of synthesis has changed during the development of the product? If so, what is the relevance of the key animal toxicology studies? What is the relevance of any changes in impurity profile to the toxicology?

Is the active stable in the finished formulation? If not, what is known about the toxicity of the degradation products — do they need to be limited in the finished product? If toxic (for example the nephrotoxic epi-anhydrotetracycline in tetracycline capsules; the 4-methyl thiotetrazole from cefamandol or moxalactam which causes hypoprothrombinaemia; the 21-dehydro derivatives of some corticosteroids which may be immunogenic; rifampicin–quinone which may be immunogenic) both the pharmacotoxicological Expert and the clinical Expert may need to contribute to the justification for the proposed limits in the pharmaceutical Expert Report.

Has the formulation changed during the development of the product? If so, have the bioavailability of the various formulations been compared and linked so that the data in the clinical trials can be pooled either to analyse efficacy or safety in man?

Is the formulation a special one (e.g. a sustained release tablet)? If so, what formulations were used in the toxicology studies — and what relevance do they have to the product which it is proposed to market?

Was the target organ toxicity seen in the animal studies investigated in the clinical trials? How do the results of the animal toxicology studies link with the results in the clinical trials?

How are the results of some of the pivotal animal toxicology studies reflected in the summary of product characteristics, data sheet, patient leaflet, etc?

11.8 THE DUTIES OF THE EXPERTS

The main duties of the Experts are discussed in the following sections.

11.8.1 To provide the Expert Report

This provides a concise, objective, and critical appraisal of the data on quality, safety, and efficacy; and a justification of the methods and limits in the Part II dossier and the proposed text of the summary of product characteristics.

11.8.2 To provide a justification for the acceptance of a product in List B ('high technology' procedure of Directive 87/22/EEC)

To gain acceptance into the high technology procedure, companies have to apply to an EC country chosen by them as the rapporteur Member State, making their arguments for the product to be admitted as a List B product. Since 87/22/EEC was brought into force in the Member States on 1 July 1987, only a small number of products have been admitted into the procedure (one in 1988/89 and three more in 1990).

If a company applies to use the List B procedure, they have to provide a case to convince the rapporteur Member State. In cases of dispute or uncertainty, the CPMP itself can be consulted by the proposed rapporteur country. As we shall see in Chapter 15, there may not be much gain for most products in using the procedure, since the concertation timetable is often prolonged, and the gain in the 'second applicant protection' from six to ten years is only in three countries — Luxembourg, Ireland, and Denmark. Since these are usually the three smallest markets in the EC, the gain may be marginal and outweighed if it is quicker to gain approvals nationally (or nationally in one or more Member States then using the multistate procedure) and the company is able to start selling in major markets earlier.

The procedure may perhaps be particularly suitable for some specialist or 'niche' products.

The arguments that seek to persuade the rapporteur will need to be included in the Expert Report (in the appropriate section). The five different sections which can be used to claim 'high technology' status are set out below, together with the section of the Report where it would normally be expected that the justification would be included:

'Other biotechnological processes... which constitute a significant innovation': pharmaceutical Expert Report.

'Products administered by means of a new delivery system... which constitutes a significant innovation': pharmaceutical Expert Report.

'Products containing a new substance or an entirely new indication... of significant therapeutic interest': clinical Expert Report.

'New products based on radio-isotopes... of significant therapeutic interest': clinical Expert Report.

'Products employing processes which... demonstrate a significant technical advance': pharmaceutical Expert Report.

The justification needs to include a careful analysis of the innovative features or the significance of the therapeutic interest to convince the rapporteur Member State. Not surprisingly, companies applying for List B status have usually had a number of meetings with officials from the rapporteur Member State to informally seek their advice before launching their valuable new product onto the relatively uncharted seas of the procedure. The justification can sometimes include several sections of List B — claims based on the use of a new delivery system and a new indication, for example. The justification needs to include a careful analysis of other products already on the market in the rapporteur Member State and other EC countries — is it really an entirely new indication in all countries?

The CPMP has indicated that it will set a high standard for what it accepts as 'significant innovation' or 'significant therapeutic interest'. In relation to a NAS, CPMP has indicated that it will normally accept the first member of a new pharmacotherapeutic class, but not normally the subsequent members unless they demonstrate some overwhelming clinical advantage to the earlier active ingredient.

11.8.3 To be available for consultation with the authorities
It is convenient if the Expert is available to explain points in his Report which are not clear to the assessors (internal or external) in the Member State concerned.

11.8.4 To participate in appeals
It is again often convenient for an Expert to be available to explain or justify the conclusions of his Expert Report in any appeal (at a hearing or as a written representation). Where the issues in the appeal are, however, related to some complex detail in a specialised part of the application, it may be more appropriate to use another 'Expert' in the appeal process.

11.9 THE PHARMACEUTICAL EXPERT REPORT: STRUCTURE, FORMAT, AND CONTENT

As previously stated, the Expert Report provides a concise, comprehensive synopsis and critical overview of all of the data on quality of the active ingredient and dosage form. It is meant to enable the reader (the assessor in the national authority of a Member State or the CPMP, the expert on the national committee) to obtain a good understanding of all aspects both quickly and easily.

11.9.1 Structure of the pharmaceutical Expert Report
The Expert Report consists of three parts.

The first is as an Appendix to the Expert Report itself, the summary of the information in the dossier, preferably using the formats in the 'Notice to Applicants' second edition (1989).

The second is as a further Appendix to the Expert Report itself, a written summary (optional and often omitted for conventional pharmaceutical products — but which may be useful where there are very extensive data in Part II such as a biotechnology product).

The third, and the most important, is the critical analysis, commentary, and justification for the proposed manufacturing methods, analytical test procedures, specification limits, etc.

The 'Notice to Applicants' includes a guideline as to the length of the evaluation section (ten pages). It should be noted that this is a guide — if the product is a complex one (e.g. a biotechnology product, a new active substance in a novel dose form), this can be exceeded. The main objective is to provide the requisite critical analysis — the Report should not be typed in microscopic script to fit in with the supposed ten page 'limit'!

The sample formats provided in the 'Notice to Applicants' are to be amended as necessary for each individual product. They are designed to be usable for the vast majority of conventional products, but they can be stretched out where the space in a section is insufficient, reduced in length where there is little relevant information to be included, or some pages may even be omitted completely. Where a special product (such as a radiopharmaceutical) is involved, the applicant can even invent his own formats to cover some of the special requirements and results. The standard formats include elements for herbal and biotechnology products, but these are likely to be amended in the third edition of the 'Notice to Applicants' — probably due for publication in 1992.

Where an applicant inserts a special format of his own, the standard heading used on each format should be included. This has been included at the specific request of the Bundesgesundheitsamt (Federal German Health Office) to enable the information on the formats to be fed into their computer.

There is no specification for length or format for the optional written summary. This is meant to provide a factual summary to complement the information on the formats. It is meant to provide a 'bridge' between the voluminous data in the dossier and the highly summarised information in the formats.

11.9.2 Contents of the pharmaceutical Expert Report
The Report should consider all of the main sections of the dossier. These are:

Part IIA: Composition of the product, container, and clinical trial formulae.
Part IIA: Development pharmaceutics.
Part IIB: Method of preparation of the dosage form.
Part IIB: Process validation.
Part IIC: Control of starting materials
- Active ingredient(s)
- Other ingredients (i.e. excipients)
- Packaging material (Immediate packaging).

Part IID: Control tests on intermediate products.
Part IIE: Control tests on the finished product.
Part IIE: Analytical validation.
Part IIF: Stability
- Active ingredient(s)
- Finished product.

Part IIQ: Additional data (e.g. summary of the bioavailability/bioequivalence data, metabolism, analytical validation of the methods for drugs and metabolites, synthesis and quality control of radiolabelled drugs used in metabolic studies).

Evaluation (conclusions).
Reference list.
Information on the pharmaceutical Expert (one page or less on the education, training, and current position(s) held by the Expert).

In the UK, if exceptionally a non-pharmacist is used as an Expert to compile and sign the Expert Report, a short additional justification should be provided. The justification would need to cover the education, training, and experience of the

Expert to write an Expert Report for the particular product concerned. This justification should be in specific terms for the product, i.e. there should not be a general justification.

11.9.3 Evaluation section of the pharmaceutical Expert Report

This section is really the kernel of the Report. The 'Notice to Applicants' gives detailed guidance on many of the aspects to be considered in the Expert Report. Also the individual guidelines on quality (e.g. that on stability) in Volume III of the *Rules governing medicinal products in the European Community* also often refer to the elements to be covered in Expert Reports.

Some of the early Expert Reports received by the authorities in 1985 and 1986 were remarkably devoid of critical comment, and often merely stated that the Expert was wholly convinced that the product was of appropriate quality and that the proposed control tests and limits were appropriate to ensure that routinely manufactured batches continued to meet this requirement. This kind of eulogy was of little use to the authorities in their assessment, and it is now emphasised that the appraisal of the dossier needs to be critical.

Cartwright & Jefferys (1987) have reviewed some of the basic elements necessary to compile an Expert Report. Goldsmith (1989) has also reviewed the general requirements for the pharmaceutical Expert and the Expert Report. Some of the detailed aspects of the pharmaceutical Expert Report have been considered by:

> Pourcelot-Roubeau (1989) — the galenical pharmacy (development pharmaceutics)
> Fournier (1989) — the active ingredient
> Bentejac (1989) — the galenical pharmacy aspects
> Bon (1989) — the analytical aspects
> Pellerin (1989) — the analytical aspects
> Veillard (1989) — stability (pharmaceutical aspects)
> Henry (1989) — chemical stability of raw materials
> Gauchon (1989) — packaging.

Some of the elements with which the pharmaceutical Expert needs to deal in the evaluation section are detailed below:

(a) Composition
Discussion of differences between the clinical trial formulae and the proposed marketing formula with a justification by reference to the work in the dossier which shows the relationships between the bioavailability of the formulations.

(b) Development pharmaceutics
Discussion of the choice of the dosage form in relation to the clinical use of the product. An explanation of the choice of the particular formulation needs to be given — the choice and concentration of additives (e.g. preservatives) need to have been shown to be optimal. Where it is not possible to use optimal levels of additives (such as less than optimal level of parahydroxybenzoate preservative mixture in an alkaline

antacid product because the bitter taste at higher levels affects patient acceptance of the product), this needs to be justified, and any other actions taken to counteract this explained (e.g. use of small packs for the alkaline antacid with a short 'use by' period after the pack is first opened). Where particular problems were encountered during the development of the formulation (such as capping of tablets during manufacture on high-speed rotary tablet presses) the steps taken to overcome these problems during future routine production needs to be stated (such as specific control of tablet hardness as part of the in-process quality control, and friability testing as part of the routine control tests on the finished product).

(c) Method of manufacture
Discussion should include information as to how the defined method will consistently yield batches of product that are acceptable and meet the specification.

(d) Process validation
Discussion as to how the proposed data show that the method of manufacture will consistently yield a product of the desired quality. Although data are only required to be provided in the dossier for critical products (such as modified release products, terminally sterilised products, low dose oral solid dose forms), it would normally be expected that the data would be available (on request) for a much wider range of products.

One particular issue which would need to be explored is where the application cites another site of manufacture to that where all the development and process development work was carried out, or where the application includes a number of alternative sites of manufacture for the product. In such a case, the applicant needs to provide reassurance that the product can be made and will meet the required standards. If the applicant has merely bought a dossier from another party data will be required in the application to show that with his equipment, the product can be satisfactorily made. Some applications which cite a number of alternative manufacturers, completely lack credibility in this respect.

(e) Control of active ingredient
Discussion as to the impurities, solid state properties, specification limits for the active ingredient. For impurities there needs to be a cross-reference to the pharmacotoxicological Expert Report for a justification of the proposed impurity limits (particularly for toxic impurities) in relation to the intended use of the finished product.

For an NAS, the impurity specification limits need to be justified by a detailed comparison of the batch analyses of material used in the pivotal toxicology studies and the clinical trials, together with an analysis of the possible effects of any impurity which is known to be toxic.

For an NAS which is chemically similar to known active(s) already the subject of a pharmacopoeial monographs, it would be useful to compare the specification with these official monographs to establish that it is in general conformity with that overall standard.

For pharmacopoeial active ingredients, it needs to be borne in mind that the purpose of such a monograph is to set a standard for any likely use of the active — for injections, suspensions, tablets, capsules, etc. For some specific uses (e.g. use in a solid oral dose form), the particle size distribution or surface area may need to be controlled and the subject of a formal specification. Thus there will need to be an additional test to those in the *European Pharmacopoeia* (Ph. Eur.) or national pharmacopoeial monograph. For pharmacopoeial actives which are made by a method of manufacture liable to leave impurities not mentioned (that is specifically limited by name) in the pharmacopoeial monograph, additional tests to limit such impurities would have to be considered — particularly if they are known to be toxic (immunogenic, mutagenic, carcinogenic, enhancing the toxicity of the active ingredient itself, etc.).

(f) Packaging material
A discussion of the packaging development trials, and justification for the stability of the pack will be required.

(g) Control tests on the finished product
The tests and limits in the finished product (release) specification should be justified by reference to:
- the results of the analytical validation studies,
- the batch analyses, and
- the results of the process validation studies.

The tests included in the specification and to be carried out routinely (that is every batch or at a specified frequency of testing) should be stated in the application. If some tests are carried out during development of the product, and this demonstrates that there is no need to carry them out thereafter on a routine basis (e.g. dissolution tests on a solid dose form containing a soluble active ingredient), this aspect needs to be brought out in the Report. The relationship of in-process tests or parametric tests to the finished product specification needs to be brought out as part of the justification for the routine finished product testing protocol.

For products manufactured outside the EC, the applicant (at least for the time being) has to include additional tests to identify all excipients in the product, and these will need to be carried out by the European marketing authorisation holder on importation into the EC.

(h) Stability
The Expert Report needs to include a detailed discussion of the stability data on the active ingredient and finished product to justify the claimed shelf life and the package storage precautions. As Cartwright (1989) has pointed out, the analysis of product stability data needs to include, wherever possible, a statistical analysis, and the shelf life then needs to be based on the stability of the least stable batch (if the batch data cannot be combined). There needs to be an attempt to consider the degradation data and the active ingredient assay data together (to attempt a material balance) to

ensure the stability specificity of the assay and to ensure that the known degradation products are sufficient to explain all of the loss of active ingredient that actually occurs. If any of the degradation products are known or suspected to be toxic, the proposed levels in the check (shelf life) specification need to be justified by cross-reference to the pharmacotoxicological and clinical Expert Reports.

11.10 THE PHARMACOTOXICOLOGICAL EXPERT REPORT: STRUCTURE, FORMAT, AND CONTENT

11.10.1 Structure of the pharmacotoxicological Expert Report

The same remarks as to the structure of the Expert Report apply as in the case of the pharmaceutical Expert Report. It can be considered as being divided into the following sections:

- the summary (using the formats supplied if possible),
- the written summary (optional),
- the Expert Report.

In the case of the pharmacotoxicological Expert Report, the recommendation for the length of the Report itself is 25 pages.

The introduction of the suggested formats for reporting the data in the 1989 (second) edition of the 'Notice to Applicants' caused considerable controversy. It was agreed that they would be included in the text as the recommended version, but that a review of the formats would be carried out before the compilation of the third (1992) edition of the 'Notice to Applicants'. The current formats are used by the Bundesgesundheitsamt for incorporation into their computer database.

The formats should also be used to summarise data from the literature where a case is being made under Article 4(8)(a)(ii) of Directive 65/65/EEC — for an abridged marketing authorisation application.

11.10.2 Contents of the pharmacotoxicological Expert Report

The contents of the Expert Report relate to the following sections of the dossier — pharmacodynamics, pharmacokinetics, toxicity, conclusions, reference list, and information on the preclinical Expert.

As with the pharmaceutical Expert Report it is the conclusions which really comprise the most important part of the Expert Report.

The information on the Expert should comprise a maximum of one page dealing with his education, training, and current work.

11.10.3 Conclusions of the pharmacotoxicological Expert Report

The Expert needs to particularly address the following issues — the effects of the active ingredient observed in the studies in relation to those expected or observed in man; the consequences of the use of the medicinal product before and during pregnancy and during lactation; mutagenic effects; the tumorigenic risk to man (if epidemiological data are available they should be taken into account); and possible irreversible toxic effects.

In general, the results of the studies need to be interpreted and to predict how well the particular results can be extrapolated to man — is the particular animal a good model for man (for example is the bioavailability and metabolism in the animal species similar to that in man)?

The Expert will need to comment and justify the wording of the statements in the summary of product characteristics which relate to the animal toxicology data (e.g. the pregnancy and lactation data, drug interactions, etc).

11.11 THE CLINICAL EXPERT REPORT: STRUCTURE, FORMAT, AND CONTENT

11.11.1 Structure of the clinical Expert Report

Again, the structure of the clinical Expert Report is similar to the pharmaceutical and pharmacotoxicological Expert Reports, and includes the study report formats on the clinical trials (ranked in order of placebo controlled studies, controlled studies with reference therapies, and uncontrolled studies); the written summary (optional but usually included in any clinically complex marketing authorisation application); and the Expert Report itself.

As with the other two sections (pharmaceutical and pharmacotoxicological), there is no limit to the length for the written ('bridging') summary. The guideline for the length of the Expert Report (the conclusions section) is 25 pages — although it is emphasised that this is a guideline, and that individual applications sometimes exceed this.

11.11.2 Contents of the clinical Expert Report

The format as laid down in the 'Notice to Applicants' includes:
- the problem statement (a summary of the different treatments which could be used for the particular condition for which the new product will be indicated, with an analysis as to how the new treatment fits into this spectrum of treatments. The problem statement needs to include a statement of the therapeutic indications for the product and the required dosage).
- clinical pharmacology
  — pharmacodynamics,
  — pharmacokinetics,
  — *in vivo* performance of the pharmaceutical forms (i.e. the bioavailability/ bioequivalence of the dosage form).
- Clinical trials
  — overall tabular presentation of all of the studies,
    — controlled trials (placebo controlled and those against reference therapy),
    — non-controlled trials.
  — assessment of individual studies,
    — the protocols
    — data concerning the patients, therapeutic efficacy, safety, and quality of the trial.
  — global analysis of efficacy

— global analysis of safety.
- Post-marketing experience.
- Other information
- Conclusions
- Reference list
- Information on the clinical Expert (one page or less).

11.11.3 Conclusions of the clinical Expert Report

As indicated in the 'Notice to Applicants', the main aspects to be covered in the conclusions include the therapeutic justification for the product; the safety (taking into account the preclinical data); the dosage regimen proposed for each treatment group; the risk/benefit ratio judged against existing clinical practice and the different treatments which are available.

The safety data need to include the adverse reactions, contraindications, interactions, warnings, and precautions for use. As Cartwright & Jefferys (1987) point out, the clinical Experts have often raised questions over drug interactions for which there were answers in the animal pharmacology data, and issues raised in the animal pharmacology have often not been addressed by the clinical Expert.

In relation to the clinical studies to establish efficacy Cartwright & Jefferys (1987) point out that the Expert Report needs to concentrate on the pivotal placebo controlled studies and not to give equal emphasis to open studies of efficacy.

The CPMP guideline on good clinical practice for trials on medicinal products in the EC was adopted on 3 May 1990 (III/3976/88 Draft No. 6) and circulated to the pharmaceutical industry. The text of this guideline was included in an Addendum to Volume III of *The rules governing medicinal products in the European Community* published in 1991. Future dossiers and Expert Reports will need to comment on the conformity of the trials with good clinical practices (GCP).

11.12 MISCELLANEOUS ISSUES IN RELATION TO EXPERT REPORTS

Some issues on which problems have arisen with Expert Reports are discussed in the following section.

11.12.1 Products outside the Directives

The legal requirement to supply Expert Reports (since it derives from Articles 1 to 3 of 75/319/EEC) applies fully only to products covered by the pharmaceutical Directives. Thus, until 1 January 1992 vaccines, serums, toxins, radiopharmaceuticals, and blood products fall outside the Directives (except for those brought in as List A or List B biotechnology/high technology products under Directive 87/22/EEC). Homoeopathic products (currently the subject of a Commission proposal for a draft Directive) are also outside the Directives since they fall in the list of exemptions in Article 34 of 75/319/EEC. Some other products in the grey area (the borderline between medicines and non-medicines, or medicines and devices, or medicines and cosmetics, or medicines and dietary aid products) may be deemed medicines in some Member States of the EC and not in others. For all of these products the applicant is still advised to include an Expert Report with the documents and particulars.

11.12.2 Clinical trial approval applications

Some EC Member States formally control clinical trials and request formal submission of data; others do not.

In the UK, most applications for approval by companies to carry out clinical trials on unlicensed medicinal products come in under the clinical trial exemption scheme. This is a negative vetting scheme (as compared to assessment of product licence applications which is a positive assessment process) and the format is a summarised one, so no Expert Report is needed in addition. Where a company applies for a clinical trial certificate (CTC) with full data, which needs positive assessment, they are encouraged to include an Expert Report.

11.12.3 Cross-referral marketing authorisation applications

In the UK and some other EC Member States, it is possible to obtain an authorisation by cross-referring to another granted licence. These applications are either transfers of authorisation from one company to another (where one company has bought the other product or company) or applications to co-market products.

In the UK, if the cross-referral application is to a recently granted licence (in the previous five years), then the Experts need only to sign a simple statement that the products are the same composition, pack, method of manufacture, and specifications for starting materials and finished product; are for the same indications; and have the same contra-indications etc. However, they need to ensure that this statement is correct — often a number of proposed changes are made to the product without these being made in any way clear. This delays processing and issue of the authorisation.

For older granted licences in the UK, a new Expert Report will be needed before the cross-referral can be processed. It needs to be borne in mind that one of the objectives of the Expert Report system is to ensure that there is always a summary of the dossier on the file.

REFERENCES

Bentejac, R. (1989). Comment le rôle du nouvel expert pharmaceutique est-il vu par un expert spécialiste de la pharmacie galénique? *S.T.P. Pharma* **5** (4), 290–293.

Bon, R. (1989). Comment le rôle du nouvel expert est-il vu par un expert analyste? *S.T.P. Pharma* **5** (4), 285–289.

Cartwright, A. C. (1989). Stability tests on active substances and finished products: new European guideline. *Drug Development Ind. Pharm.* **15** (10), 1743–1757.

Cartwright, A. C. & Jefferys, D. B. (1987). Expert Reports for product licence applications in Europe — a regulatory review. *Pharmaceutical Med.* **2**, 229–237.

Fournier, J-P. (1989). Comment le rôle du nouvel expert est-il vu par un expert spécialiste de la chimie thérapeutique? *S.T.P. Pharma* **5** (4), 281– 284.

Gauchon, M. (1989). Rôle de l'expert dans le cas d'un changement de conditionnement pharmaceutique. *S.T.P. Pharma* **5** (4), 309–313.

Goldsmith, J. (1989). Y a-t-il uniformité de vue au niveau européen sur le rôle de l'expert pharmaceutique? *S.T.P. Pharma* **5** (4), 297–299.

Henry, J. (1989). Rôle du nouvel expert dans les études de stabilité chimique. *S.T.P. Pharma* **5** (4), 303–304.

Pellerin, F. (1989). Le rôle du nouvel expert pharmaceutique par rapport à l'expert analyste. *S.T.P. Pharma* **5** (4), 276–280.

Pourcelot-Roubeau, Y. (1989). Comment le rôle du nouvel expert est-il vu par un rapporteur galéniste? *S.T.P. Pharma* **5** (4), 294–296.

Veillard, M. (1989). Rôle de l'expert dans les études de stabilité pharmacotecnique. *S.T.P. Pharma* **5** (4), 305–308.

12

Defects in applications — an analysis

12.1 INTRODUCTION

In this chapter consideration is given to deficiencies encountered in applications for product licences (marketing authorisations) submitted to the United Kingdom (UK) Medicines Control Agency (MCA) and its predecessor (the Medicines Division of the Department of Health). In addition some discussion is included on quality-related deficiencies in applications referred to the Committee on Proprietary Medicinal Products (CPMP) under various EC procedures for considering applications for marketing authorisations.

It is indicated in Chapter 17 that in the UK it is usual practice for all novel products, especially those containing new active ingredients, to be referred to the advisory committees (the Committee on Safety of Medicines (CSM), and the Committee on Dental and Surgical Materials CDSM). In addition, it is necessary for applications about which the MCA or the Licensing Authority has doubts to be referred to the advisory committees if it is wished to grant the product licence other than in the terms included in the application or if it is wished to reject the application. The reference to the committees gives the applicants the right of appeal.

To put into perspective the information on deficiencies in applications, it may be useful to give some idea of the scale of the licensing activities undertaken by the MCA. The numbers of applications received for product licences in 1987, 1988, and 1989 were 1169, 838, and 1376, respectively. These include 77 national new active substance applications and a further 17 applications submitted through the European Community (EC) CPMP procedures in 1987; 62 and 22 in 1988; and 121 and 2 in 1989. The numbers of national and CPMP abridged applications submitted were 984 and 10 (1987), 709 and 14 (1988), and 906 and 20 (1989).

Submission of an application does not mean its acceptance automatically as valid in terms of an application containing all the necessary information for an assessment to be undertaken, of course. In 1988, 277 applications required additional data before they could be accepted for processing, and 93 applications were rejected at

Sec. 12.1] Introduction 191

this preassessment stage. In 1989 the figures were 308 applications requiring additional data and 331 rejected applications.

The numbers of other types of application received which relate to product licensing functions of the MCA in 1987 to 1989 are included in Table 12.1.

Table 12.1 — Numbers of applications etc. submitted to the Medicines Control Agency in the UK

Type of application	1987†,‡	1988	1989
Product licences			
New actives	94	84	123
Abridged	994	723	926
Clinical trial certificates (CTCs)	12	4	1
Clinical trial exemptions (CTXs)	213	257	261
Changes to approvals			
PLs, CTCs, PL(PI)s§	10 569	7 980	7 527
CTXs¶	2 154	2 026	2 320

† Numbers relate to calendar years.
‡ Numbers relate to the numbers of individual dosage forms and strengths of dosage forms. An NAS application may consist of a number of different product licence references, each covering a single strength of a single dosage form, for example.
§ Parallel import product licences.
¶ Includes reports of adverse events and reactions.
Source: MCA data.

The numbers of product licences granted in a similar period is given in Table 12.2.

Table 12.2 — Numbers of product licences granted from 1987 to March 1990

Type of application	Number of licences granted†		
	1.87 to 12.87	1.88 to 12.88	4.89 to 3.90
Product licences for products containing new active ingredients	41	47	79
(Number of substances)	(18)‡	(27)	(40)
Abridged applications referred to committees	60	52	56
Other abridged applications	564	487	528

† The numbers relate to product licences granted in the period. These do not necessarily relate to applications submitted in the same period.
‡ The numbers in parentheses relate to the numbers of new active substances approved in the respective period.
Source: Medicines Act Information Letter (MAIL).

One area of deficiency which applies in many applications is the inadequacy of cross-references to relevant information in any of the three parts of the dossier or the Expert Reports. It is pointed out that such cross-referencing is considered to be particularly useful by assessors and members of advisory bodies.

The chapter consists of four parts. In the first, the nature of the defects found in the clinical dossier of applications seen by the CSM is discussed (DBJ). In the second, the problems found with the pharmaceutical parts of the submission are discussed for products considered by the CSM and the CPMP (BRM). The third part reviews the points still outstanding after consideration of additional data by the CSM and the CPMP. The fourth part considers deficiencies in the preclinical section of applications (JCR).

12.2 THE CLINICAL DOSSIER

12.2.1 Introduction

The production of the clinical dossier is arguably both the most difficult and the most important part of the registration process.

When one considers that it may have cost up to £150 million to develop a new active substance and that the final licensing decision will depend on the demonstration of clinical efficacy and the reassurance of clinical safety, then one can see that the clinical dossier should be compiled with great care and attention to detail. Unfortunately, this is not always the case, and regulatory authorities are often faced with inadequate and poorly presented dossiers. It is frustrating for drug regulators to see good science spoilt by a poor dossier.

In this section of the chapter the defects in the clinical dossier will be considered, and the defects in applications will also be discussed in detail.

12.2.2 Structure of the dossier

As indicated in Chapters 3 to 6 the second edition of the CPMP 'Notice to Applicants' sets out the basic structure for the submission of an application throughout the EC. This document centres principally upon the requirements for the Expert Report (see Chapter 11), and the section addressing the clinical dossier is considerably briefer than that for the clinical Expert Report. It will be necessary in the third edition of the 'Notice to Applicants' for the section relating to the clinical dossier to be considerably expanded to offer more information and guidance to applicants. It has to be recognised, however, that there is a wide range of products which necessitate different sorts of dossiers. For example, a particular niche product may have a relatively small clinical database, whereas an anti-infective agent to be used as a broad spectrum antibiotic may have a large clinical database with patients largely drawn from open studies.

In a recent analysis of applications submitted in the UK between 1987 and 1989 it was noted that the number of patients included in efficacy studies range from 41 to 4906 patients, with a mean of 861, whilst in the safety database the range was from 43 to 15962 with a mean of 1171 patients.

The 'Notice to Applicants' sets out the elements which are required in the clinical dossier. The most important of these is the clinical Expert Report which will be considered later. The summary of product characteristics, whilst not in itself a part of the clinical dossier, is nevertheless a most important item which needs to be carefully considered in relation to the dossier and to the Expert Report.

At present a written 'bridging' overall clinical summary is regarded as an optional item. The MCA has always considered that the written summary is a very important and helpful document standing between the Expert Report and the individual summaries of the clinical studies, and it is one which is commonly found in successful clinical dossiers. In the autumn of 1989 the Association of the British Pharmaceutical Industry (ABPI) published a guidance booklet on the content of the clinical section of an application for marketing authorisation for a new active substance (ABPI, 1989). This document analyses the requirements for a marketing authorisation and should be closely read together with the 'Notice to Applicants'.

Above all, it has to be remembered that an assessor in a regulatory authority has to be able to read the dossier. Thus, it is very important that there should be a brief introduction explaining clearly where to find the relevant data and how the clinical section has been organised and presented. In this context it is important that a complete index should be provided which is relevant to the application as a whole and will enable an assessor to track data down to an individual report if that is considered necessary. It is also essential that there is clear and unambiguous volume and page numbering of the dossier. In the past, assessors have often had difficulty in finding their way through a dossier and locating particular references.

12.2.3 The clinical Expert Report

The clinical Expert Report is perhaps one of the most important items in the dossier. The requirement for an Expert Report is that the Expert should have undertaken a critical analysis of the data. Moreover, it is expected that the Expert will have been closely involved in the development of the drug and will have sought to ensure that any deficiencies have been resolved by further research before the application is submitted. If a premature application is submitted, then the Expert may not have done the job adequately.

It is not sufficient for the report to be written after the completion of the clinical research. Ideally, the Expert should be involved at the very early stages of research, but should at least be involved from one year before submission of the dossier. The Expert is not required to summarise the data, but it may be appropriate for a degree of summarising of relevant issues to be included in the report so that the document can be free-standing. In the past, this differentiation between a summary and the critical analysis which is actually required has caused considerable problems, and meant that in the first two years following the introduction of the Expert Reports they were extremely lengthy documents which were of no particular help to the regulatory authorities.

An Expert Report should not be a testimonial, but rather should address the potential problems with an application whilst advancing the arguments as to why the product should still be marketed.

It is a requirement that the clinical Expert Report addresses issues raised by the pharmaceutical and by the preclinical expert. For example, if target organ toxicity is seen in the preclinical studies, then the clinical Expert needs to consider this issue and to seek reassurance from the clinical safety database that the target organ toxicity seen in animals is not seen in man.

The Expert is also required to consider the summary of product characteristics and the proposed data sheet in the report. This consideration should reflect the critical analysis contained in the Report. Too often Experts ignore this duty, and items raised in the Expert Report are not reflected in the summary of product characteristics. Particular examples apply to drug interaction statements and precautions and warnings which are often inadequate in the data sheet when related to the clinical database for the product.

It is worth remembering that the Expert Report was introduced both to improve the quality of the application and also to be a help to the regulatory authorities. A good Expert Report focuses the attention of the assessor on the important issues concerned with a particular application, and either parts of it or the whole Report can be placed before an advisory committee. Expert Reports for new active substances were introduced in November 1985. During the first two years the Reports were of a low standard, and few, if any, could be presented to the CSM or CDSM. Since then the standard has improved, and most Reports can now be placed before the committees. This is important for the applicant, because it means that the company's views are directly placed before the committee in the form of a self-contained critical review.

In a limited study in the UK it has been shown that there may be a threefold difference in the assessment times comparing a bad with a good Expert Report. Over recent years both the Secretariat of the MCA and CSM in the UK have attempted to give feedback to companies to enable them to improve the standard of their Expert Reports.

Companies often ask how they may judge the Expert Report and the work of the Experts. One suggestion is that the Expert should produce a list of all the potential problems which can be foreseen in the assessment of the product. If a deficiency or Section 21(1) letter is received for the product (that is, a provisional refusal), this may be compared with the original deficiency list produced for the company. If the Expert has performed a good assessment, then the two lists should contain nearly identical items. If there are major differences, there can be a number of conclusions: for example, the Expert and his Report were inadequate or a perverse decision may have been made by the committee. If the latter is the case, then appeal mechanisms exist.

Clearly, there will be differences in interpretation of the data between a licensing authority and its advisory committees compared with the assessment made by the company and its Experts. Nevertheless, it would be expected that similar issues should be raised and considered by both groups.

The Expert Report is thus one of the most important items in a dossier. The 'Notice to Applicants' gives a guide to the content of the Expert Report. There is considerable freedom in how the report may be constructed, and this is appropriate, given the large number of products for which Expert Reports are required. Different formats suit different types of application.

12.2.4 Overall summary

The overall written summary is described as a bridging document between the Expert Report and individual clinical reports. The EC 'Notice to Applicants' currently states that the summary report is optional. However, as mentioned earlier, the view of the MCA is that this is a very important document, and it is hard to produce a good dossier without such a summary. A good overall summary allows the Expert to focus on important elements of the data in the knowledge that the exhaustive summary is contained in a separate document which is not constrained by the 25 pages of text which are the limit for the clinical Expert Report.

The summary should relate to all data which have been submitted by the applicant, and it is often of help if the data are suitably tabulated with clear cross-referencing so that an assessor can trace a particular item through to the original data. It should be remembered that an assessor will normally consider the summary of product characteristics, then read the Expert Report, and then consider the summary before proceeding through a detailed assessment of the individual summary clinical trial reports. It is very important that a complete safety analysis is included in the application.

For a new active substance the complete experience of exposure in man should be presented. Thus, data obtained from studies in different indications should be brought together so that the maximum safety data are made available to the regulatory authorities. It is also important that safety data from clinical volunteer studies, etc., are brought together in an overall analysis.

12.2.5 Clinical pharmacology

The clinical pharmacology of most drugs is usually well conducted and assessed. Particular problems arise with the establishment of the safe starting dose for the drug and the establishment of the true maintenance dose. Often inadequate dose titration studies are presented, and there are few attempts to undertake back-titration analyses to demonstrate that a true maintenance dose has been established. From recent experience we are aware that inappropriate starting doses have been defined for α-blockers, for ACE inhibitors, and for the oral contraceptive. Too often a dose has been chosen for the clinical studies with inadequate establishment, and then large-scale studies have been undertaken at this dose.

Another item in the clinical pharmacology which is frequently poorly considered is that of drug interaction studies. Often, little regard is paid to the preclinical data in the consideration of drug interaction potential. Studies, when undertaken, involve small numbers of patients or volunteers and are often of poor design. If a drug is likely to interfere with the metabolism of the oral contraceptive, then it will be necessary to undertake an appropriate study. Careful consideration should be given to the range of drugs which are likely to be given concomitantly to patients with the agent under study. Where studies are undertaken they should be of adequate power.

Increasingly attention needs to be paid to active metabolites and to stereo-isomerism.

If a particular adverse drug reaction pattern is seen, then further investigations may be necessary to see whether this is a dose-related phenomenon in certain individuals and whether it has a metabolic or indeed a primary pharmacological basis. It is equally the case that some adverse drug reactions are predictable from a careful consideration of the secondary pharmacology of the drug. It is interesting that in some summaries of product characteristics considerable attention is paid to speculative suggestions concerning the primary pharmacology of the drug, with no regard being paid to the more definite secondary pharmacology which may be of relevance to potential toxicity. A more detailed consideration of individual issues is given below.

12.2.6 Reports of individual clinical trials

The summary should be followed by clinical research reports. These should be free-standing, and it is hoped that they are each prefaced by a one to two page summary in a tabular format. The ABPI document on tailoring the clinical dossier (ABPI, 1989) makes clear that it is helpful to structure reports in a modular format so that appendices can be made available on request. Tabulated individual listings of data by patient should be included for all adverse events.

Over recent years, the clinical dossier has grown dramatically in size. Dossiers have grown too voluminous and contain unimportant and repetitive data. In 1988 the average number of volumes supporting a new active substance application submitted in the UK was 170 volumes. This led to extensive discussions with the pharmaceutical industry, and a significant reduction in the size of the dossiers was recorded during 1989. It is hoped that this trend will continue. It is clear that some of this data could be held by the company and made available on request by the national authorities. However, the dossier should make it clear that such data are available, and they should be listed in the documentation which is submitted for licensing.

It is important that the dossier is focused and that this approach also extends to the Expert Report. In the United States of America the great increase in data volume has been one of the factors which has led to the introduction of the computer assisted new drug application (CANDA). It is still not clear whether such electronic filings improve the assessment process or whether they save time and resource in the regulatory authority. A limited experiment has been conducted in the UK with an electronic submission. It is unclear whether the CAPLA (computer assisted product licence application) will achieve much prominence in the EC. Perhaps more appropriately the technology and facilities will be adopted and held by the applicant companies such that additional data can be requested by the use of electronic mail. This would allow companies to respond rapidly to requests for data from regulatory authorities, but would allow the control and manipulation of the database to remain with the company. Such an approach would have the advantage that it would reduce the amount of data which is submitted with the initial filing and might improve the standard of applications.

It should be noted that a different approach to the assessment of applications exists in Europe compared with the United States. The European application centres around the role of the Expert and the Expert Report with appropriate summarising of the data.

The initial rejection rate for a new active substance application remains worryingly high across the leading regulatory agencies. During the period 1987–1989 the

CSM in the UK considered 118 new active substances, and of these the committee was only able to advise the Licensing Authority to grant 40 per cent of the licences on first consideration of the data. Even when the committee advised the grant of a product licence there were frequently major conditions attached to the advice. These major conditions included restrictions to the licence indications, the satisfactory completion of additional studies, and important modifications to the data sheet. This figure of 60 per cent initial rejection corresponds well with an earlier analysis undertaken by Griffin and Diggle (1981) during the years 1977–1980.

In the most recent survey 56 of the applications over the three-year period were rejected on grounds including inadequate evidence of efficacy. In the majority of these cases there was inadequate evidence of overall efficacy of the product for the indications claimed. Frequently, the problems centred upon inadequate establishment of the proposed dosage. In a few instances there was uncertainty about the products' long-term efficacy or a failure to demonstrate efficacy throughout the dosage interval.

It is also of interest that fully innovative products were more likely to be successful than semi-innovative products (categorised by the Lund and Dukes classification), and that the successful applications had more patients evaluable for safety and efficacy than unsuccessful applications. The difference in the average number of patients evaluable for efficacy was 1126 compared to 785 evaluable for the unsuccessful applications. This difference was statistically significant at the $p=0.05$ level.

Poorly designed studies rank as one of the most common reasons for a failure to establish efficacy, along with inappropriate choice of outcome measures and inappropriate primary analyses. There was also a tendency for efficacy to be demonstrated in only some of the indications being sought.

There were also major deficiencies in applications concerning clinical safety. There are several recurring issues in the rejection of an application on safety grounds. These include an inadequately defined safe starting dose and an inadequate demonstration of long-term safety. An overall safety analysis was frequently missing and could have provided reassuring data. Trend analyses were also lacking from some safety assessments. Of particular concern is the failure to follow through target organ toxicity seen in the preclinical studies. This may suggest that some preclinical studies are being undertaken as a matter of routine, rather than to provide an alerting signal which should trigger further investigation in man. Thus, if cataracts are seen in animals, then prudence would dictate that careful follow-up should be undertaken in a cohort of patients to look for lens abnormalities during clinical exposure.

Similarly, the assessment of at-risk groups is often a source of difficulty. This is surprising since there are extensive guidelines making it clear that a drug should be fully investigated in representative groups of the final target population. Thus, if a drug is to be used in the elderly there is a requirement that studies are undertaken in elderly patients and that a careful investigation is made of the handling of the drug in renal failure.

Appropriate drug interaction studies need to be undertaken and the results related to statements in the summary of product characteristics. If adverse reactions are encountered, then these need to be investigated. Frequently a pharmacokinetic or metabolic cause can be found for the reaction, which may lead to the safer use of the drug.

On occasions the rejection of an application is because of an inappropriate risk-to-benefit ratio for the drug. It is clearly to be expected that there will be such differences in scientific opinion between an innovative company and an advisory committee which is concerned above all with protecting public health. Too often, however, inadequate dossiers are presented which are clearly premature and have insufficient data either to demonstrate convincing evidence of efficacy or to provide adequate reassurance as to the safety of the drug in long-term clinical usage.

A successful drug licensing application needs to combine carefully planned and executed clinical research with the production of a clear and well-ordered dossier. In some companies there seems to be the need for a better integration of the research and development function with the regulatory affairs and registration departments. It can be readily evident to the drug regulator when such close integration has occurred within a company, and this leads to the production of a high standard dossier which reflects well-conducted and well-designed clinical research.

12.3 THE PHARMACEUTICAL DOSSIER

12.3.1 Introduction

The requirements for the pharmaceutical parts of the dossier are described in Chapter 3 for new chemical active substances and Chapter 6 for abridged applications.

The Expert Report on the pharmaceutical aspects of the dossier should consist of three parts: a short product overview, a data summary (ideally using the recommended formats), and a critical assessment of the dossier. Due account is expected to have been taken of any relevant points included in the Expert Reports on the preclinical and clinical data. If a drug master file has been referred to or submitted as part of the supporting data the Expert Reports for both the marketing authorisation and the drug master file should have discussed common key areas, and the information included should be mutually compatible. The Expert is expected to take a defensible position on the dossier in the light of the current state of pharmaceutical science.

The information in the dossier should be presented in an easy to assimilate form — it is not helpful for large numbers of standard operating procedures or large numbers of pages of undigested computer printout from stability studies to be included when it is perfectly easy for the applicant's regulatory affairs staff to have prepared a good summary document, for example.

All parts of the dossier should be in English (or a full translation provided), and should be adequately (and intelligibly) paginated with an index. Any chromatographic traces or photographs should be capable of interpretation in all copies of the dossier.

These are all comments of a general nature. A large number of the applications submitted do not meet all of these expectations and hopes.

12.3.2 Analysis of deficiencies in UK applications

An analysis of the deficiencies in the pharmaceutical part of the dossier for applications submitted to the CSM was undertaken in early 1990. The applications considered were those submitted to the CSM between January 1987 and December 1989. 118 new active substance applications and 107 abridged applications were considered by the Committee during this period. The analysis reported below does not include products containing a biological, biotechnological, or immunological active ingredient — it relates only to chemical active ingredients.

12.3.2.1 Deficiencies relating to the drug substance

The major areas in which problems were found are listed in Table 12.3

Table 12.3 — Major areas of deficiency in drug substance data

Area of deficiency	Application type	
	New drug	Abridged
Evidence of structure	12	4
Synthetic route	103	31
Stereochemistry	22	1
Physical characteristics	1	1
Polymorphism	3	5
Synthesis of radiolabelled material	7	—
Impurity profile	10	24
Specifications	126	33
Compliance with pharmacopoeial requirements	10	9
Authorisation for access to drug master file omitted	2	—
British Approved Name needed for drug	6	—
Application grossly deficient	4	5

The deficiencies in the information on the synthetic route included inadequate details of the synthesis (for example scale of synthesis, reaction conditions and yields), poor discussion of synthetic intermediates and in-process controls, and inadequate information on the synthesis of the starting materials. The largest area of deficiencies, however, relates to the specifications for starting materials and intermediates. This is often accompanied by an inadequate discussion of the influence of impurities on the synthetic process and potential resulting impurities or related substances in the synthetic material (which should be included in the development chemistry part of the application). The distribution of the problem areas is illustrated in Fig. 12.1.

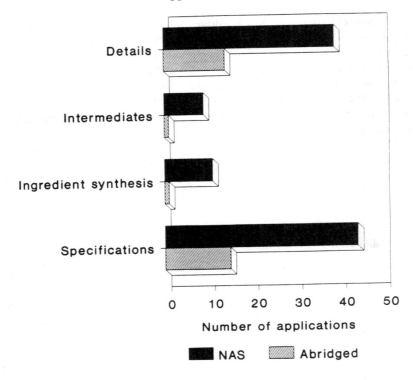

Fig. 12.1 — Deficiencies in synthetic route information submitted.

The evidence of structure should establish unequivocally that the material to be included in the product is what it is stated to be, and that the synthetic procedure is capable of ensuring that it is consistent from batch to batch. In some cases the stereoselectivities of key stages of the synthetic procedure need to be fully established, for example. Adequate batch analysis data should be submitted for the proposed synthetic route to help show that the synthetic product is consistent.

The stereochemistry of molecules is receiving increasing attention as evidence of *in vivo* metabolic, pharmacokinetic, drug interaction, or pharmacological differences between different isomers becomes more widely reported. This is an area which is commonly discussed between pharmaceutical and preclinical assessors. It should be borne in mind that the stereochemical purity of a drug in some biological studies may be affected by a number of factors, including species-dependent metabolism and the stability of the drug to light or in the medium used to administer the material in toxicity studies.

Impurity profiles are also gaining importance. These may be of particular significance in the case of abridged applications relating to products for which claims of essential similarity are made. Adequate evidence is expected of the nature and quantity of impurities present in several typical full-scale production batches of the material prepared by the requested synthetic route.

The drug substance specification is important and is the subject of frequent comment. What is wanted is a package of tests which will ensure adequate quality and safety and efficacy in the finished product. In many cases, inadequate thought has been given to the items to be included in the draft specification and a large number of objections to the company proposals are of a general nature — along the lines of 'inadequate specification'.

The largest single problem area is the control of impurities including related substances, reaction byproducts, and degradation products. The proposed controls should be realistic and not designed to allow any batch of material onto the market without regard to its qualitative and quantitative impurity profile and to any relevant toxicological safety considerations. Particular attention is paid to the impurity profiles of the batches used in the toxicity testing, and to those reported in the batch analyses for the production synthetic process. Excessively wide limits in the proposed specification are likely to result in objections from the advisory committees. It is increasingly expected that impurity controls relate to named impurities rather than allowing the presence of unlimited numbers of unspecified materials.

Fig. 12.2 gives a breakdown of the major areas of difficulty found in 'specifications' of drug substances in the applications examined.

If an application is so poor that the advisory committee feels that the applicant has not taken sufficient heed of the published data requirements it can recommend refusal to grant a product licence on the grounds that the application was not in accordance with the Guidelines.

12.3.2.2 *Deficiencies relating to the finished product*

The major areas of deficiency in applications with respect to the finished product (or dosage form) are given in Table 12.4.

The development pharmaceutics section of the dossier should include information to justify the choice of the formulation ingredients and to establish that the optimal concentration of each is present. Factors likely to affect bioavailability or bioequivalence should be discussed. For some solid dosage forms *in vitro* dissolution studies should be reported. The choice of dissolution medium may need to be justified fully if non-aqueous solvents or surfactants are used, for example. Any procedures necessarily applied to the product before it is given to the patient (such as reconstitution or dilution) should be investigated and justified as being suitable. In the case of products intended for intravenous infusion due account should be taken of compatibility with diluents or other co-administered materials. Consideration may also need to be given to the type of containers (glass or particular plastics) with which the product should or should not be used, or to syringe or giving set compatibility.

The manufacturing methods and their control are of great interest. Where a novel process or product is concerned, particular attention will be paid to reports on process validation. In all cases adequate information is expected which the assessors and the advisory committee can consider. The amount of information expected may be greater for a product not made in the EC.

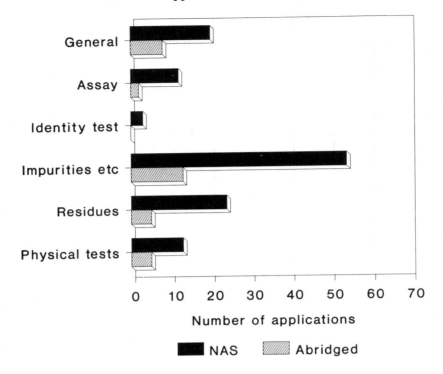

Fig. 12.2 — Deficiencies in drug specification information.

Table 12.4 — Deficiencies relating to the finished product

Area of deficiency	Type of application	
	New drug	Abridged
Development pharmaceutics	38	45
Pharmacokinetics, bioavailability, and bioequivalence	22	30
Manufacture and in process controls	35	14
Finished product specification	111	81
Labelling	9	1
Trade name	4	6
Import testing	3	1
Legal status	1	2

Details are required of any critical processes, particularly sterilisation methods. This is especially the case where the applicant has requested a reduced frequency of sterility testing or perhaps parametric release. Parametric release will normally require considerable process validation data to show that the process is fully understood and under control, as well as additional routine in-process controls such as bioburden monitoring. Any request for parametric release will result in additional attention being paid to such aspects of the application. In addition, the Medicines Inspectorate will be asked to comment specifically on requests for parametric release. Whether or not a reduced frequency of sterility testing is agreed, the finished product specification will be required to include at least a requirement that the product will comply with the sterility test if tested.

The requirements included in the finished product specification will need to be reviewed for other cases of parametric release, as will the stated frequency and type of in-process controls applied.

The finished product specification will be expected to include basic tests required by the *European Pharmacopoeia* general monographs. In addition, compliance with the requirements of the pharmaceutical Directives (especially those in the Annex to Directive 75/318/EEC), are required unless deviation can be justified. Some of the basic tests to be included in a specification will therefore include identity test(s) for the active ingredient and certain excipients; assays for active ingredients (with release limits of nominal ±5 percent unless otherwise fully justified and acceptable shelf-life limits), preservatives and essential excipients; dissolution or disintegration tests for tablets, capsules, etc.; controls on related substances, impurities, and degradation products; necessary pharmaceutical tests (for example friability, rheological controls, particulate contamination controls, resuspendability of suspensions, dimensional controls, weight controls, uniformity of content, etc.).

Recommendations to refuse the grant of product licences on grounds related to safety have been made based on the proposed trade names for products. Guidance is now included in the latest edition of the *Guidance notes on applications for product licences (MAL 2)* (MCA 1989) on the construction of pharmaceutical trade marks and trade names. Applicants should ensure that there is no possibility of confusion of the proposed product with existing products when the name is written or spoken.

12.3.2.3 *Points of general applicability*
In addition to the specific points discussed above and illustrated in the tables and figures, there are some points which apply generally to the pharmaceutical dossier.

Analytical validation is often the subject of questions from the advisory committees. The survey reported here relates to applications submitted before the CPMP guideline for validation studies was published. The problem areas identified in the cases examined are summarised in Table 12.5.

The validation of the analytical methods used for different purposes may need to be addressed in different ways. This was discussed in Chapter 2.

It is sometimes proposed to use a limulus amoebocyte lysate test for endotoxins in the finished product specification for an injectable product rather than a rabbit pyrogens test as described in the *European Pharmacopoeia*. The acceptability of such a proposal will depend on the submission of suitable validation data for the

Table 12.5 — Deficiencies relating to analytical validation

Deficiencies identified	Type of application	
	New drug	Abridged
Limulus test validation	4	—
Dissolution method validation	5	11
Biostudy analytical method validation	4	11
Stability test method validation	8	12
Specification test method validation (drug or dosage form)	26	18
Impurity control method validation	5	5

method for use with the product. Furthermore, it is unlikely that the use of thelimulus test will be allowed as an alternate to the rabbit test: one or the other is to be applied and the result used for product release purposes, not both.

The validation of methods of analysis used in stability studies is often particularly difficult. It is not only necessary to show that the methods have sufficient specificity, accuracy, and precision for their intended purpose, but also that the method is sufficiently robust to enable numerous analysts to use it reproducibly over a period of months or years on a variety of instruments, etc.

Another major area in which problems are encountered is that of stability studies. 46 objections were raised in the applications analysed relating to stability studies for new active ingredients or their dosage forms, and 28 for these aspects of abridged applications. One particular area of difficulty is the applicant proposing too long a shelf life on the basis of limited data.

Impurity control methods are required to be adequately validated, and the increasing attention being paid to the impurity, related substances, and degradation product profiles of both drugs and products adds to the significance of these data.

Applications are frequently deficient in adequate batch analysis data. This was cited in the case of 42 new drug applications and 28 abridged applications. It is normally expected that five batch analyses at production scale will be provided for both the drug substance and, if possible, the dosage form. If the required numbers of analyses are not available the company might wish to consider offering to provide the missing data on an on-going basis.

It should not be forgotten that reference standards used in analytical methods should be adequately characterised and reported. The lack of this information was on the basis of objections in 9 new drug applications and 11 abridged applications.

12.3.3 Deficiencies in applications referred to CPMP
An analysis has been made of the deficiencies in the first 55 applications submitted to the CPMP, and a more recent survey has been carried out on 12 applications considered by CPMP between September 1988 and May 1989. The following summary is based on these data (Cartwright 1990).

The main areas of deficiency in the applications are indicated in Table 12.6.

A more detailed breakdown of some areas of the data on the 55 earlier applications is also available. In the case of deficiencies in the area of active ingredients particular problem areas were found for assays and limits, impurities, and controls, manufacture of the active ingredient, quality checks during manufacture, development chemistry, batch analyses, and reference materials.

Weaknesses in the finished product control information included identity tests for active ingredients and excipients, method validation, batch analyses, assay limit justification, preservative limits, dissolution tests and limits, impurity degradation product and related substances controls, microbial contamination, and the limits proposed for the release and shelf life specifications.

Additional information is included in Fig. 12.3.

12.3.4 Objections remaining after consideration by advisory committees
12.3.4.1 Introduction
This section of the chapter is concerned with the outcome of consideration of additional information. It consists of two parts. The first considers the outcome of consideration of additional information within the CPMP procedure. The second is concerned with the outcome of the consideration of appeal data by the CSM.

12.3.4.2 The outcome of additional data consideration of applications routed via the CPMP
The following data were provided by Cartwright (1990).

Table 12.6 gives an analysis of the deficiencies identified in applications considered by CPMP. Table 12.7 gives information on the outcome following consideration by the CPMP of the initial objections and the applicants' responses.

These data indicate that the deficiencies in the pharmaceutical parts of applications can be reasonably quickly addressed and satisfactory data provided in a large proportion of cases. The need to provide additional information after the submission of an application always results in additional delays and difficulties. It would be far better if the information could be included in the original application.

12.3.4.3 Applications considered by the CSM
In addition to the analysis of outstanding points in applications considered by the CSM in 1987 to 1989, an analysis has also been undertaken of the pattern of objections included in the section 21(1) letters issued and of the remaining points in appeals (written representations and hearings) considered during the same period. The numbers of appeals considered by the CSM in these years were 32, 40, and 58 respectively (as stated in the committee's Annual Reports). The following analysis includes all but 8 of the appeals.

The grounds on which applications may be rejected under the UK Medicines Act 1968 are those relating to quality, safety, and efficacy. The distribution of the initial grounds for refusal for those appeals considered in 1987, 1988, and 1989 are given in Table 12.8a, and the position following the consideration of the appeal are included in Table 12.8b.

Table 12.6 — Deficiencies in applications referred to the CPMP

Defect	Applications	
	55 older	12 recent
Part IIa		
Composition	31	8
Container	22	0
Clinical trial formulation	1	0
Development pharmaceutics	21	10
Part IIb		
Manufacturing formulation	25	4
Manufacturing process	57	7
Process validation	13	0
Part IIc		
Active ingredients	227	79
Other ingredients	192	33
Packaging	—	7
Part IId		
Intermediate controls	42	0
Part IIe		
Finished product controls	377	74
Part IIf		
Stability	209	29
Part IIq		
Other information	—	1

These data indicate that not all appeals are successful before the CSM. Information in the CSM Annual Report indicates that the number and type of unsuccessful appeals considered in these years were:

7 hearings unsuccessful in 1987, 4 in 1988, and 4 in 1989;
6 written representations unsuccessful in 1987, 5 in 1988, and 11 in 1989.

For comparison the CDSM considered 12 appeals in 1987, 12 in 1988, and 33 in 1989. Of these, 12 were unsuccessful in 1987, 9 in 1988, and 23 in 1989.

For information a summary table of the cases considered by all the advisory bodies under the UK Medicines Act 1968 is given in Table 12.9.

It was indicated earlier that to go through an appeal procedure causes problems. One of these from the applicant's point of view is that delay will occur while new data are being generated or reports are prepared for submission to the advisory body. A further delay will also occur while the application is assessed by the MCA professional staff, and a free slot found in the timetable of the advisory body where the

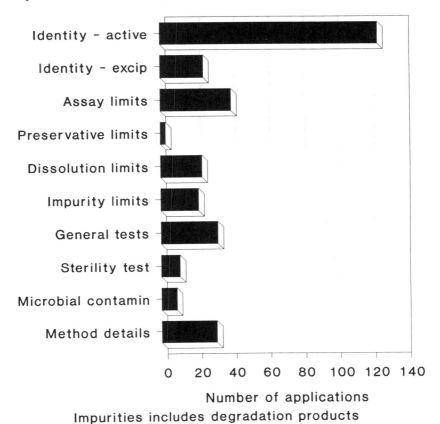

Fig. 12.3 — CPMP finished product information deficiencies.

appeal can be taken (which can be quite difficult in the case of a hearing if a large number of other applicants have requested hearings for their appeals).

For the CSM appeal cases analysed, the time between the first consideration of the application by the committee and the second consideration (that is, the appeal) has been calculated.

In the case of written representations, the average time taken for all appeals considered in 1987 was 18.2 months, while the average time for successful appeals was 16.3 months. In 1988 the figures were: overall mean = 24.1 months; successful appeals = 23.5 months. In 1989 the figures were: overall mean = 19.8 months; successful appeals = 14.7 months.

For hearings the average times were as follows: 1987 all hearings = 19.7 months (16.6 months for successful cases); 1988 hearings = 25.4 months (22.4 months for successful cases and 24.2 months for those considered as writtren representations prior to a hearing); and 1989 hearings: all cases 18.0 months (18.0 months for successful cases, and 20.5 months for those considered as written representations prior to any hearing).

Table 12.7 — Numbers of objections remaining on quality points following consideration of additional information by the CPMP

Defect in part of application	Objections	
	Before†	After‡
Part IIa Composition, etc.	65	21
Part IIb Manufacture, etc.	95	11
Part IIc Active ingredients	227	37
Other ingredients	192	39
Part IId Intermediate controls	42	13
Part IIe Finished product controls	377	103
Part IIf Stability	209	59
Other objections	5	3

† Summarised from Table 12.6.
‡ That is, after the additional information has been considered by the committee.

Table 12.8a — Initial grounds for proposed refusal of applications subject to appeal to CSM in 1987, 1988, and 1989

Year	Grounds for refusal						
	QSE	QS	QE	Q	SE	S	E
1987	13	5	3	1	4	4	2
1988	23	7	1	1	5	1	2
1989	32	9	0	1	4	3	1

Notes:
Q = quality grounds for refusal.
S = safety grounds for refusal.
E = efficacy grounds for refusal.

From this it can be seen that the delays in marketing are considerable if the original application does not comply with the data requirements.

12.4 THE PRECLINICAL DOSSIER

12.4.1 Introduction

In the past, defects have been identified in all areas of the preclinical section of product licence applications. However, defects are more common in certain areas than in others. It is the aim of this section to focus the reader's attention on those areas which, for whatever reason, repeatedly cause regulatory problems. Defects in each of the areas of the preclinical sections are discussed below.

Table 12.8b — Outcome of appeals to CSM considered in 1987, 1988, and 1989

Year	Grant etc.		Grounds for refusal						
	G	GOC	QSE	QS	QE	Q	SE	S	E
1987	4	14	5	3	0	0	3	0	3
1988	6	22	1	0	1	0	1	1	3
1989	13	23	7	1	0	0	5	0	1

Notes:
G = grant of product licence according to current application recommended.
GOC = grant of product licence according to current application recommended subject to compliance with conditions.
Q = quality grounds for refusal.
S = safety grounds for refusal.
E = efficacy grounds for refusal.

Table 12.9 — Cases considered by the advisory bodies appointed under the UK Medicines Act 1968 in 1987, 1988, and 1989

Year	Advisory body (numbers of cases)				
	CSM	CRM	CDSM	VPC	MC
Applications not previously considered					
1987	131	52	43	150	†
1988	171	45	30	100	†
1989	200	51	29	75	†
Appeals					
1987	32	34	12	19	25
1988	40	27	12	39	21
1989	58	39	33	33	16

Notes:
† Not applicable: Medicines Commission does not consider applications other than at the appeal stage.
CSM = Committee on Safety of Medicines.
CRM = Committee on the Review of Medicines.
CDSM = Committee on Dental and Surgical Materials.
VPC = Veterinary Products Committee.
MC = Medicines Commission.
Source: Annual Reports of the advisory bodies.

12.4.2 Pharmacology

The pharmacology section of product licence applications does not generally present any major problems for regulatory authorities. In particular, the pharmacological actions of the proposed medicinal product related to its intended therapeutic use are usually perfectly adequately investigated. This is not surprising since in the development process the decision to further investigate a candidate compound, or not, requires a detailed and thorough knowledge of a compound's primary pharmacological activity.

Secondary pharmacology screens on the other hand are not always performed to an adequate standard. The usual requirement is that a general pharmacological profile of the product is obtained, with particular attention being paid to the major body systems. The most common defect in this area is the omission of some or (rarely) all of these studies from an application.

Although an omission by itself may not result in an application being refused it may make interpretation of the animal toxicology findings or adverse reactions in patients much more difficult and thus impede the assessment and approval process.

12.4.3 Pharmacokinetics

Defects in the preclinical pharmacokinetics section of product licence applications are most commonly related to inadequacies in characterising exposure of animals to the product in toxicity studies. However, defects may range from a complete absence of any pharmacokinetic data in a species used in toxicity testing to simply inadequate investigation of exposure in a study where the drug is given *via* a particular route or method. A common example is where adequate pharmacokinetic data are provided for oral gavage but no evidence of exposure is provided when the drug is given in the diet. Thus, the exposure in chronic toxicity studies (usually performed by gavage) is known, but the exposure in carcinogenicity studies (usually performed by dietary incorporation) is not. These data are necessary to validate the studies (that is to show that the animals were exposed to adequate amounts of drug) and also to allow the clinical relevance of any toxic effects seen in these studies to be assessed.

Comparative pharmacokinetic tables are an extremely helpful way of presenting the animal pharmacokinetic data, both for the purposes of rapid assessment and for indicating whether or not a problem might exist in the exposure of the animals to the drug. Applicant companies are encouraged to draw up such tables and include them in their applications, usually in the Expert Report.

Where an exposure (or any other) problem has been shown to exist, the issue should be fully discussed in the Expert Report and the company's development strategy defended by scientific argument.

12.4.4 Toxicology

Defects in a single dose toxicity study are extremely rare in product licence applications, and it is difficult to envisage a situation in which such a defect would represent significant grounds for objection to an application.

The package of repeat dose toxicity studies on the other hand frequently has defects which represent grounds for objection. Common defects include inadequate exposure of animals to the drug, inadequate characterisation of pathological changes, inadequate discussion of pathological changes and their significance for the clinical use of the drug, and inadequate evidence to support proposed mechanisms for toxicity.

A further problem, which is not uncommon, is for the impurity profile of the drug substance used in toxicity studies to be different (qualitatively and quantitatively) from that proposed for clinical use. Where this results in an impurity to which patients will be exposed not having been adequately tested, an obvious problem exists.

It is intended that the Expert should play a major role in eliminating these defects in applications before they reach the regulatory authorities. Where this cannot be done the Expert should identify the defects, discuss the scientific aspects of the problem, and present rational scientific arguments to support the course of action taken by the applicant.

12.4.5 Reproduction studies

Reproduction studies are generally adequately performed to internationally recognised protocols. The most common defects in this section of the application arise not from the performance of these studies but in the animal findings in terms of the clinical use of the product.

Prescribers of the drug need to be made aware (through the product literature) of the animal data on the drug, any human experience with the drug, and finally given advice on prescribing.

The preclinical Expert Report should consider the animal data and make recommendations as to whether any restrictions should be imposed on the type of patient who may be exposed to the product. These recommendations may then be taken up by the clinical Expert Report author and form part of the considerations leading to the proposed product literature, Unfortunately this does not always happen, and inaccurate (or sometimes no) information is provided on the animal data in the product literature.

12.4.6 Mutagenicity

There are three types of defect which commonly occur in the mutagenicity section of applications. First, there may be a complete absence of a mutagenicity package with no adequate explanation. Second, a package of mutagenicity studies may be submitted, but the package differs from that recommended in the EC guideline (Council Recommendation 87/176/EEC) and no adequate explanation provided. Third, a package of mutagenicity data may be submitted, some of which have positive findings, but again no adequate discussion provided of those positive findings and their significance in the clinical use of the product.

The common factor in each of these defects is the lack of adequate discussion and scientific justification from the applicant as to the reasoning behind the selected approach to investigating the mutagenic potential of the product. It may be perfectly reasonable and scientifically justifiable, in certain circumstances, not to perform any mutagenicity studies at all, or to perform a different package of studies from those recommended in the guidelines, or to obtain positive findings in some tests, and still to consider that a positive risk to benefit ratio exists for use of the product in patients.

However, it is critical that the applicant sets out very clearly the scientific reasoning behind the approach taken to assessing the mutagenic potential of the proposed medicinal product. Of course the regulatory agencies may not agree with the scientific rationale put forward by the applicant and this would then be a matter for scientific debate, but at least the issues would be clearly defined in the application and a rapid regulatory decision could be reached.

12.4.7 Carcinogenicity

Problems with carcinogenicity studies are one of the commonest type of defect in the preclinical sections of the product licence applications. This is perhaps not surprising when the sheer size and complexity of the studies is considered.

The first type of defect concerns the question of whether carcinogenicity studies should be performed or not. The EC guidelines (Council Recommendation 83/571/EEC) state the circumstances in which carcinogenicity studies may be required. However, there are a few grey areas — for example the interface between a proposed clinical use involving a few short term exposures during a lifetime (where studies may not be required) and chronic intermittent use (where studies probably would be required). Where doubt exists about whether these studies should be performed, the issues should be discussed with regulatory authorities during the development of the product.

When carcinogenicity studies have been performed a number of technical defects in the studies commonly occur. These include inadequate survival of animals, inadequate exposure of animals to the drug, inadequate characterisation and discussion of pathological changes and their significance for the clinical use of the product, and inadequate evidence to support the proposed mechanisms resulting in the pathological changes.

Given the complex nature of these studies it is inevitable that problems will arise. However, it is extremely important that companies identify and discuss the shortcomings in their own studies so that the regulatory authorities are in a position to make the best possible judgement on the overall issues of carcinogenicity.

REFERENCES

ABPI (1989) *Guidance on the content of the clinical sections of an application for marketing authorisation for a new active substance.* London.

Annual Reports of the Advisory Bodies, published by HMSO: London.

Cartwright, A. C. (1990) Personal communication.

Griffin, J. P. & Diggle, G. E. (1981) A survey of products licensed in the UK from 1971–1981. *British Journal of Clinical Pharmacology,* **12** 452–463.

Medicines Act Information Letter (MAIL), MCA: London.

Rawlins, M. D. & Jefferys, D. B. (1990) unpublished data and (1991) *Brit. Med. J.,* **302**, 223–225.

13

CPMP and the Pharmaceutical Committee

13.1 THE COMMITTEE FOR PROPRIETARY MEDICINAL PRODUCTS (CPMP) AND ITS ACTIVITIES

The CPMP was established by Council Directive 75/319/EEC which was adopted on 20 May 1975. The Directive was brought into force on 20 November 1977.

13.1.1 The original functions of the CPMP

The main function of the CPMP as defined in 75/319/EEC was to facilitate the issue of marketing authorisations to place the same medicinal product on the market in two or more of the European Community (EC) Member States.

The original role of the CPMP was stated to be to give an opinion as to whether a particular product complies with the requirements of 65/65/EEC, and to recommend measures to abolish any remaining barriers to the free movement of products, particularly in the light of experience gained in the CPMP.

13.1.2 The chairmanship and vice-chairmanship of the CPMP

The first meeting of the CPMP was held on 27 and 28 September 1976.

Mr Léon Robert (Luxembourg) was elected as the first Chairman (President) at the meeting of 11/12 November 1976. He served two consecutive three-year terms of office and retired at the meeting held on 7/8 September 1982.

Dr E. L. Harris (UK) was elected Vice-Chairman. However, after his appointment to other duties, Professor Duilio Poggiolini was elected as his successor.

A second CPMP Vice-Chairman is appointed by the Commission of the European Communities (CEC). Mr D. J. Devine (Director) was appointed Vice-Chairman, but he withdrew and was replaced by Mr Nicolaas Bel, the Head of Division (Pharmaceuticals, veterinary medicines) in Directorate-General III.

At the meeting on 7/8 September 1982 Dr Claudius A. Teijgeler (Netherlands) was elected as Chairman to succeed Mr Robert. He also served for two successive terms of three years until 13/14 September 1988.

Mr Bel retired from the CEC in July 1986 and was replaced as the second Vice-Chairman by Mr Fernand Sauer, the new Head of Services of Directorate-General III/B–6 (now redesignated as DG II/C-3).

On 13/14 September 1988 Professor Duilio Poggiolini (Italy) was elected Chairman of the CPMP. The elected Vice-Chairman (by now responsible for scientific affairs and to act as deputy to the Chairman) was Professor Jean-Michel Alexandre (France).

13.1.3 The current role of the CPMP
The current role of the CPMP is to:

- Consider applications made under Directive 75/319/EEC (the 'multistate procedure' — see Chapter 14), where reasoned objections are made by one of the concerned Member States.
- Consider applications made under Directive 87/22/EEC (the 'concertation procedure' — see Chapter 15) for biotechnology and high technology medicinal products.
- Consider applications referred to it under Article 12 of 75/319/EEC as being of Community interest.
- Consider questions relating to the safety of already issued authorisations for medicinal products (pharmacovigilance issues).
- Consider policy questions raised by the Member States in considering marketing authorisation applications.
- Consider proposals for harmonising requirements for testing of products — issues relating to safety, quality, efficacy, and biotechnology.
- Produce guidance on procedures and technical requirements (the texts of the four volumes of *The rules governing medicinal products in the European Community* which concern marketing authorisation applications for human pharmaceutical products).

With regard to multistate and concertation applications, the CPMP produces an Opinion, which is handed down to the Member States. This Opinion is persuasive, but is not binding. In relation to concertation applications, the Opinions have with very few exceptions been agreed by all Member States, and the text of the summary of product characteristics (SPC) has been accepted by all. However, in relation to multistate applications the opinions are not binding, and the texts of the summaries of product characteristics agreed nationally by the individual Member States have often been divergent — to fit in with national guidelines or the precedents set nationally for similar products.

1990 has seen an increasing use of Article 12 of Directive 75/319/EEC for applications for products which are felt to be of significant Community interest — to arrive at a common view wherever possible. This fact has been seized on by commentators in the press, and it will be interesting to see whether use of this Article increases further in the run up to 1993.

13.1.4 The future role of the CPMP
The CEC's proposals for a 'future system' which would create a Single Market in pharmaceutical products are set out in Chapter 21 of this book. They envisage an adaptation of the CPMP to make it less of a group of delegates from the national

authorities and more of an expert body in its own right, with a balance of the scientific and technical expertise necessary to form an independent judgement on applications made directly to it (the 'centralised procedure' applications) or referred to it for arbitration ('decentralised procedure' applications). After 1 January 1993 the Opinions of the CPMP will be able to be transformed into decisions which will effectively create 'Euro-licences'. To this end a strengthened Secretariat will start to be recruited in 1991. It is likely that some of the ideas and procedures which will need to be introduced in 1993 and later, will be tested and evaluated in the current CPMP.

13.1.5 The CPMP working parties

In the period 1977 to 1978 three expert panels were set up under Article 13 of the CPMP rules of procedure. Their task was to harmonise the technical requirements for marketing authorisations in the Member States. The panels were the 'Safety of Drugs' panel chaired by Dr John P. Griffin (UK), the 'Efficacy of Drugs' panel chaired by Dr M. N. G. Dukes (Netherlands), and the 'Medicinal Products of Plant Origin' panel chaired by Professor Bernard Schneiders (Federal Republic of Germany).

By 1979, the Safety Working Party had completed its work on the major toxicology guidelines which covered single dose toxicity studies, repeated dose toxicity studies, reproduction studies, carcinogenicity studies, inhalation toxicity studies, and pharmacokinetics.

The Efficacy Working Party had similarly completed the drafting by 1979 of the guidelines on fixed combination products and anti-inflammatory preparations.

The above guidelines were formally adopted subsequently as Council Recommendations.

Subsequently both Drs Griffin and Dukes moved away from work in the national regulatory agencies. Professor Jean-Michel Alexandre (France) succeeded to the chairmanship of the Efficacy Working Party and Professor Rolf Bass to the chairmanship of the Safety Working Party.

In 1985 a new Quality Working Party of the CPMP was set up under the chairmanship of Mr Anthony (Tony) Cartwright (UK).

The three main working parties of the CPMP have continued their work of harmonising requirements for marketing authorisation applications, and particularly in producing proposals for new guidelines. As mentioned earlier, all the guidelines on quality, safety, efficacy, and biotechnology which had been adopted by the CPMP up until March 1989 were published in Volume III of *The rules governing medicinal products in the European Community*. Subsequent guidelines which have been adopted have been issued to the companies via the European and national pharmaceutical industry trade associations (the European Federation of Pharmaceutical Industry Associations (EFPIA) and the Associations Européens des Societés Grands Publics (AESGP)). The new guidelines will be collected together in new supplementary volumes, the first of which appeared in late 1990. This new volume included the Efficacy Working Party guideline on good clinical practice, the Quality Working Party guideline on analytical validation, and the Biotechnology/Pharmacy Working Party guideline on cytokines.

From the beginning, the working parties have involved the industry in their work of elaborating new guidelines, and each final draft guideline has been the subject of detailed comment and usually discussion with the European industry as well as with the national authorities. From 1988 onwards, each final draft has also been sent to the Japanese Ministry of Health and Welfare (MH) in an attempt to harmonise international requirements and to prevent the unnecessary repetition of work by companies. Since 1989, drafts have also been sent to the United States Food and Drug Administration (FDA) with the same objective.

Guidelines represent a statement of the requirements for the industry (an interpretation of the legal statements in 75/318/EEC), and an agreed consensus view from the authorities on the way they will assess marketing authorisation applications. They include (see Chapter 19) a definition of the major areas of policy; a statement of the minimum requirements (e.g. the number of batches of product which need to be tested in a stability test); and a statement of test methods in broad principle (but without going into such detail that it would inhibit companies from using suitable alternative methods).

In addition to the formal working parties, several have been created in response to specific needs. In 1985, in response to the requirements of Directive 83/570/EEC for an Expert Report for a new active substance marketing authorisation application, an *ad hoc* working party was set up under the chairmanship of Professor Duilio Poggiolini. This working party produced the 1986 first edition of the 'Notice to Applicants', which included guidance on the (then) new multistate procedure, the requirements for Expert Reports and the dossier.

The second edition of the 'Notice to Applicants' was drafted by the same *ad hoc* working party and published in 1989. It now included details of concertation and multistate procedures, a revision of the requirements for Expert Reports (see Chapter 11) and for the dossier.

Ad hoc drafting groups and informal meetings of experts have taken place increasingly frequently since 1988 to deal with specific topics. A drafting group on radiopharmaceuticals (with Dr Knud Kristensen (Denmark) as its chairman/rapporteur) met in 1989 and 1990 to devise a guideline on the special requirements for marketing authorisation for radiopharmaceuticals, and to draft a special section of the 'Notice to Applicants' as well as to propose amendments to the Annexe to Directive 75/318/EEC. In addition, the group has commented on the text of a guide to good manufacturing practices (GMP) for radiopharmaceuticals, and has contributed to a guideline on radiolabelled monoclonal antibodies. This drafting group started as sub-group of the Quality Working Party, but has now been taken over by the CEC as one of its own *ad hoc* groups.

Similarly, an *ad hoc* drafting group on quality of herbal remedies with Dr F. Hefendehl (Federal Republic of Germany) as its chairman/rapporteur met to develop a new guideline. This drafting group was again a sub-group of the Quality Working Party. Whereas Professor Schnieder's 1977 working party was unsuccessful in looking at all aspects of herbal medicines (and particularly in devising harmonised criteria for safety and efficacy), the new guideline succeeded in attaining its more limited objective. The guideline was published in Volume III of *The rules governing medicinal products in the European Community*.

In addition to work on guidelines, *ad hoc* meetings of experts have met to consider specific applications or groups of applications. In June 1989 a group of regulators and acquired immune deficiency syndrome (AIDS) experts met to consider questions in relation to new indications for existing products, or new therapies. This group was chaired by Professor Alexandre in his role as Vice-Chairman responsible for scientific coordination. It is likely that such meetings will be more frequent in future, and that after 1992 they will become a regular means of achieving a Community scientific consensus view which can be recommended to the CPMP on the approvable indications or recommended contraindications and warnings for major innovatory new active substances.

In 1989 an *ad hoc* Pharmacovigilance Working Party was set up under the provisional chairmanship of Professor René Royer (France) to consider adverse drug reaction reporting (ADR) systems used in the Member States, to produce proposals for a Community system of ADR reporting for after 1992, and to advise on pharmacovigilance issues in relation to individual products already approved in one or more of the Member States. This working party has met in parallel to the CPMP.

Also in 1989 a new operational working party was set up under the chairmanship of Dr Claudius Teijgeler (Netherlands), the retired CPMP Chairman. Its remit was to consider general operational tasks for the CPMP, to produce procedural guidelines (for example on the role of the rapporteur in the multistate and concertation procedures), and to consider future revision of the 'Notice to Applicants'.

13.1.6 The Commission working parties

The CEC has created a number of working parties to provide advice directly to it. The areas of advice include revision of the text of technical Directives (and particularly 75/319/EEC); on the text of new guidelines; and advice on new procedures needed for regulation of the testing, inspection, and distribution of medicinal products.

In 1986 the Biotechnology/Pharmacy Working Party was created under the chairmanship of Dr Geoffrey Schild (UK). Its first guidelines were included in Volume III of *The rules governing medicinal products in the European Community*. This working party has considered the quality aspects of all of the List A biotechnology concertation applications which have been received, and has produced recommendations for consideration by the CPMP.

A Commission working party on inspection has met over several years and is now devising a system for coordinating national inspections by the Member States in the post-1992 'Future System'. Mr Fernand Sauer (CEC) has chaired this group. A drafting group under the chairmanship of Mr Bryan Hartley (UK) has devised the text of Volume IV of *The rules governing medicinal products in the European Community* — the European good manufacturing practices guide, published in 1989.

13.2 THE PHARMACEUTICAL COMMITTEE

The Pharmaceutical Committee was established by a Council Decision of 20 May 1975. It is chaired by a senior representative of the CEC, and its membership consists of 'senior experts in public health matters from the Member States administrations'. It formally consists of one representative from each Member State, but each is also allowed one deputy who is allowed to participate in the meetings of the committee.

The functions of the Pharmaceutical Committee are stated in the council Decision. They are that the committee shall be consulted on any new proposals for Directives on proprietary medicinal products (and in particular any amendments to Council Directive 65/65/EEC), and should examine any question relating to the application of the Directives which is brought to it by its chairman or a representative of a Member State, and should examine any other question on medicinal products brought up by its chairman or a representative of a Member State.

In practice, the representatives of the Member States consist of the director or one of the senior management of the national agencies.

The primary role of the Pharmaceutical Committee is to consider any new legal proposals brought forward by the CEC (although the CPMP is nearly always informally consulted on technical aspects as well). They also consider any broad policy issues on licensing and control of medicinal products (for example the working of the national schemes for regulating parallel imports in accord with the Commission Communication).

The Pharmaceutical Committee first met in January 1976. It now meets once or twice in each year (depending mainly on the complexity of the current legislative programme being prepared by the CEC.

13.3 THE COMMITTEE FOR THE ADAPTATION TO TECHNICAL PROGRESS

Council Directive 87/19/EEC was adopted on 22 December 1986 and implemented in all Member States on 1 July 1987. It amended Directive 75/318/EEC, and one of its provisions was to create a mechanism where rapid amendment of the technical provisions of the Annex of Directive 75/318/EEC could be carried out. A new committee — the 'Committee for the adaptation to technical progress of the directives on the removal of technical barriers to trade in the proprietary medicines sector' was created. The details are set out in the new Article 2 of 75/318/EEC.

The new committee will consist of a representative of the Member States with a representative of the CEC as chairman. At the time of writing, the first meeting of the committee had still to take place, but it will do so in early 1991 to consider the draft Commission Directive amending 75/318/EEC to bring in the special requirements for radiopharmaceuticals, blood products, and immunologicals, and to update the Directive with other changes recommended by CPMP and Commission working parties (for example to introduce the possibility of separate submission of data on the active ingredient — the European drug master file procedure, see Chapter 7).

The procedure to be followed by the committee is as follows:

(a) Matters are referred to the committee by the chairman or by the representative of a Member State.

Sec. 13.3] The Committee for the Adaptation to Technical Progress

(b) The representative of the Commission delivers a draft of the measures to be adopted. The committee delivers its Opinion on the draft within a time limit set by the chairman, having regard to the urgency of the matter. The Committee acts by qualified majority, the votes of the Member States being weighted as provided in Article 148(2) of the Treaty of Rome.
(c) The CEC adopts the measures where the committee (with a qualified majority vote where necessary) agrees.
(d) Where the measures are not agreed by the committee, the matter is referred to the Council of Ministers. The Council of Ministers can again decide by a qualified majority.
(e) If the Council has not acted on a set of proposals within three months, the CEC can adopt the measures.

14

CPMP multistate procedure

14.1 INTRODUCTION

Council Directive 75/319/EEC was adopted on 20 May 1975 and implemented in the Member States on 21 November 1976. Articles 9 to 11 of 75/319/EEC set up the so-called 'CPMP procedure', whereby having obtained an authorisation in one European Community (EC) Member State, an applicant could then apply simultaneously in at least five other Member States by asking the authorities in the authorising country to send a copy of the dossier (containing the authorisation and the documents and particulars specified in Article 4 of Directive 65/65/EEC) to all of the other countries where it wished to obtain an authorisation (the 'concerned' Member States). This procedure was not very popular with the pharmaceutical industry, and only 41 applications were made in the eight years that it operated. The applications were for a mixture of different types of product — one or two new active substances, but mostly for 'abridged' (second applicant or generic or 'me-too') products.

Council Directive 83/570/EEC was adopted on 26 October 1983 and implemented in the Member States on 1 November 1985. This Directive made a number of important changes to the procedures laid down for the Committee for Proprietary Medicinal Products (CPMP). Amongst these were substantial changes to the previous 'CPMP procedure'. The new procedure was named the multistate procedure. In the five years since it was implemented it has become increasingly popular with companies. In the early years it was mainly used by smaller companies with limited resources who wished to obtain an authorisation in a number of Member States, often to 'sell on' the authorisation to a distributor or a licensee in that country. Latterly the procedure has been used by a wider variety of companies, who often use it to circumvent national delays in registration — since if the Member State does not send in reasoned objections within 120 days of the application having been accepted as a valid one, it has to grant the authorisation. More recently the major multinational companies have used the procedure in an increasingly sophisticated way — sometimes submitting national applications, but withdrawing them if there are long delays and then submitting a multistate as soon as they have an authorisation in at least one EC Member State. This aspect is described in greater detail in Chapter 16. The managements of some of the larger companies have also now identified that the use of a regulatory strategy including the multistate procedure enables them to carry out the international submission of major new product authorisation filings without the need for regulatory staff in each of the major EC countries. They have therefore an ability to reduce the staff costs of filing submissions in a number of countries, as well as speeding up the process.

In the last year or so, as the Single Market from 1 January 1993 looms closer, companies have been anxious to get experience of the existing procedures, since it is clear that the post-1992 future procedures (and particularly the decentralised procedure which is described in Chapter 21) will be modelled closely on, and developed from, the multistate procedure. Thus, there has been a considerable increase in the number of applications submitted that use the multistate procedure.

14.2 THE FORMER CPMP PROCEDURE

As pointed out above, the former CPMP procedure, where it was necessary to make applications in five or more Member States after the initial authorisation, was not popular with the industry. From 1976 to 1985 only 41 applications were made. The number of applications increased from 1980 to 1983, but declined thereafter.

The sources of the 41 applications were as shown in Table 14.1.

Table 14.1 — Source countries for CPMP applications: former multistate procedure (1976 to 1985)

Member state	Number of applications received	Percentage
United Kingdom	16	39
France	7	17
Denmark	7	17
Germany	5	12
Belgium	5	12
Ireland	1	2

The recipient countries were most frequently the Benelux countries (Belgium, the Netherlands, and Luxembourg); all involved countries are listed in Table 14.2.

It should be noted that owing to the date of their accession to the EC (1986), Spain and Portugal were not involved with this procedure, and Greece was only involved from 1981 to 1985.

The applications came from companies with their origins in the USA (11 dossiers), France (7 dossiers), Denmark (11 dossiers), Germany (3 dossiers), Sweden (3 dossiers), Belgium (3 dossiers), the Netherlands (1 dossier), Switzerland (1 dossier), and United Kingdom (1 dossier). Only 9 of the applications (22%) came

Table 14.2 — Recipient countries for CPMP applications: former procedure (1976 to 1985)

Member state	Number of applications received	Percentage
Luxembourg	37	14.5
Netherlands	35	13.7
Belgium	33	13.0
Italy	28	11.0
Denmark	28	11.0
Germany	25	9.8
Ireland	24	9.4
United Kingdom	18	7.1
France	14	5.9
Greece	12	4.7

from major multinational companies; the majority came from small or medium sized companies.

Of the 41 applications, 28 (70%) received a favourable opinion. The remaining 13 (30%) received an unfavourable opinion, of which 5 were unanimous.

The above applications led to 175 marketing authorisations and 63 final refusals (that is, refusals after all the national appeal stages).

14.3 THE NEW RULES OF THE MULTISTATE PROCEDURE

Directive 83/570/EEC introduced in 1985 a number of changes to the previous 'CPMP procedure':

- The minimum threshold is reduced from five to two Member States.
- Applicants have direct access to the CPMP at a hearing (this right is not available nationally in some Member States).
- The recipient Member States are given the approved summary of product characteristics (SPC) in addition to the assessment report of the first Member State.

The changes to the procedure have made it much more attractive to the industry, although as we have seen in the Introduction to this chapter, there are a number of other factors which have influenced this too.

14.4 WHAT AUTHORISATIONS CAN BE USED IN THE MULTISTATE PROCEDURE?

The multistate procedure can only be put into operation when an authorisation has already been obtained in one or more EC Member States. What kind of authorisations can be used?

Any full marketing authorisation (product licence) for a product granted in one of the EC Member States can be used in the procedure. Thus, an application may be made on the basis of either a full authorisation granted in accord with the current provisions of the Directives (65/65/EEC and 75/318/EEC as amended), or on the basis of a reviewed marketing authorisation (i.e. an old authorisation granted in accordance with previous national provisions and fully reviewed in line with current requirements as part of the review of 'old' medicines).

In the case of a full authorisation, the product could be either a new active substance (NAS) product or an 'abridged' product authorisation where the active ingredient has been previously authorised in another product.

It is important to check whether the active substance has been previously authorised in all of the Member States in which marketing is envisaged. If the active ingredient is well established, causing the product to be regarded as an abridged application in the Member State where the product is authorised (i.e. the 'outgoing' Member State) but an NAS in one or more of concerned ('incoming') Member States, this will cause considerable difficulties. A very well-known active ingredient may be licenced in a number of products and its therapeutic properties may be well documented in the first country because of its long period of use. If the same active ingredient is unknown in one or more of the other Member States, then they will be tempted (not unreasonably) to treat it as an NAS, and to demand a complete package of pharmacology/toxicology and clinical trials data. It is possible to overcome these problems by ensuring that the multistate application includes Expert Reports (particularly the pharmacotoxicological and clinical Reports) which address such issues. The adverse drug reaction experience in the first EC country should also be summarised in the clinical Expert Report to provide supportive evidence on the safety in use of that product or similar ones.

Some EC Member States have taken the view that the procedure should be mainly used for therapeutically important new products, and not 'me-too' second applicant products with no particular therapeutic innovation. Thus they may be unwilling (particularly if they have only limited professional resources) to act as the rapporteur for such products. Intending applicants need to discuss such matters with the authority that granted the authorisation to ensure that they are willing to act as the rapporteur (outgoing) country.

14.5 WHAT AUTHORISATIONS CANNOT BE USED IN THE MULTISTATE PROCEDURE?

Authorisations which cannot be used in the procedure include unreviewed old authorisations (e.g. unreviewed product licences of right in the UK); products currently excluded under Article 34 of Directive 75/319/EEC — vaccines, serums, immunologicals, blood products, radiopharmaceuticals and homoeopathics; and products which are outside the scope of the Directives as strict medicinal products but are controlled as medicines under national legislation (such as contact lens products brought under control in the UK by an order under Section 104 of the 1968 Medicines Act).

In relation to the 'exempt' products, the 'extension' Directives (89/342/EEC, 89/343/EEC, and 89/381/EEC) will bring immunologicals, radiopharmaceuticals and blood products into the framework of the pharmaceutical Directives after 1 January 1992, any full authorisation for any of these products will be able to be used in the multistate procedure. Also, existing authorisations for these categories of product (that is, granted before 1 January 1992) are required to be reviewed before 31 December 1992. As soon as they have been reviewed, these. licences can be used in the existing multistate procedure (or its eventual successor, the decentralised procedure).

It should be noted that there have been cases where a product which falls into the 'exempt' category would have also been considered as falling into either List A (biotechnology) or List B (biotechnology/high technology) of Directive 87/22/EEC. In one or two cases such a product had already been approved in one EC Member State before Directive 87/22/EEC came into force (i.e. before 1 July 1987). In these cases it was accepted that the extension of the product authorisation to other EC countries could proceed via the multistate procedure rather than the concertation procedure, since the concertation procedure would be inappropriate where a product had already been authorized in one country.

14.6 SUITABILITY OF PRODUCTS FOR THE MULTISTATE PROCEDURE

As well as the legal acceptability of products into the multistate procedure, as discussed above, there is also the question of their suitability in terms of indications, contraindications, etc. for a number of other EC countries. The fact that a product has been authorised in one EC country with a particular SPC, does not mean that it will be readily approved in other countries. Often the same active ingredient is used in different products in different ways across the Community. The use of products can differ owing to differences in the practice of medicine in the Member States (for example hypotension is a very widely diagnosed and treated condition in Germany but is very rare in the UK); owing to different traditions in the use of particular drugs in the Member States (a drug may be used for several indications in some EC Member States but only one in others); to differences in the access to sophisticated facilities (such as hospitals and clinics); and to differences in access to or use of other treatment regimens which may constitute an alternative to the product (such as surgery, radiotherapy).

The prospective multistate applicant is well advised to research carefully his likely chances of success in the procedure. Do other similar products exist (with full authorisations, not unreviewed old authorisations) on the markets in question? If so, what are their accepted indications and contraindications listed in the various publications (*Rote List* in Germany, *Dictionnaire Vidal* in France, the *Repertorio* in Italy, etc.)? If the product has major new indications not previously accepted by the authorities, are there sufficiently convincing recent clinical data to support these new indications? If the dossier does not include sufficient clinical data to support the claimed indications, the applicant will have to rely on the scientific literature, and then the role of the clinical Expert and the quality of his Expert Report is crucial.

Between now (1991) and 1992 a major effort will need to be made to harmonise what will be accepted as the major clinical indications and contraindications for the most important pharmaco-therapeutic groups of active ingredients. In this interim period there will also have to be an increasing effort made to agree an EC text for the SPC. Thus, the price to be paid for using the multistate procedure in the future, to gain authorisations in a number of EC Member States, may be the risk of the loss of some cherished indication in the first approving (outgoing) Member State, so as to get an agreed EC set of indications. It will be up to the applicant after he has done all his research to consider whether that risk is one he wants to take. One cynical observer in the industry has called this the 'product de-launch'!

At the moment, if there are differences in the views of the national authorities they will often be represented in a positive Opinion, but one where the national positions are maintained. In such a case, the applicant can usually go on to agree a different SPC with the authorities in the Member States concerned.

14.7 SECOND APPLICANT (ABRIDGED) PRODUCTS

If a so-called 'abridged' application is made in the multistate procedure (that is, an application for a product containing an established active ingredient), the application needs to carefully document the section of Article 4 of 65/65/EEC under which it is made. An application may be made without full information on pharmacology-toxicology and clinical data by one of three different routes specified in Article 4, and the legal route must be stated. The three possibilities are:

Article 4(8)(a)(i): consent of the first applicant to refer to his data on pharmacology/toxicology and clinical studies;

Article 4(8)(a)(ii): detailed reference to the published scientific data on efficacy and safety;

Article 4(8)(a)(iii): that the product is 'essentially similar' to a product authorised within the EC for ten years (six years in the case of applications made to Denmark, Ireland, and Luxembourg) and marketed within the Member State concerned.

Where reference to Article 4(8)(a)(iii) is used, the applicant needs to provide evidence that the product has been authorised within the EC for at least ten years. Suitable proof of this authorisation may be provided by reference to the official publications in the various EC countries where the authorisations are published. In some countries where the records of authorisation dates may not be accurate or complete (for example in Denmark where in the past the date published has been the date of offer of a licence 'subject to' the provision of satisfactory data, and in the UK where the date published has been the date of marketing and not the date of grant of the authorisation), the authorities have agreed to provide this information on request to prospective applicants.

The above information (on date of authorisation of an earlier originator product), must be provided in Part 1A, Administrative data (Point 2(a)); and in the Product Profile (Point (a) Type of application).

It should be noted that the three possible routes described above for an abridged application do not apply to Spain, Portugal, and Greece until 1 January 1992. In the case of these countries, the previous provisions of Article 4(8)(a) of Directive 65/65/EEC apply — a list of published references should be provided to show that the product has an established use, and it has been adequately tested on human beings so that its effects, including side effects, are already known and are included in the published references.

14.8 CHANGES TO THE ORIGINAL AUTHORISATION ('VARIATIONS')

Applicants are encouraged to bring their file up to date to the current Directive requirements before submission in the Member States. Further information may also have become available since the date of the first authorisation (e.g. more stability data, more clinical data). Any changes made to the first authorisation must be approved by that authority before the multistate application is submitted — particularly if they affect the specifications for starting materials and finished products, method of manufacture, the composition, the proposed clinical indications, the contraindications etc.

Applicants should avoid making changes ('variations') during the multistate procedure to either the product as authorised in the first Member State or to the application going through the multistate procedure, since this will cause difficulties and delays in processing the multistate application.

Where an authorisation has been amended, the Expert Report will need amendment and updating. Some countries (e.g. Germany) prefer to see the original Report with an updating addendum; others prefer to see a new Report referring to all the new information.

Any additional clinical experience with the product (for example trials finished since the first authorisation was granted) should be included and documented in the covering letter accompanying the application — even if the original indications are unchanged. The same is true of any new pharmaceutical data (such as new stability data) or toxicology data.

Where new clinical data are submitted, there needs to be a complete revision of the global analysis of the human safety data submitted in the clinical Expert Report — particularly if these new data include results of postmarketing surveillance (PMS) studies.

14.9 MULTISTATE APPLICATIONS FOR PRODUCTS WHOSE AUTHORISATIONS WERE GRANTED IN THE ORIGINATING (OUTGOING) MEMBER STATE SOME YEARS PREVIOUSLY

Applications can be made for such products, but the original file needs to be systematically reviewed and brought into line with current requirements as stated in the Directives, the guidelines, and the 'Notice to Applicants'.

Where the original submission was made before the requirement to provide Expert Reports (that is before 1985), the new multistate application must include such Reports.

In the UK, if an 'abridged' application was made for an authorisation, there may not be an assessment report available to send to the other (concerned) Member States unless the product had been considered by an advisory committee (such as the Committee on Safety of Medicines). This is not a barrier to using the multistate procedure, but in this case, the quality of the Expert Report is even more crucial.

14.10 THE MULTISTATE PROCEDURE AND TIMING

The procedure is as follows:

(1) Preliminary consultation with the rapporteur
The applicant consults the rapporteur in the outgoing Member State as to the suitability of the product for the procedure, the need for updating the original file, the need for changes ('variations') to the original authorisation and about the timing of the submission to the other (concerned) Member States.

(2) Notification of impending submission
The applicant notifies the rapporteur in the outgoing Member State about the impending submission (say three to four weeks before it is made). This alerts the rapporteur to obtain the assessment report, so that it can be sent out as soon as the application is accepted by all of the concerned Member States.

(3) Sending of the assessment report to the concerned Member States by the rapporteur
The assessment report is sent to all the concerned Member States and the Commission of the European Communities.

(4) Filing of the application
The application is filed simultaneously in all of the concerned Member States, with a copy to the Directorate-General III/C-3 Secretariat to the CPMP. Careful attention needs to be paid to the number of copies needed of the different parts of the application (see the table in the 'Notice to Applicants'), and the languages needed. The national application fees should be paid with the application, since any delays may delay the acceptance of the application into the procedure.

(5) Start of the 120-day period
Each of the concerned Member States notifies DGIII/C-3 that it has received a valid application. Once a month after the last acceptance, the DG III/C-3 Secretariat notifies Member States by telex or telefax of the start of the 120-day consideration period for all applications accepted that month.

(6) The 120-day period
Each of the concerned Member States has 120-days to notify reasoned objections to grant of an authorisation. If no objections are raised within 120-days, they are obliged to grant an authorisation. All reasoned objections are sent to:

- DGIII/C-3 Secretariat (the CEC),
- the rapporteur, and
- the applicant company.

(7) The appeal process
After receipt and translation of reasoned objections into English (for a UK rapporteur), these are then discussed with the rapporteur. The applicant needs to have evaluated the objections and to know which are the most difficult to answer, which will need further work, etc. The applicant, after consulting the rapporteur, then decides whether to go for an appeal in writing only (written representation) or for a hearing in front of the CPMP. The applicant advises how long it will take to prepare the appeal, and the rapporteur advises which meeting of the CPMP would probably be suitable. The applicant then requests from the DGIII/C-3 Secretariat an Opinion at the CPMP meeting which he and the rapporteur have agreed. The applicant needs to discuss his appeal strategy with the rapporteur — what Experts he may need at a hearing, etc.

(8) Lodging the appeal document
At least 30 working days before the CPMP meeting nominated for the Opinion, the written appeal document is lodged. If it contains very substantial new information, or the 30-day period is just before a major holiday period (such as August or Christmas), it is wise to allow more than 30 working days. This will ensure that the appeal is fully considered by the concerned Member States.

(9) Notification to the company of outstanding issues after consideration of the written appeal data
Approximately five to seven days before the CPMP meeting, the concerned Member States notify the rapporteur about the outstanding points. The rapporteur then notifies the company so that they can consider their final appeal strategy (including the final choice of Experts to address the CPMP at a hearing).

(10) The rapporteurs meeting
The day before the CPMP meeting, the Member States hold a meeting of all of the rapporteurs to brief the chairman of the CPMP. There is an opportunity to clarify and discuss objections which remain.

In the case of a written appeal, the DGIII/C-3 Secretariat and the rapporteur start to write the Opinion to present to the CPMP.

(11) Briefing the applicant before a hearing
After the rapporteurs meeting before the CPMP, the rapporteur confirms the outstanding issues which the company needs to address at the hearing. The applicant and the rapporteur can discuss the final strategy for the hearing.

(12) The CPMP meeting
The company presents its appeal. The CPMP then advises its Opinion and considers the SPC for the product.

(13) Notification of the Opinion
The CPMP Opinion is notified to the applicant and to the concerned Member States.

(14) Acting on the CPMP Opinion
The Member States notify the CEC as to what action they will take on the Opinion. If there are outstanding issues, these need to be resolved by the applicant as soon as possible (e.g. national labels and leaflets) so as to expedite issue of a national authorisation.

(15) National appeal against an unfavourable (negative) Opinion
In the event of a negative (unfavourable) Opinion or a divided Opinion (one or more of the Member States not in favour of the authorisation), the subsequent appeal uses national appeal mechanisms (to the Dutch College, to the UK Committee on Safety of Medicines etc).

The final national decision is notified to the CPMP.

14.11 THE ROLE OF THE RAPPORTEUR AND CO-RAPPORTEUR

The term 'rapporteur' is used in several different ways in the context of the various procedures. It is often a nominated person from the outgoing Member State who assists an applicant company to get the product through the procedure. Since no single person can be knowledgable about all aspects of the safety, quality, and efficacy of a product, he is responsible for coordinating the help of other administrative and professional colleagues in his own Member State to advise the company — that is, he acts as a facilitator. He is also the link between the CPMP and the company, ensuring at each stage that the applicant is fully aware of all issues, and he answers these points as fully as possible.

In the context of the multistate procedure, the role of the rapporteur is:

- to advise the company on the suitability of the product for the multistate procedure,
- to advise the company on the need for file updating, revision of their Expert Report, etc.,
- to initiate preparation of the assessment report,
- after the end of the 120-day period to discuss the reasoned objections and help the company to decide whether to reply only in writing, or to have a hearing in addition,
- to discuss the timing of their appeal with the company,
- one week before a hearing, to discuss the outstanding points, so that the company can make a final decision on the Experts they will need at the hearing,
- one day before the hearing (after the rapporteurs meeting), to discuss the outstanding points with the company,
- at the CPMP meeting, to present the outstanding issues to be answered by the company,
- to follow up any problems with the Opinion which the company encounters at a national level.

In each of the concerned Member States a 'co-rapporteur' is nominated as a contact person, who advises on outstanding issues at each stage of the consideration of the application. In theory, the co-rapporteur is also someone with whom the rapporteur can discuss points raised, so that minor points can be dismissed. However, in practice, the reasoned objections often do not come in until at least day 118 or 119, so this leaves very little time for the points to be informally resolved.

14.12 THE ASSESSMENT REPORT

The assessment report consists of the documentation sent by the rapporteur country (the outgoing Member State) to the concerned Member States. It details all of the stages of consideration of the application before the original authorisation, and any subsequent major changes to that authorisation. It consists of some or all of the following items:

- the original Expert Report of the applicant,
- the comments of the assessors in the Member States (either internal assessors or external experts or a combination of both) on the application,
- the advice of the official committee in the Member State (such as Kommission A in Germany, the Commission d'AMM in France, the College in the Netherlands, the CSM in the UK) on the application,
- any appeal data from the company,
- the advice of the national official committee on the appeal,
- the approved SPC,
- details of any major changes ('variations') to the marketing authorisation,
- an analysis of national adverse drug reaction (pharmacovigilance) reports on the product,
- a note of any postmarketing surveillance (PMS) studies, and the results obtained to date.

In the UK, there will be no advice from the advisory committee (such as the CSM) if the product was not considered by them — if, for example, it was a simple abridged application.

Some Member States write an assessment report especially for an outgoing multistate application. In such a case (for example in France), the authorities should be advised at the time of first submission of the marketing authorisation (MA) application, that if it is successful, the MA will be used as the basis of a multistate.

14.13 LABELS AND LEAFLETS

Part V of the application includes labels and leaflets. For a multistate application it is permitted to draft these in accord with national requirements for content, languages, etc., and to include them in the national multistate application. However, all of the labels and leaflets must be compatible with the approved SPC of the rapporteur (outgoing) Member State.

14.14 SAMPLES OF THE STARTING MATERIALS AND DOSAGE-FORM

Eight Member States (Belgium, Spain, Greece, Ireland, Italy, Luxembourg, the Netherlands, and Portugal) require samples of the finished product to be provided systematically for analytical checking by the national (state) control laboratory. The other four EC countries (Denmark, Germany, France, and the UK) may request such samples to be provided (they should be kept ready to send).

Five Member States require samples of the active substance to be provided (Greece, Ireland, Luxembourg, the Netherlands, and Portugal). The other countries may request such samples.

14.15 APPLICATIONS TO PORTUGAL

Portugal has a derogation from the full implementation of the Directives until 1 January 1991. It has stated that it is willing to receive a national application for any product going through the multistate procedure.

14.16 THE FORMAT AND LANGUAGE OF MULTISTATE APPLICATIONS

The format of applications is the same for national, multistate and concertation (high technology/biotechnology) applications. Thus, an application which has received a national authorisation can readily be adapted to use in the multistate procedure.

The application may need to be translated, however, for subsequent use in the procedure. This factor is one which has undoubtedly contributed to the popularity of the UK as the rapporteur country — since only Spain requires the Part II data in Spanish, and Spain, France, and Portugal require the summaries (including the Expert Reports) to be in Spanish, French, and either French or Portuguese respectively. Thus, most countries now accept the major part of the application in English.

The format of applications is shown in Table 14.3.

National application forms are required in some countries (e.g. Germany and the UK). Where these are used, they should accompany the multistate application, since otherwise this may delay its acceptance by those authorities.

14.17 HEARINGS

Hearings are a procedure intended to allow the applicant to answer any remaining concerns of the concerned Member States after they have reviewed the written appeal data. A hearing is not an opportunity to make a long formal presentation.

The rapporteur will have briefed the applicant on the outstanding issues before the meeting, enabling the company to have suitable Experts present to address the outstanding issues. The company usually addresses those issues by means of a short presentation (about ten minutes).

The choice of Experts is crucial, and Experts need to be present to be able to answer all outstanding issues. If there are clinical issues which are unresolved, it is often useful to use an outside independent Expert who has been involved in the clinical trials or has used the product in his own clinical practice. Such an Expert can testify to the risk/benefit of the product from his own experience.

The use of visual aids (overhead transparencies and slides) can help to emphasise particular points. However, the use of visual aids needs to have been arranged with

Table 14.3 — The format of applications

Part reference	Contents of part
Part I	Summary of the dossier.
Part I(A)	Administrative data.
Part I(B)	Summary of product characteristics.
Part I(C)	Expert Reports (including the product profile).
Part II	Chemical, pharmaceutical, and biological documentation.
Part III	Pharmacological/toxicological documentation.
Part IV	Clinical documentation.
Part V	Special particulars.
Part V(A)	Label/carton text, patient and/or practitioner leaflet.
Part V(B)	Samples of active ingredient and dosage-form.
Part V(C)	Manufacturing authorisation.
Part V(D)	Marketing authorisation from the rapporteur Member State with the approved SPC; details of authorisations in other EC Member States; details of authorisations in other (non-EC) countries.

the CPMP Secretariat beforehand to ensure availability of equipment. Hard copies of such material also need to be available for the delegates, the Secretariat of the CPMP, and the interpreters who will be present.

The procedure in a Hearing is as follows:

- the Chairman asks the applicant company to introduce their Experts (normally between two and six in number),
- the Chairman asks the rapporteur to summarise the outstanding issues,
- the company makes a presentation on those issues only,
- delegates from the concerned Member States ask supplementary questions,
- the company is invited to make any final remarks,
- the company leaves.

14.18 THE 'EURO-SPC'

In the past the CPMP Opinions have been generalised ones where many of the issues have been unresolved. During the last three years, there has been an increasing tendency to try to come to a common position on applications on which all the concerned Member States can agree. Also, the text of the SPC is now routinely appended to the Opinion. The SPC can be that of the rapporteur country, attached as a model example, or it can be a text agreed by all of the concerned Member States and the rapporteur. As the Community nears 1993, there will be an increased emphasis on trying to achieve such an agreed text so that the product can be marketed throughout the EC with one set of indications, dosage, contraindications, etc.

The attempt to agree such an SPC means that even where there are no reasoned objections from one country, they will still wait until the SPC has been discussed in the CPMP before granting the national authorisation.

However, at the moment most SPCs are agreed nationally between the applicant and the authorities after the Opinion, and these invariably differ to a smaller or larger extent (depending on national custom and practice for the active or class of active concerned).

14.19 ANALYSIS OF MULTISTATE APPLICATIONS (1986 TO 1989)

The multistate procedure has gained considerably in popularity in recent years. The numbers of new applications made in each year were:

1986	1987	1988	1989
2	20	31	53

The average delay in months between the end of the 120-day period and the CPMP Opinion in each year was as follows:

1986	1987	1988	1989
3.0	3.25	4.36	4.48

The overall success rate (positive Opinion) in the period 1986 to 1989 was 94%, and 6% of applications in that period received a negative Opinion.

The mean time taken from receipt of the Opinion to completion of the national procedures (i.e. grant of an authorisation or the end of all national appeals resulting in final refusal) was 9 months (varying nationally from 4 to 24 months).

In the period 1985 to November 1989 the countries listed in Table 14.4 were the

Table 14.4 — Source countries for multistate applications

Country	Number of applications	Percentage
United Kingdom	36	34
France	28	26
Ireland	9	8.4
Denmark	8	7.5
Germany	8	7.5
Italy	7	6.5
Netherlands	6	5.6
Belgium	5	4.6

main sources of multistate applications.

In the period 1985 to November 1989 the countries listed in Table 14.5 were the main recipient countries.

The percentage quoted in Table 14.5 is the percentage of the possible occasions when a Member State could have been used. In the period reported there were 105

Table 14.5 — The multistate recipient countries

Country	Number of applications	percentage
Germany	70	66
Belgium	57	54
Luxembourg	54	51
Netherlands	53	50
Greece	51	49
Spain	48	46
Denmark	44	42
Ireland	39	37
United Kingdom	36	34
France	30	28

multistate applications, and if any country had been involved in all applications their percentage score would have been 100.

REFERENCE

Poggiolini, D. & Donawa, M. E. (1990). EEC pharmaceutical regulation: the multistate procedure and the CPMP. *Pharm. Technol.* **2**, 104, 106, 108, and 110.

15

The concertation (high technology/biotechnology) procedure

15.1 INTRODUCTION

Directive 87/22/EEC was adopted on 22 December 1986 and implemented by the Member States on 1 July 1987. It obliged the competent authorities in the Member States to consult each other before deciding to authorise, refuse, or withdraw a medicinal product produced by biotechnology. At the request of the applicant company, this consultation procedure can also be used for certain high technology medicinal products, provided that the competent authorities in the rapporteur and concerned Member States agree.

This requirement on the authorities to consult each other ('concertation') was designed to ensure that the European Community (EC) pooled its technical resources when considering these novel and technologically complex products. It was meant to ensure that there was a uniform decision throughout the EC. It was also felt that the market for many of these products would be rather small and specialised, and that rapid access to the whole EC market might make them more commercially viable — thus encouraging the development of a strong EC biotechnology industry.

15.2 PROTECTION OF INNOVATION

One of the objectives of Directive 87/22/EEC was to create a favourable regulatory environment in the EC for high technology and biotechnology medicinal products. Products which use the Concertation procedure gain a certain type of protection from a second applicant coming onto the market.

For pharmaceutical products, the 20-year protection offered by the Münich Convention on the European Patent is often insufficient because of the time taken to carry out the toxicological, pharmacological, pharmaceutical, analytical, and clinical studies. The time taken to obtain a marketing authorisation also reduces the time. In addition, the protection offered to biotechnology products under patent law is often uncertain.

The protection offered to the originator under Directive 87/22/EEC is to require that for any product authorised under this procedure (either a high technology or a biotechnology product), a second applicant must either obtain the consent of the originator to refer to his package of pharmacological/toxicological and clinical data, or he must wait until at least ten years from the date of the first Community authorisation and then show that his product is essentially similar, or he must show by detailed reference to the published scientific literature that the constituent or constituents of the product have a well-established medicinal use, with recognised efficacy and an acceptable level of safety.

The alternative to these approaches is for the second applicant himself to provide a sufficient pharmacology/toxicology and clinical trials dossier. In fact this has (so far) been the only approach, with each applicant making an independent application. It seems difficult (at least for the moment) to visualise a 'generic' biotechnology product, since in practice their quality is not fully defined by their active ingredient specification, the finished product specification, etc. The control of the method of manufacture and also its validation is regarded as being a vital part of the definition of the product quality. In essence, each biotechnology product is being treated as a product containing a new active (biological) substance, requiring a full data package.

The second applicant protection (particularly for the high technology products) has not proved to be particularly successful, and very few companies have applied to use the voluntary high technology procedure. Thus, the problem of inadequate patent protection for pharmaceutical products remains, and the Commission of the European Communities (CEC) (following national initiatives in France and Italy) has now proposed another Directive to give supplementary patent certificates. In essence this would extend the patent protection to 15 years from the date of grant of the first marketing authorisation of the product in the EC.

15.3 EARLY EVALUATION OF THE PROCEDURE

In anticipation of the coming into operation of the new procedure, France introduced an application for a monoclonal antibody biotechnology product indicated for the prevention of renal graft rejection, and this received a favourable opinion in June 1986. As mentioned above, the procedure came into operation formally in July 1987.

15.4 BIOTECHNOLOGY PRODUCTS — AN OBLIGATORY PROCEDURE

Directive 87/22/EEC contains two separate lists of products — List A (the biotechnology products) and List B (the high technology products). The use of the concertation procedure is obligatory for all List A products.

List A products are those developed by means of the following biotechnological processes — recombinant DNA technology; controlled expression of genes coding for biologically active proteins in prokaryotes and eukaryotes, including transformed mammalian cells; and hybridoma and monoclonal antibody methods.

The obligation is on the first Member State (the rapporteur) to receive the application to refer it to the Committee for Proprietary Medicinal Products (CPMP), or the Committee for Veterinary Medicinal Products (CVMP) for veterinary products).

The Directive states (Article 2(2)) that it applies to 'a medicinal product developed by means of new biotechnological processes'. The CPMP, in considering this statement, has accepted that this means that any biotechnological manufacturing process which is in any way different from one previously used, triggers the procedure. Thus a broadly similar process of manufacture of a product using the same organism (*E. coli* or yeast cell line) would still trigger the procedure because the detail of the process, or the subsequent purification steps, will differ (that is the process is a 'new' one). Thus, any application for a recombinant insulin product or new mixture of recombinant zinc insulins comes into the procedure automatically.

The new procedure extends to products otherwise exempt from the Directive requirements until after 1 January 1992. These include vaccines, serums, blood products, and radiopharmaceuticals. Thus, a recombinant DNA vaccine would automatically come into the procedure as a List A product.

15.5 EXEMPTION FROM THE OBLIGATORY BIOTECHNOLOGY PROCEDURE

A company can claim exemption from the procedure for products that are only of interest in one EC country. In such a case it has to certify that it has not applied for an authorisation to place a product containing the same active ingredient on the market of another EC Member State within the last five years, and that within the next five years it does not intend to seek an authorisation to place a product on the market of another EC Member State.

If, within the five year period, another application is lodged with the authorities of another EC Member State, the product must then be automatically referred to the CPMP (or CVMP in the case of a veterinary product) for an Opinion.

15.6 THE HIGH TECHNOLOGY PROCEDURE

For products in List B of the Annex to Directive 87/22/EEC, the use of the Concertation procedure is not obligatory, but it can be used on request from the applicant company, and where the authorities agree. The categories of product concerned are:

- products from other biotechnological processes (that is, other than those in List A), which constitute a significant innovation;
- products administered by means of new delivery systems which constitute a significant innovation;
- products containing a new substance or an entirely new indication, which is of significant therapeutic interest;
- products based on radioisotopes, which are of significant therapeutic interest;
- products the manufacture of which employs processes which demonstrate a significant technical advance.

In each case, the applicant produces an argument to support the significance of the innovation/therapeutic interest/technical advance. The authority chosen as the rapporteur then considers the arguments and accepts or does not accept the product as being high technology. Because of the very limited experience with the procedure, companies intending to use the procedure have invariably undertaken wide-ranging discussion and consultations with the officials from the competent authority, before submitting the application, to find out their likely views on the significance of innovation etc. In relation to new active substances (NAS), the CPMP has stated that they will normally accept the first member of a new pharmaco-therapeutic group as being of significant therapeutic interest, but not normally the second or third in the series (unless they have some particular and clear therapeutic advantages).

The arguments on the significance of innovation etc. are advanced in the Expert Report. The relevant sections for each of the categories of high technology products are as follows:

For 'other biotechnological processes', 'new delivery systems', and 'technically advanced processes' the justification would be provided in the pharmaceutical Expert Report.

For a 'new substance/new indication' or 'radioisotope' the justification would be provided in the clinical Expert Report.

Some products may fall into more than one of these categories, such as for example a new delivery system being used to deliver an active ingredient for a new indication. In such a case, the arguments will need to be presented in both sections of the Expert Report.

Applicants need to make their case as to a delivery system etc. being a 'new' one, in relation to a complete survey of all of the products which have been approved in all of the EC Member States, and not just the rapporteur country.

The EC Member States have been anxious to maintain a consistent attitude with this new requirement. Thus, if there is any doubt about whether the product is of significant therapeutic interest etc, the matter is usually referred to the CPMP for discussion and decision. This may add a month or two to the processing of such an application.

If an application is refused 'high technology' status, the application is then added to the national assessment queue for that particular category of product in the countries concerned.

There have been a great number of enquiries from companies about using the new procedure but very few have chosen to use it. Those who have chosen to use the procedure have been mainly smaller companies trying to gain marketing authorisation for products for particular specialised 'niche' markets.

15.7 THE CONCERTATION TIMETABLE

The legal timescale for processing applications is the same as is laid down in Directive 65/65/EEC for national applications, but subtracting 30 days for consultation of the CPMP (or CVMP). The timescale is therefore 120 days (the normal period allowed for assessment) +90 days (exceptional additional period allowed for assessment of complex cases) −30 days (period for consulting the CPMP) = 180 days. However, there is provision for 'stopping the clock' according to Article 4(c) of Directive 75/319/EEC to ask the applicant to 'supplement the particulars accompanying the application' (that is, to provide further information or explanation).

The formal timetable is usually preceded by a period of four to six weeks' extra time to allow the rapporteur Member State to produce their initial assessment report. This period is sometimes referred to as the 'pre-assessment' period.

The timetable is proposed by the rapporteur country (usually in discussion with the applicant) and agreed by the CPMP at the first meeting after receipt of the application. It will usually include the following elements:

(a) the date of filing of the application in all of the Member States;
(b) the date of sending out of the assessment report by the rapporteur, with a proposed list of points on which further information or comment is needed from the applicant;
(c) the date by which comments are needed from the other concerned Member States, with any additional points on which further information etc. is needed from the applicant;
(d) the date of CPMP working party (e.g. the Biotechnology/Pharmacy Working Party) meeting at which any special aspect of the issues relating to the product would be discussed to arrive at a consensus and a consolidated list of points;
(e) the date of the CPMP meeting at which a consolidated list of points (relating to safety, efficacy, and quality issues) would be presented; and
(f) the tentative date for any appeal (written representation with optional hearing).

As soon as the applicant receives the consolidated list of points it usually discusses these with the rapporteur, and then agrees a timetable for the appeal process. The written data must be received at least 30 working days before the meeting at which an Opinion will be given, to allow the Experts in the countries concerned sufficient time to evaluate any new data.

In the case of a biotechnology application, the quality/manufacturing issues are often discussed with the applicant at an informal hearing of the Biotechnology/Pharmacy Working Party.

The total length of time needed for a concertation procedure is quite lengthy — typically over a year from the initial filing to the formal Opinion. However, this period includes the period during which the 'clock is stoppped' under Article 4(c) of Directive 75/319/EEC. It should be noted, however, that many of the early biotechnology applications were from companies with limited pharmaceutical and regulatory expertise, where the clinical data were severely restricted, and where the data on manufacturing and process validation were also incomplete. Not surprisingly, the applicants then took a considerable period to answer the concerns raised by the CPMP — often needing to generate further clinical data to support the human safety and efficacy of the product.

15.8 APPEALS

Appeals may be either written representations only, or written representations and then a hearing.

As with the multistate procedure, hearings are an opportunity for the applicant company to present information on issues which remain after the consideration by the Member States of their written representations. The rapporteur advises the company of the outstanding issues about five to seven days before the CPMP meeting, to enable them to arrange for suitable Experts to be present at the hearing, and for them to prepare their case. About six Experts is the maximum that should be needed to present the information at such a hearing.

The total length of a typical CPMP hearing on a biotechnology product is about 45 minutes to one hour. The hearing is unlike some national appeals where the company is allowed to give a long formal presentation (often recapitulating material given in their written representation), and only about ten to fifteen minutes is allowed for the formal presentation on the remaining issues. The rest of the time is taken up by questions from the individual national CPMP delegates and Experts to the company.

15.9 THE SUMMARY OF PRODUCT CHARACTERISTICS (SPC)

Wherever possible, an agreed SPC text (a 'Euro-SPC') is appended to the Opinion, representing the indications, contraindications, warnings, etc. that have been accepted by all of the concerned Member States. It is easier to agree this for a concertation application, because the product has not been licensed in any Member State previously, and the nature of the products considered in the procedure means that national medical custom and practice is much less likely to be a barrier to devising such a common text.

15.10 CHANGES TO THE MARKETING AUTHORISATION ('VARIATIONS')

When a new product has been approved through the concertation procedure, the specifications for starting materials and the finished product, method of manufacture, indications, contraindications, etc. will all have been agreed by all of the concerned Member States. It is, therefore very important, that these are not allowed to diverge as the applicant company wishes to make changes to the product details. Thus, any applications to change the authorisation must be made to all countries, and the rapporteur used to provide a timetable for the consideration of the variation. Simple variations may only need to be notified by the rapporteur to the other countries, and then it would only be if they disagreed with his approach that there would be any need to discuss the matter in the CPMP. More complex variations may need the rapporteur to prepare an assessment report and allow a lengthier timetable for consideration in the CPMP and its working parties.

Some biotechnology products were approved before Directive 87/22/EEC came into force on 1 July 1987. When it is necessary to vary these authorisations, an attempt is made to review all the existing indications as approved in the different countries and to harmonise them. If this attempt succeeds, the major biotechnology products will (in the end) have one set of EC indications and contraindications.

15.11 EXPERIENCE WITH THE BIOTECHNOLOGY PROCEDURE

By the end of July 1990, about 25 biotechnology products had been considered. Some of these were new strengths and new mixtures of existing products (such as insulins), whilst others were innovatory new active substance products. About 12 Opinions had been delivered, and the majority of these were agreed positive Opinions in favour of grant of an authorisation. However, in at least one case there had been a divergent Opinion leading to a preliminary refusal in at least one Member State. Overall, however, the experience with these products has been very acceptable to the companies concerned.

15.12 EXPERIENCE WITH THE HIGH TECHNOLOGY PROCEDURE

As mentioned in section 15.6, the experience with this part of the procedure has been much more limited. One early new active substance product marketing authorisation application was withdrawn from the scheme after considerable technical problems with the data had been revealed. More recent applications have tended to be from smaller companies for specialised 'niche market' products. It is as yet too early to say whether it will be possible to process this category of applications faster than the technically more difficult biotechnology applications. It is likely that more of the major multinational companies will wish to explore the use of this procedure as 1993 approaches, since it is likely to provide useful experience of a procedure which will be replaced with the very similar 'centralised procedure' in 1993.

16

Regulatory strategy: the EC, EFTA, the PER scheme

16.1 REGULATORY STRATEGY

The introduction of new pharmaceutical products onto the market of even one country is a complex undertaking and always involves the development of a marketing strategy — research into competitive products, consideration of what type of advertising and promotion will be needed, deciding what budget will be allocated to the advertising and promotion, etc. Where the product contains a major new innovatory active ingredient (new active substance), which will have cost over $100 million to have developed from the discovery chemistry stage to clinical evaluation in man, it will be necessary to try to market the product in as many countries as possible to try to repay this enormous R and D investment. It is surprising, therefore, that companies often seem to concentrate on filing the marketing authorisation applications for a product in their major markets; the success or otherwise of such filings often seems a matter of luck, not judgement. The success rate of an international regulatory affairs department ought to be judged on the speed with which they obtain authorisations, not on how speedily they file the applications with the authorities. It is as important, therefore, to have a regulatory strategy as to have a marketing or financial strategy — if there are no new products approved there will be none to sell, and the company will suffer a period of 'product drought' where sales of old products are likely to reduce before the new ones come on stream.

Where the very largest companies can seemingly afford to have regulatory staff either in all of the major European markets or specifically to deal with them, the same is not true of the medium or smaller companies. As competition grows in the developing post-1992 Single Market in pharmaceutical products, they will less and less be able to relax in the haven of safe and secure home markets. The future of these medium or small companies is likely to depend on direct sales in other countries or on commercial links with other companies in the other EC Member States who can sell their products for them. These companies will increasingly need to consider how they can use authorisations granted in one country to gain approvals in others. Thus, a thorough knowledge of all of the procedures available to them — national application, multi-state, concertation, is essential. Increasingly, companies are now using the multistate procedure because it gives them experience of the type of 'decentralised' procedure that is likely to be introduced in the post-1992 'future system' (see Chapter 21).

16.1.1 Regulatory strategy in national applications

As with all applications (but see Chapter 12 for further discussion of this question), the most effective regulatory strategy is to submit legible, complete, technically sound, well-documented, indexed, and presented applications with well-argued Expert Reports to highlight and explain the resolution of any problems. However, even if all of this is done, further steps can be taken to improve the success rate of applications.

New active substance (NAS) product marketing authorisation applications are generally given priority over other types of application in nearly all Member States. In some countries, if a suitable case is made, an application can (very exceptionally) receive medical 'fast-tracking'. The clinical case would need to be made to the Director of the national agency, showing, for example, that the new treatment was for a life-threatening condition, and that effective alternative treatments did not exist. In other countries (e.g. Germany), products are sorted into assessment streams or 'baskets', and important new active ingredient products are allocated into the 'fast basket'.

Applications may be sorted nationally into different types, and it is important to know the speed of national agencies in assessing the different types of product. Several countries (e.g. UK, France) assess new active substance applications quickly. Others assess abridged applications more slowly in general. In the UK the 'simple abridged' applications (e.g. applications cross-referring to an existing authorisation to allow another company to market the same product — the so-called 'piggy-back' applications) are processed more quickly, and it would be speedier to use this route rather than to reapply separately, using the same dossier as the first company. If applications are made for additional strengths or line extensions of a new active substance product, and these are filed before the original product is granted, it may be possible to link the files so that they can all be assessed together. In this last case, if the application for the additional strengths had been made after the grant of the authorisation for the NAS, it would be treated as a separate abridged application — with whatever waiting time was necessary in that national abridged queue.

There may be special quirks of national procedure, and these should be known to the astute company regulatory official. In the UK, for example, there is no right of appeal against a refusal for a variation to add a new indication. The device of the 'medically targeted' abridged application has been invented to overcome this problem. In this case, the company makes an application for an abridged licence for the new indication, it is given priority in assessment, and if granted the new licence is 'rolled back' into the existing licence.

16.2 REGULATORY STRATEGY IN CONCERTATION APPLICATIONS FOR BIOTECHNOLOGY PRODUCTS

The factors which influence success have been enumerated by Cartwright (1990):

- quality of the dossier,
- completeness of the data,
- choice of rapporteur country,
- liaison with the rapporteur,
- choice of the three Experts to compile their Expert Report in the application, to critically explain and, justify the methods used, any omissions, etc.
- quality of written responses to the questions raised,
- speed of response to the questions raised,
- quality of response of the company experts at any CPMP hearing,
- speed of response to remaining 'subject to' points after the issue of a favourable CPMP opinion.

These points can be analysed in more detail.

16.2.1 Quality of the dossier

Some of the early biotechnology applications were filed by small inexperienced companies without adequate experience of developing and testing pharmaceutical products. Some of these applications were incomplete, with insufficient numbers of patients to convincingly demonstrate either safety or efficacy, and with inadequate validation of the production methods or the analytical test procedures. Some of these products have now been approved — but only after considerable extra data had been provided, and after waiting for a considerable time to generate these data to give to the CPMP in the appeal.

16.2.2 Choice of the rapporteur country

The rapporteur country does the first assessment and then provides a report with a list of the important objections to give to the other concerned Member States. It is essential to choose a rapporteur who:

- has the capacity to carry out the assessment at that time,
- has the technical expertise to carry out the assessment (i.e. someone who can deal with the complexity of the product involved), and
- who will set a realistic timetable for the other Member States to follow; an unrealistic timetable may leave important issues which remain to be resolved after the CPMP opinion and which delay issue of the authorisation.

If a non-English speaking country is used as rapporteur, there may sometimes be some delay (and additional costs) when the assessment report is translated into other Community languages.

16.2.3 Liaison with the rapporteur
The rapporteur provides the link between the company and the CPMP and gives advice on technical and procedural matters. The company needs to nominate a single person to be their contact point for an application.

16.2.4 Choice of Experts for the Expert Report
Suitable Experts are needed to explain and justify the choice of manufacturing methods, specifications, toxicological tests, etc. These will be particularly crucial in a rapidly changing and developing technology.

16.2.5 Quality of the written response to questions
The company needs to be organised to translate any questions into their own working language and to be able to respond quickly and completely. All questions should be answered. There should be no attempt made to tailor answers or to do deals with individual Member States, since the purpose of the concertation procedure is to end with a single agreed dossier, test procedures, specifications, and text of the summary of product characteristics (SPC). However, if there is any ambiguity in any of the questions raised by any of the Member States it would be reasonable for the applicant company to seek clarification directly, or to ask the rapporteur to do so on its behalf.

16.2.6 Choice of the Experts for hearings
Experts may be needed to address quality issues at informal hearings before the Biotechnology Working Party, or to review the safety and efficacy data before the CPMP. A small number of Experts (up to six) should be used who are able to answer any questions raised.

At a hearing, the rapporteur is normally asked by the chairman of the CPMP to enumerate the outstanding issues (those which have not been completely answered in the written representation), and then the company answers those points only. Member States may then ask supplementary questions to clarify matters.

16.2.7 Response to remaining 'subject to' points
Issues may be outstanding after the hearing. These points should be discussed with the rapporteur after the hearing and then answered as quickly as possible after receipt of the written opinion from the CPMP Secretariat. This will help to expedite issue of the authorisation in all of the concerned countries.

16.3 REGULATORY STRATEGY IN HIGH TECHNOLOGY APPLICATIONS
The factors which influence success in this procedure include the following:

- preliminary liaison with the rapporteur country to determine whether the product is high technology or not;
- choice of a product which fits in well with the criteria defined in List B of Directive 87/22/EEC;
- choice of rapporteur country to act as advocate in the CPMP for the product as being a high technology one according to the criteria, and an Expert Report which

argues a convincing case in relation to the products available in the concerned Member States (e.g. if the product is supposed to be a new delivery system, is this true in all of the countries?);
- completeness of the dossier;
- choice of the three Experts to compile their Expert Report in the application;
- quality and completeness of any written response;
- choice of Experts for any hearing;
- speed and completeness of any response to remaining 'subject to' points in the CPMP Opinion.

16.4 REGULATORY STRATEGY IN THE MULTISTATE PROCEDURE

The factors which influence success in the procedure include the following:

- choice of product and its suitability for registration in a number of EC Member States;
- other similar products approved in those markets and the precedents set in national monographs, guidelines for the approved indications and contra-indications for products with full licences is those countries;
- whether the product is regarded as a licensable medicinal product in those Member States;
- whether the product contains an active regarded as well established in all of the EC countries concerned;
- whether the product is a single active or combination product;
- quality of the dossier (and particularly whether it has been effectively updated since the grant of the original authorisation to the currently accepted EC requirements);
- choice of Experts to write the Expert Report;
- effective liaison with the rapporteur before submission of the application, after receipt of reasoned objections, and before the CPMP meeting at which the Opinion will be given;
- quality of written responses to the reasoned objections;
- choice of experts for the hearing and effective presentation at the hearing;
- prompt follow-up to any outstanding 'subject to' points after the CPMP.

16.5 OVERALL REGULATORY STRATEGY FOR THE PRODUCT

The method of making optimal use of all of the relevant national and CPMP procedures constitutes the strategy for the product. From the point of view of the company, it is effective if it results in grant of as many authorisations as possible in as short a period as possible.

The possible stategies include:

- simultaneous national applications in all of the major EC markets;
- obtaining an approval in one or more EC countries and then using the first approval to make subsequent multistate applications in the other major EC markets;

- simultaneous national applications in most of the major EC markets, and (after seeking approval from the authorities to do so) substituting a multistate application in any EC country which has not picked up the application for assessment at the time the first authorisation is obtained.

Factors influencing the choice of strategy include:

- whether the applicant has regulatory staff in all countries (the multistate procedure is particularly suited to the needs of the small/medium companies);
- whether the application will be full or abridged;
- if the product contains an NAS, whether it will be 'fast-tracked' or receive 'fast stream' treatment;
- the likely processing times for national applications in the Member State(s) concerned for the type of product concerned.

16.6 THE PER SCHEME

The product evaluation report (PER) scheme was started on 13 June 1979 with Austria, Norway, Finland, Sweden, and Switzerland as the founding members. It is a scheme for the mutual recognition of evaluation reports on pharmaceutical products. The objective of the scheme is to facilitate trade in pharmaceutical products by eliminating, through the exchange of evaluation reports, the unjustified re-evaluation of data for registration.

The scheme works by the regular quarterly circulation of lists of new active substance products approved in the member countries. If another country has received an application for the same product, it can ask for a copy of the evaluation report (identical for practical purposes to the EC 'assessment report'). The report is drawn up either in English or in the official language of the issuing country. If translation of the report is needed, this can be done at the expense of the registration holder. The evaluation report is sent to the registration holder for comments and approval within thirty days. If consent is refused, the withholding of consent is notified to the requesting country. The scheme is administered by the European Free Trade Association (EFTA) secretariat in Geneva.

The work of the scheme is coordinated by the PER committee. Their task is to:

- consider measures for achieving the effective operation of the scheme,
- secure the more effective implementation of the scheme with a view to achieving mutual recognition of the previous authorisation.
- promote international cooperation in the field of registration of pharmaceutical products, and
- discuss the participation of other authorities in the scheme.

Other countries have joined the scheme since it began. Germany and Italy joined, and more recently the United Kingdom in March 1988, and the Netherlands in May 1990

Canada and Australia formally joined the scheme in 1990. Hungary has been invited to participate as an observer, and has now formally applied to join the scheme.

Since it joined the scheme, the UK has become the major donor of reports — approximately 67%.

The PER scheme has sometimes been found to be beneficial to companies who have found an expedited issue of an authorisation from one of the countries who participate in the scheme. From the viewpoint of the company, it is also very useful to have the access to the written evaluation report of one of the major authorities. It can learn from this and improve the presentation and analysis of future new active substance applications.

The EFTA Secretariat (who administer the PER scheme) is based in Geneva.

REFERENCE

Cartwright, A. C. (1990). Company strategies in Europe: successful use of the CPMP procedure. *BIRA Journal* **9** (2), 9–11.

17

The United Kingdom's system for licensing pharmaceutical products

17.1 INTRODUCTION

In Chapter 1 the history of the licensing of pharmaceuticals was discussed, including the background to the introduction of the Medicines Act 1968. The United Kingdom's (UK) system of licensing of pharmaceutical products has developed from this major piece of framework or 'enabling' legislation.

In this chapter the system in use during summer 1990 will be outlined as it relates to pharmaceuticals for use in humans. This will include a detailed consideration of the process through which a product licence application (or marketing authorisation application in European Community (EC) parlance) passes before a licence is issued which enables the marketing company to place the product on the UK market.

A brief discussion will also be included concerning certain other procedures which are called upon during the life of the product licence such as that required to introduce changes into existing licensed products and the renewal of product licences.

However, before coming to the market in the first place a company may wish to undertake clinical trials in the UK, and a section is included on the procedures by which authorisation to carry out such trials may be obtained.

There are certain other aspects of the licensing activities of the UK regulatory authority which will not be considered in this chapter: these relate to manufacturers' licences (for UK-based manufacturers) and the scheme associated with changes to them, and to wholesale dealers' licences.

17.2 SOURCES OF INFORMATION

The UK regulatory authority uses as the basis of its pharmaceutical licensing operations the provisions of the Medicines Act 1968, and the Regulations and Orders made under it are also taken into account. A list of relevant Statutory Instruments relating to UK pharmaceuticals regulation is given as Appendix 1. In addition, the provisions of the EC pharmaceutical Directives (65/65/EEC *et seq.*) and the guidance notes and 'Notice to Applicants' issued under their aegis via the Committee for Proprietary Medicinal Products (CPMP) are taken fully into account. To be fully aware of the legal basis of the licensing of pharmaceuticals, interested parties should therefore obtain copies of the primary legislation and of relevant subsidiary documents whether of EC or UK origin.

The regulatory authority also takes into account information included in national guidelines in areas where there are no EC guidelines. For the UK these are usually included in Medicines Advice Leaflets (MALs). Those MALs relating to human medicines are published by or for the Medicines Control Agency. A list of the current MALs is given in Appendix 2.

17.3 PRODUCT LICENCES AND CLINICAL TRIAL CERTIFICATES FOR PHARMACEUTICALS FOR USE IN HUMANS

17.3.1 Introductory remarks

Before describing the stages through which an application passes it is first necessary to discuss briefly the stages of a product's life in which the Medicines Control Agency has a direct interest of one sort or another.

In the very early experimental stages of the development of a product there is no 'official' interest for the Medicines Control Agency. In the UK there is no control over the performance of volunteer studies, although local ethics committee involvement and approval is probably a necessity, and adequate provision for insurance against claims arising from the studies would be prudent.

At some stage it is necessary to start using the product in a clinical situation. In the UK there are three options open for this. The first is the clinician-initiated request for materials to be made available so that the clinician may carry out a trial. In this case the clinician should obtain ethics committee approval and should, in the case of a new ingredient or new dosage form (or for a placebo to be used with marketed products), apply for a Doctors and Dentists Exemption (DDX). Provided that the Medicines Control Agency is not aware of any problems associated with the material or the proposed trial the trialist may continue, but under his own responsibility. (It should be noted that in the UK it is the right of any clinician to use any material for any purpose in the treatment of his own patients, but that he does so on his own responsibility.)

The DDX scheme is for those trials where the pharmaceutical company was not the originator of the trial. For those cases where this is not the case — for example, where the company wishes to organise the trial — there are two other schemes available. These are the clinical trial certificate scheme (CTC) and the clinical trial certificate exemption scheme (CTX).

In most cases the company applies in the first instance for the CTX scheme. This involves negative vetting of the summary of data provided. The advisory committees are not consulted on CTX applications. (The nature of the data requirements will be outlined later.) Objections to the approval of a CTX application have to be raised by the Medicines Control Agency within a very short period following the receipt of the application (35 days, with the option of extending by a further 28 days).

There are no types of application automatically debarred from using the CTX scheme. If a particular application is considered to be unsuitable for the CTX scheme owing to a lack of information, the company is free to resubmit a corrected application under the CTX scheme or to submit an application under the CTC scheme. It is not permissible to submit an application under both the CTX and CTC schemes at the same time. There are applications where the Medicines Control Agency will consider that the CTX scheme is not suitable, for example where it is considered that full data assessment is needed or where advisory committee advice is considered necessary. There is no appeal against the refusal to grant a CTX approval.

The CTC scheme involves a full (positive) assessment of complete data to show that the product is of adequate quality for the intended purpose, and that it is sufficiently safe. It is not necessary to show efficacy at the CTC stage since the clinical trial applied for is presumably intended to demonstrate both efficacy and safety in man.

The quality and preclinical safety data requirements for a CTC and a product licence (PL) are similar, and the processing of the applications is the same. For this reason the processing of CTCs and PLs will be discussed together.

17.3.2 Purpose of an application
The purpose of an application is presumably to gain an authorisation in as short a time as possible. To do this the applicant company should submit adequate information to demonstrate that the product is of adequate quality for its intended use; that it is sufficiently safe; and in the case of a PL that it is efficacious. This may seem to be self-evident, but from the experience of those who work in the regulatory agencies it would seem that it is an aim that is often overlooked. In the licensing of human pharmaceutical products it is noteworthy that the Licensing Authority may not take into account matters other than those relating to quality, safety, and efficacy. Comparative efficacy cannot be taken into account; comparative safety may be.

17.3.3 Application forms
Whenever an application is to be submitted to the Medicines Control Agency the appropriate application form must be completed. For a product licence submission this is MLA (Medicines Licence Application) 201. For a clinical trial certificate it is MLA 202.

These forms are modified from time to time, and it is worth checking that the latest version is available before the company submits its application, since using an out-of-date edition may result in delays in the processing of the application because necessary information may be omitted if earlier editions are used. Information and copies of updated application forms are provided in the Medicines Act Information Letter (MAIL) which is issued by the Medicines Control Agency from time to time, or may be obtained from the Agency.

It is essential that the information included in the MLA forms be very carefully checked since it is against this that the whole application is assessed.

17.3.4 Before submitting the application

Before the application is submitted, the company will of course have checked that the data and Expert Reports required are all available, that the necessary forms have been completed, and that the appropriate number of copies of all documents have been made.

About 10 to 30 days before the company intends to submit the application and supporting data, the Medicines Control Agency should be asked to allocate reference numbers to the applications. A unique reference number will be given to each strength of each dosage form (and also to items such as constituting media or diluents provided with the product) in the case of a PL application. To minimise the opportunity for error (and to speed the registration process) the company should apply the appropriate reference number to each copy of the relevant file. The reference numbers will eventually become the clinical trial certificate (CT) or product licence (PL) numbers.

Before submitting the application it would also be advisable to check that the copies of the document are properly paginated (using an intelligible system) and that the photoprinting quality is adequate: someone will have to read the data in your application!

17.3.5 Submitting the application and supporting data

The number of copies of an application required may vary according to the type of application. In the case of a novel active ingredient a larger number of copies of some parts is required than is the case with an abridged application — for example, because of the reference of such applications to the advisory committees and subcommittees. The requirements vary from time to time, and announcements of changes are given in MAIL. If insufficient numbers of copies of applications are provided, additional copies will be required in due course, and may be requested at short notice.

The address to which the copies of the application and supporting data should be delivered has changed on a number of occasions over the years, and applicants should be certain that they are submitted to the correct address. (Again, notification of changes is included in MAIL.)

17.3.6 Registration

Having been received safely by the Medicines Control Agency, the application will be registered. The unique reference number will be applied to each volume of each copy of the relevant application if this has not already been done by the applicant company. It will be appreciated that this process can be quite slow in the case of a new active substance application which may be accompanied by several copies of up to two hundred volumes of supporting data. This is why it was suggested above that the applicant could accelerate the process by applying the reference number before submitting the application.

A file is raised for the application at this stage, and a copy of the data is attached. This is then sent to the validation section.

17.3.7 Validation

As the name implies, the validation section is responsible for ensuring that the application is valid. It does not undertake an assessment of the data, which is the work of professional assessment staff.

The MLA forms are checked for completeness (including a signature: the application is invalid without a signature). The supporting data are checked for pagination and for the presence of information in English. If data are included in a foreign language a full translation — not a summary — must be provided in English as well as the original paper.

An early task for the validation section is to identify the type of application that has been submitted. This is done from the information included in the application form by the applicant company. On page 1B of MLA 201, under question 10, it is necessary for the applicant company to identify the type of application from amongst a number of different options, such as new active substance (that is, one not previously seen by the Medicines Control Agency); high technology or biotechnology products as defined in the EC 'high tech' Directive; new salts or esters of known drugs; novel delivery systems; a new route of administration for the active material or a new clinical indication; a surgical or dental product; a new source or synthetic route for the active ingredient; a new sterilisation method; a modified release product; etc.

The information on the type of application is used to route it to the appropriate 'Business' (see section 17.3.8) in the Medicines Control Agency where the professional assessment will take place.

In the case of an abridged application submitted under Article 4 (8) (a) of Directive 65/65/EEC (the significance of which is discussed in Chapter 6 [abridged applications]) various additional checks are necessary at validation. Depending on the part of Article 4 (8) (a) under which the application has been submitted, the following information may be required: (1) an authorisation to access data relating to another product licence (or in some cases a drug master file) in which case the authorisation must be in the form of an original communication (not a fax transmission or a photocopy) on the relevant company's official letterhead and bearing a signature known to the Agency; or (2) the identity of a product with which essential similarity is claimed together with the name of its manufacturer and the country and date of first authorisation within the EC, with evidence that the comparator product has been authorised and marketed in the UK in the same pharmaceutical form and strength.

Where reference is made to a drug master file it is essential that the data be held by the Medicines Control Agency. Where this is not the case the application may be returned as invalid. Reference has been made in the past to United States Food and Drug Administration drug master files!

A check is made that the data submitted in support of an application is in general conformity with the requirements of the pharmaceutical Directives data requirements, although no assessment is undertaken at this stage. Compliance with relevant MALs is also checked.

Applications which involve a new active substance are expected to be accompanied by full chemical and pharmaceutical data (or possibly to include a cross-reference to a clinical trial certificate application or to a drug master file). A reference to a CTX application is not normally acceptable for a product licence application since the information provided in support of the CTX is in the form of limited summaries. New active ingredient applications are also expected to be accompanied by full toxicological and pharmacological data and by clinical data.

In the case of other applications, it is always expected that adequate chemistry and pharmacy data will be provided except where an authorised cross-reference is made to a full product licence granted after 1976 or to a recently-reviewed product licence of right. Information will be expected on the drug substance in most cases: exceptions may be made with simple salts and with particularly well-known substances (such as aspirin (acetylsalicylic acid) and paracetamol (acetaminophen)). In the case of a pharmacopoeial material, if the monograph to which reference is made is not in English a translation of the monograph and any relevant methods, general requirements, etc., will be required. It may be necessary to provide evidence of the relevance of the pharmacopoeial specification quoted with reference to the adequacy of control of material made by the synthetic route used by the supplier(s) to be used. In the case of abridged applications the toxicology and pharmacology aspects may be discussed in the clinical Expert Report if no separate report is provided.

In terms of the quality data the validation process includes a check that certain key pieces of information are included, such as stability data (on three batches of finished product for an adequate duration of testing), and antimicrobial preservative efficacy test data in appropriate cases.

Where a new type of formulation is proposed, or for unusual or special products, data are normally expected on aspects relating to bioavailability (and in some cases bioequivalence between different dosage forms or even strengths of the same dosage form). Such data will also be expected where there have been documented cases of bioinequivalence in the literature; or for the first application for a generic version of a product just coming off patent. In some cases it may be felt necessary, usually on clinical grounds, for such data to be provided for all generic versions of a particular drug.

The validation section checks that the Expert Reports have been signed by appropriately-qualified persons, and will seek further advice of professional assessment staff if the Expert does not seem to be acceptable. A check will be made for the superficial completeness of the application, that is that it contains information under all the parts of the application identified in the 'Notice to Applicants' or that justifications are provided for the omission of data.

If deficiencies are identified in the application for which the applicant has not put forward justification, an opportunity is usually given for the missing information to be provided within a reasonable period — usually taken to be within 15 working days. In some cases the application is considered to be too extensively deficient for this period of grace to be allowed, or the missing data may not be forthcoming in a reasonable period. In either case the application is returned as invalid. An accompanying letter explains the deficiencies.

During the validation process, appropriate enquiries are instituted of the Medicines Inspectorate on matters relating to the acceptability of the manufacturing sites named in the application; and of the Agency's trade marks adviser on the acceptability of the proposed proprietary name for the product (if any).

If the application is found to be valid it is now referred for professional assessment. Depending on the type of application it is placed in a chronological queue of applications of the same type which will be assessed by one of the dedicated assessment teams.

17.3.8 Professional assessment

The Medicines Control Agency includes amongst its staff a number of professionally qualified staff whose task is to assess applications. Until recently these staff were formed into pharmaceutical and medical secretariats. This has now changed, and professional staff are allocated to 'Businesses', together with administrative and support staff. Each 'Business' has a defined area of responsibility. The main Business areas of relevance to applicants are those dealing with new products, applications routed via the Committee for Proprietary Medicinal Products (CPMP), and 'biological' — which includes biotechnology — applications (Business A); abridged applications, variations, renewals, applications for reviewed product licences, and applications for dental, surgical, and related products including contact lens care products and ophthalmic products, and radiopharmaceuticals (Business B); and pharmacovigilance (Business C). (Business D is concerned with manufacturers licensing and inspection and enforcement of the Medicines Act; and Business F relates to the British Pharmacopoeia, its secretariat and laboratory. Business E is an 'administrative' business.)

Each of the Businesses responsible for the assessment of applications has allocated to it a number of pharmaceutical and medical assessors. In the case of business A there are also suitably qualified staff who undertake the toxicology and pharmacology assessments. (If another Business requires the services of one of these assessors, they 'contract' for the assessment time needed.)

The assessment of applications is influenced by a number of factors. First and foremost are the requirements of the EC pharmaceutical Directives, the 'Notice to Applicants', and the notes for guidance developed by the CPMP. Included in these provisions is a requirement that applications shall be determined within 120 days (with exceptionally an extension by a further 90 days).

In addition to the EC requirements there are also a number of national guidelines which have to be taken into account in appropriate cases. There are also differences in professional practice between different Member States of the EC which may be of some significance, especially where matters such as diagnosis and treatment are concerned.

When an application for a product licence has been validated it is placed in a queue for professional assessment. As indicated above there are several different queues in practice. There is one for applications submitted through the CPMP (other than specialist cases such as biotechnology and ophthalmic products). A second queue contains new chemical active substance applications. The third is for abridged applications. The fourth is for biological and biotechnological products, blood products, and immunological products. The fifth queue is for dental and surgical products, including medicated toothpastes, contact lens care products, non-oral contraceptive products, and ophthalmic products. Separate queues are also kept of product licence applications for parallel imported products and for applications to change product licences (commonly known as 'variations')

In the case of abridged applications a special scheme of 'triage' has been operated whereby experienced pharmaceutical and medical assessors take a look at the information gleaned during the validation process and try to identify those cases that will obviously require additional data — for example, where a bioavailability study will required but has not been submitted — so that these may be returned to the applicant quickly for the deficiencies to be remedied. Other types of application that will require minimal assessment — for example, cross-references to a recently granted product licence — are also identified and processed rapidly. This is also true of the pharmaceutical assessment of abridged applications for products where the only reason for the application is to gain some additional clinical indications.

Having been allocated to a list, the application will await an assessor being free to begin the assessment. In the case of an application for a new active substance or a CPMP application it is likely that the assessment will be undertaken in parallel by the pharmaceutical, toxicological/pharmacological (or 'scientific'), and medical assessors. Most other cases will be subject to sequential assessment, with the medical assessment following on from the pharmaceutical assessment.

The role of the assessors is to determine whether, in their professional opinion, the applicant company has made an adequate case for the quality, safety, and efficacy of the product described in the application, taking into account the claims made in the application forms. If the assessors are satisfied they can advise that the product licence be issued. To get to this stage may, of course, involve a process of discussion with the applicant, and possibly requests for additional information. Such requests for information may be made relatively informally — for example, in a telephone conversation — or by using a formal procedure described in Section 44 of the Medicines Act 1968, thus giving these formal communications the title 'section 44 letters'. Provided that any additional information satisfies the assessors, this interim process need not delay the grant of the licence unduly — the delays are most likely to be due to the response time of the applicant in dealing with the points raised.

17.3.9 Reference to advisory bodies

If the assessor(s) are not content that the information provided is adequate for a product licence to be granted, or if the terms in which the application is drafted are not acceptable (for example, imprecise or unacceptable clinical indications), it is obligatory that the application be referred to the advisory committees, where a report is presented summarising the application and the original data, submitted as necessary to some or all of the committee members. It is normal practice for all new active ingredient applications to be referred to the advisory committees, as are certain other categories of application including novel delivery systems and the first application for a generic version of a product just coming off patent. All committee consideration is carried out under strict confidentiality. Section 118 of the Medicines Act makes this obligatory.

There are three levels of advisory committee available to the Medicines Control Agency. The first of these is the expert subcommittees: the chemistry pharmacy and standards subcommittee (CPS); the safety efficacy and adverse reactions subcommittee (SEAR); and the biologicals subcommittee, which are the most commonly used. The membership of these subcommittees is drawn from academia and the hospital service of the United Kingdom. In addition to the normal membership, individuals with specialist knowledge may be appointed as members for a particular meeting at which a relevant application is to be discussed.

The next tier of advisory committees is those bodies set up under Section 4 of the Medicines Act 1968, and thus known as 'section 4 committees'. These are the Committee on Safety of Medicines (CSM), the Committee on Dental and Surgical Materials (CDSM), and the Committee on the Review of Medicines (CRM). In addition, the British Pharmacopoeia Commission (BPC) is a section 4 Committee (although it does not deal with product licensing matters) as is the Veterinary Products Committee (VPC) (which is operated through the Veterinary Medicines Directorate rather than the Medicines Control Agency). Membership of these bodies is drawn from academia and the hospital service with the exception of the BPC which includes industrialists among it membership in addition to those employed in the government service or academia or the hospital service. Each of the section 4 committees has a defined remit.

The final tier of advisory committees is the Medicines Commission, which is set up under the terms of Section 2 of the Medicines Act 1968. The composition of the Medicines Commission is laid down in the Medicines Act, and includes representatives of the pharmaceutical industry and the professions (including lawyers, doctors, and pharmacists).

In the past there have been other advisory bodies — such as the subcommittee on ophthalmic products (SCOP), and the Committee on Radiation from Radioactive Medicinal Products (CRRMP). These have been disbanded.

If an application is referred to the advisory committees it is usual for it to be referred first to the relevant subcommittee(s). The members of the subcommittee(s) consider a summary of the application and relevant parts of the original data, and make recommendations. These recommendations are referred with the summary paper to the section 4 committee relevant for the application. The committee will make a recommendation which is then considered by the Licensing Authority.

Under the terms of the Medicines Act 1968 the Licensing Authority consists of the Ministers of the government responsible for health matters. In practice, most of the powers are delegated by the other health Ministers to the Secretary of State for Health. In turn, most of the day-to-day matters are dealt with by his staff, usually under the responsibility of the Director of the Medicines Control Agency.

The advice that can be offered by the advisory committees includes: grant the licence as requested; grant the licence if certain conditions are met (and the conditions might be quite far-reaching); or that the committee has it in mind to recommend that the application should be refused on grounds related to quality or safety or efficacy or any combination of those grounds.

When the advice is considered by the Licensing Authority there are two options open. The advice can be accepted, or not: this is why the committees are described as 'advisory'. In practice it is unlikely that a committee recommendation would be overturned without very good reason.

If the advice is that the licence should be granted it would be usual for this to be done as quickly as possible. If the Licensing Authority decides that this cannot be done for some reason, then the normal appeal procedures — described below — do not apply. A special process known as the 'person appointed' procedure comes into play. This is discussed later.

If the advice is that the licence can be granted provided that certain conditions are met, then a letter is raised in which the conditions are laid out. This letter must be replied to in general terms within 28 days. If the company is not able to accept one or more of the conditions or if any additional information submitted in response to the conditions (which need not be submitted within 28 days) is felt not to be acceptable, then a letter will be sent which converts the 'grant subject to' letter to a 'minded to advise that the application be refused' letter, stating the reasons. This communication is sent under the terms of Section 21(1) of the Medicines Act 1968 and is usually known as a 'section 21(1) letter'. A section 21(1) letter will also be sent if the advice of the committee is that the licence should not be granted.

When a section 21(1) letter is received it that the company has the right to appeal against the committee's advice. This appeal can take the form of the provision of additional written information (a 'written representation') or by means of a personal appearance before the committee (a 'hearing'). The company is required to state within 28 days whether or not they wish to take up the right of appeal, and which form the appeal is to take.

Even when a hearing is chosen it is likely that a large percentage of the information to answer the committee's points will be available in hard copy. This can usefully be submitted for advance consideration by the committee. It is not unusual for the written evidence alone to satisfy the committee, thus eliminating the need for a hearing.

In the case of a written representation the company submits its written data, and these are assessed by the appropriate professional staff. In the case of pharmaceutical assessment it has been normal practice to use the same assessor for the first assessment and the appeal to the section 4 committees. Medical assessments are usually undertaken by a different assessor at each stage. The small number of scientific assessors limits the flexibility in terms of who undertakes the appeal assessment.

A committee paper is prepared and copies of the written evidence are submitted with it to the subcommittee members, and then, with the subcommittee's recommendations, to the section 4 committee. After consideration of the evidence and the advice from the subcommittees the committee will make a recommendation. This might be to grant the product licence; to grant the product licence if certain conditions are met; or to refuse the application on grounds relating to those of the original objections as laid down in the section 21(1) letter. If any new concerns or grounds are identified as a result of the appeal it is open to the committee to raise those objections in a new section 21(1) letter.

If the Licensing Authority accepts the advice the appropriate action will be taken as before, giving the right of a further appeal stage if the recommendations are not acceptable to the applicant company.

In the case of a hearing it is advisable for the appellant company to submit as much information as possible in written format in advance of the hearing. The written information will be professionally assessed and usually referred through the appropriate subcommittees to the section 4 committees together with provisional recommendations from the subcommittees. They are provisional because the subcommittees will not have had the opportunity to hear what is said at the hearing itself, which might put a completely different light on the written information.

The committee will consider the written evidence and the advice of the subcommittees. It might be that many of the points raised in the original section 21(1) letter will have been satisfactorily answered by the written information alone. If all of the initial objections to the grant of the product licence have been answered satisfactorily, then the committee might advise that the licence be granted in the terms now applied for without actually progressing to a hearing. If all of the major points have been satisfied but there are certain minor points or conditions still to be agreed, the committee may recommend that the product licence be granted if certain conditions are met. The hearing may or may not be needed in such cases, depending on the acceptability of the conditions to the appellant company. The third possibility is that only some of the points have been satisfactorily addressed, and the committee may advise the company to attend the hearing but to base their presentation on the outstanding points of concern.

When attending the hearing the company representatives are ushered into the committee meeting room. The members of the committee sit along one side of a long table with the chairman and members of the committee secretariat on the other. The team making the company's presentation is shown to a raised area at one end of the table. The chairman introduces himself and the members of the committee and asks whether the company has any objections to the presence of the Secretariat. Even if the company does object, certain members of the staff have to remain to ensure the smooth running of the proceedings and to prepare a note of the appeal. Next the chairman explains the procedures and asks the company representatives to give an assurance that all relevant information, for and against the product, has been made available to the licensing authority. Assuming that the answer is affirmative, then the chairman asks the leader of the presentation team to introduce his colleagues. The company is then free to make its presentation (possibly restricting this to any outstanding points) as it wishes. Overhead projection and 35-mm slide projection equipment is available, but the room shape is not amenable to good use of such presentation aids, and hard copy should be provided for those present at the meeting.

At the conclusion of the company's presentation there is an opportunity for the members of the committee to ask questions with a view to clarifying the information presented. However, there is no obligation for members to ask questions: it is for the company to make its own case. If no questions are asked, the company may have answered all of the objections of the committee or none of them!

After any questions from the committee members the company has a further opportunity to sum up before being ushered from the room. Once they have left, the members of the committee discuss the evidence made available to them both in any written submission and verbally at the hearing. A recommendation is made to the Licensing Authority. As before, the advice might be grant; grant on condition; or refuse on grounds relating to those originally included in the section 21(1) letter. If any new grounds have been identified they may have to be included in a new section 21(1) letter.

The Licensing Authority considers the advice as before. If the advice is that the grant of a licence cannot be recommended, then a letter is raised under section 21(3) of the Medicines Act to give further rights of appeal to the Medicines Commission.

In the case of a 'grant subject to' recommendation the company has the usual opportunity to accept or reject the conditions and to provide supporting evidence as necessary before the product licence is issued or the notification of the committee's findings is converted to a letter under section 21(3) of the Medicines Act.

The final appeal on scientific grounds is to the Medicines Commission. The assessment of any written evidence is usually undertaken by different assessors. The procedures are similar to those described above for written representations or hearings. The Medicines Commission does not seek advice from the expert subcommittees except in very exceptional circumstances, and does not refer cases back to the section 4 committees. The outcome is advice to the Licensing Authority that the licence should be granted, granted if certain conditions are met, or refused on relevant grounds.

There is no further appeal after the Medicines Commission on scientific matters.

17.3.10 Other appeal procedures

The committee appeal procedures apply only in the case of matters relating to applications for product licences or clinical trial certificates, and then only for matters relating to quality, safety, and efficacy.

Where the Licensing Authority does not accept the advice from its advisory committees (section 4 committees or the Medicines Commission) a different procedure comes into play. This is the 'person appointed' procedure. The 'person' will usually be a small panel of experts in the relevant field. Servants of the Minister can be members of the panel only if the applicant does not object to their presence.

The person appointed procedure is also used for non-product licence related matters (for example, manufacturers licences) and for matters not related to quality, safety, and efficacy (for example, legal status).

The Statutory Instrument which lays down the procedure is the Medicines Act 1968 (Hearings by persons appointed) Rules 1968. This requires a notice to be sent to the applicant 28 days before the hearing. The applicant has the option of the person appointed hearing being held in public. A copy of each document to be considered at the hearing must be supplied to the applicant. The procedures adopted at the hearing will be determined by the person appointed, but in practice are likely to be similar to those described above. The applicant has the right to appear in person or be represented by any other person, to call witnesses, and to address the person appointed. In addition, any member of the Council on Tribunals may attend.

At the conclusion of the hearing the person appointed prepares a report including findings. This is sent to the Minister, and a copy is sent to the applicant.

For applications that have followed the normal appeal procedures but have been unsuccessful, there are no further grounds for scientific appeal. However, the company is able to appeal to the High Court if it considers that procedural irregularities have occurred, such as a decision being made which is outside the powers of the Medicines Act or a failure to comply with the requirements of the Act or its Regulations.

Finally, the company is free to seek a judicial review under Order 53 of the Rules of the Supreme Court, for example if it feels that the rules of natural justice have not been observed.

17.3.11 The issue of a product licence or clinical trial certificate

Having come through the assessment procedure (and possibly the appeal procedures) the application is, one hopes, found to be satisfactory — although the terms in which the approval is to be given may be rather different from those in which it was originally submitted, of course. The last operation to be undertaken is to prepare and issue the licence or certificate documents.

These are prepared from the original MLA forms submitted with the application, as amended by any later modifications. It is important that whenever the applicant company makes a change to the application which affects any of the information on the MLA forms, they should also submit revised copies of those forms.

The licence or certificate is then issued. The company should examine this carefully to ensure that no errors have accidentally crept into the document. Any errors should be referred to the Medicines Control Agency for correction and for the corrected document to be reissued.

17.3.12 Processing of applications routed *via* the Committee for Proprietary Medicinal Products

These applications are subject to very tight deadlines: the EC 120-day deadline is rigidly applied with respect to the submission of the Member States' objections. If any Member State fails to submit objections within the period of 120 days it is assumed that that Member State has no objections and that the marketing authorisation will be issued in that Member State.

The clock starts when the CPMP Secretariat sends a telex confirming that all relevant Member States have received a valid application. Within 120 days all Member States concerned must have identified any objections. For this timescale to be met it might not always be possible for the UK advisory committees to be involved before the case is considered by the CPMP. In any case, the application will be referred back for consideration by the advisory committee in the UK once the CPMP opinion is available in appropriate cases (such as new drugs or applications about which the licensing authority has doubts). The advice of the CPMP will be taken into account when the advisory committees come to their recommendations.

17.4 THE CLINICAL TRIAL EXEMPTION SCHEME

17.4.1 The scope of the scheme

The clinical trial exemption (CTX) scheme was introduced as a rapid process which would allow a negative vetting procedure to be applied to summarised applications prior to a clinical trial being undertaken. It can apply to any type of application for clinical trials from an existing product being investigated for new indications to a totally new product.

17.4.2 How the procedure works

When an application under the CTX scheme is submitted it is normally processed within a period of 35 days from the receipt of a valid application, although this period may be extended by a further 28 days for stated reasons. The application is required to contain a summary of information on the quality and the safety of the product. Guidance on the information requirements is given in the *Guidance notes on applications for clinical trial certificates and clinical trial exemptions (MAL 4)* and the first supplement to those guidance notes. Additional guidance is included in certain other MALs — for example MAL 39 on products containing herbal ingredients, MAL 41 on biological medicinal products, in the annex on contact lens care products in MAL 2, and MAL 61 for intrauterine contraceptive devices.

The data requirements depend on the status of the active ingredients (pharmacopoeial, previously licenced, or novel); the intended route of administration; the dosage, frequency of administration and duration proposed for the clinical trial; and the inclusion of any novel excipient or the use of a known excipient for a new route of administration.

The application should be accompanied by the appropriate application form (MLA 164), fully completed. A single reference number will be allocated on receipt which covers all dosage forms and strengths of the trial product requested together with comparator products and placebos.

The application is not validated in a formal sense. It is referred immediately for assessment as soon as a file has been raised.

Applications for new active substances will be assessed in parallel by a pharmaceutical assessor, a scientific assessor, and a medical assessor. (Where necessary, specialist advice will be sought.) Such applications are discussed at regular meetings. Other applications are usually assessed sequentially but will not normally be discussed at the meetings unless some particularly difficult issue is identified.

After assessment, a recommendation is made by the professional assessors. This results in a letter being sent to the applicant. The letter will either state that there are no objections to the proposed trial(s) continuing, or that there are stated objections. The letter may also include remarks on specific aspects of the data or assumptions on which the assessment is based on the part of the professional assessors.

There are no appeal rights associated with the CTX scheme. If an application is unsuccessful the company can submit another application for a CTX when any deficiencies have been made good. Alternatively, an application can be made for a clinical trial certificate (CTC), with full data being submitted and full appeal rights.

17.5 CHANGES TO LICENCES, CERTIFICATES, AND EXEMPTIONS

17.5.1 Scope

Once a product licence or clinical trial certificate or clinical trial exemption has been issued it is probable that at some time it will be necessary to change details of the product or its indications, specifications, name, container, shelf life, etc. To do this it is necessary to submit an application to change the details of the licence or certificate or exemption. There are certain types of change that cannot be made by this procedure: the most common one is the change of a licence/certificate/exemption holder. (The licences, etc., are not transferrable, and a new application must be submitted in order to change the holder of the authorisation.)

17.5.2 The procedures

Changes to product licences are dealt with by Business B; CTX changes and clinical trial certificates changes are dealt with by Business A. The application must be on the correct form (depending on whether a PL, CTC, or CTX is being changed) and be accompanied by relevant supporting data as well as amended pages for the MLA 201, MLA 202, MLA 164, etc.

Applications for changes are not validated. They are linked with the appropriate files and referred on for assessment as required. The routing of a change application will depend on the nature of the change requested: it might involve administrative staff, pharmaceutical and/or medical assessors, the Medicines Inspectorate, or the Agency's trade marks adviser. During assessment the assessors may contact the company with requests for clarification or additional data or assurances.

After assessment the assessors will advise whether the application should be approved or not, and in relevant cases will comment on the fee indicated as appropriate in the application form.

Applications for changes may be approved or refused (with reasons being stated). There are no appeal rights. Very few such applications are referred to the advisory committees, but even where this is done there are no rights of appeal to the advisory committee. To obtain appeal rights it is necessary to submit an abridged application for a product licence or an application for a clinical trial certificate which incorporates the requested change.

17.6 RENEWALS

17.6.1 Scope

All product licences are granted for a period of five years from the date of issue. Before the end of the five years the company holding the product licence must apply for it to be renewed. Clinical trial certificates and exemptions are granted for a period of two years, and again the holder is responsible for applying for a renewal before the expiry date.

EC pharmaceutical Directives require that applicants take due account of developments during the lifetime of the product. It may therefore be appropriate for certain information to be updated at the time of renewal.

17.6.2 The procedures

The application for renewal should be provided on the appropriate forms, be accompanied by any necessary data, and be accompanied by the appropriate fee. If any changes are to be introduced at the time of the renewal it is necessary to submit at the same time separate applications for approval of those changes.

After professional assessment, applications for renewal may be referred to the advisory committees. Full appeal rights apply in such cases.

17.7 LEGAL STATUS AND RELATED TOPICS

17.7.1 Introduction

The legal status of a product with a full product licence is determined by the ingredients contained in it and, in some cases, by its pharmaceutical form or route of administration. Part III of the Medicines Act makes the normal legal status for medicinal products 'pharmacy sale' — that is, they should be sold or supplied through community or hospital pharmacies by or under the supervision of a pharmacist.

Provision is made for certain products to be made available only on the prescription or order of an appropriate medical, surgical, or dental practitioner.

Certain other categories of persons may have access to prescription only or pharmacy medicines under certain circumstances.

Further provision is made for certain products to be made available without any professional supervision, that is through general sales outlets.

There are also some categories of product controlled under the Medicines Act to which Part III was not applied. Such products do not have a legal status. Examples are absorbable surgical products and products used in connection with contact lens care.

17.7.2 Proposed method of sale

In an application form for a product licence there is a section asking for details of the proposed method of sale or supply for the product. This should be consistent with the legal status of the product. Due account may also be taken of other factors such as the pack size or the claimed indications or other factors which may argue against the product being supplied direct to the public. Thus the labelling of what would be a general sales list (GSL) product could indicate that a particular product should be restricted to supply through a pharmacy by applying the 'P' symbol; or it could be indicated that a pharmacy sale product should be supplied only on the prescription of an appropriate practitioner. Such labelling is, of course, advisory: it does not of itself change the legal status of the product.

In addition, there are some examples where the Licensing Authority has taken advice from the relevant section 4 committees and has adopted a policy that certain products should be restricted in their proposed method of sale. An example of this is with contact lens care products, which should be supplied only through professional (optician or pharmacy) outlets.

17.7.3 Prescription only medicines
It was indicated earlier that the natural status of all products with a full product licence is as a pharmacy or 'P' medicine. In deciding which products are to be made available on prescription of an appropriate practitioner a number of factor are taken into account. These include whether the product represents a known or potential hazard; whether its use could give rise to an adverse ratio of risk to benefit; whether its use could give rise to physical or psychological dependence; and whether the product is capable of endangering the health of the community if it is not properly safeguarded.

A product is made prescription only (POM) by the inclusion of its active ingredient or ingredients in a Medicines (Prescription Only) Amendment Order. In some cases specified products are named in the Orders, thus making them specifically POM. Any product administered parenterally is a POM, except for insulins which are pharmacy medicines.

It is possible for exemption from POM restrictions to be granted for certain ingredients subject to certain restrictions such as a maximum permitted single dose or daily dose not being exceeded, or limitations on the indications that may be promoted to the public. An example of this is the provision of products containing small quantities of codeine phosphate in combination with aspirin in tablets or on its own in a linctus, subject to a maximum single dosage and maximum daily dosage restriction. There are also provisions for the supply of a limited amount of a POM product in an emergency.

There are specific provisions for the sale, supply, or use of POM products by certain people who would not otherwise have access to them. Examples of these include registered ophthalmic opticians (who can sell or supply ophthalmic products containing mafenide propionate, up to 30 per cent sulphacetamide sodium, up to 4 per cent of sulphafurazone as its diethanolamine compound, or atropine sulphate, bethanecol chloride, carbachol, cyclopentolate hydrochloride, homatropine hydrobromide, hyoscine hydrobromide, naphazoline hydrochloride or nitrate, neostigmine methylsulphate or salicylate, pilocarpine hydrochloride or nitrate, or tropicamide, provided that the sale is in the course of their professional practice and in an emergency), the Royal National Lifeboat Institution (so far as is necessary for the treatment of sick or injured persons), or the owner or master of a ship not carrying a doctor as part of the ship's complement (so far as is necessary for the treatment of those on board the ship), or the operator or commander of an aircraft (for the immediate treatment of sick or injured persons carried on the aircraft, on the basis of a written order signed by a doctor and excluding parenteral products).

17.7.4 General sales list products
The Medicines Act indicates in section 53 the conditions under which a medicinal product may be supplied through general sales outlets. A major requirement is that the product shall have been manufactured and packed other than at the retail site, and that it shall be sold in unopened containers. To be acceptable for supply through

general sales outlets there may be restrictions on the maximum single or maximum daily dosage, the maximum amount of active ingredient in the dosage form, the dosage form itself, the proposed uses, the route of administration, and the pack size. Any product which does not comply with the restrictions becomes a pharmacy medicine.

The following types of product cannot be supplied through general sales outlets: eye drops and eye ointments; enemas; parenterally-administered products and irrigations for wounds, bladder, or rectum; products containing aspirin (acetylsalicylic acid) or aloxiprin for administration to children; and anthelminthics.

Products for external use (that is application to the skin, hair, teeth, mucosa of the mouth, throat, nose, eye, vagina, or anal canal) may be suitable for general sales outlets where only local action is intended and where systemic absorption is unlikely to occur. Throat sprays, pastilles, lozenges, or tablets; nasal drops, sprays, and inhalations; and babies' teething preparations are not considered to be suitable for general sales.

17.7.5 The determination of legal status

Legal status of a product may be controlled by its ingredients or its dosage form. It is possible to make a product general sales list (GSL) for a period of two years by means of a product licence. It is also possible to allow a product to become GSL for a period of one year through a change to the terms of the product licence (a 'variation'). In both cases it is necessary to issue a Medicines (General Sales List) (Amendment) Order to make the change permanent.

For a product containing a previously unlicensed active ingredient it is possible to make the product POM through its licence for a period of five years. During this five-year period it is necessary to issue a Medicines (Prescription Only Medicine) (Amendment) Order, or the product will revert to pharmacy medicine status on the first renewal of its product licence. It is not possible to change the status of a licensed product to POM by using a change to the terms of the licence.

When the Medicines Act came into force in the UK in 1971 there were a large number of medicines already on the market. These were allowed 'product licences of right' (PLRs), all of which were due to be reviewed in due course. In practice, because of requirements in the EC pharmaceutical Directives, the review of all PLRs was to be completed by May 1990. The review process involves the company submitting a dossier to show the adequacy of the quality, safety, and efficacy of the product and the assessment of the dossier. Where necessary, applications have been submitted to the Committee on the Review of Medicines (CRM) or the Committee on Dental and Surgical Materials (CDSM).

An application for a reviewed product licence includes a request for a specified legal status. Up to the issue of a reviewed product licence PLR products with a GSL status are listed in Schedule 2 to the General Sales List Order; once a reviewed licence has been issued the product is transferred to Schedule 1 to maintain its GSL status. The review process includes a consideration of the appropriateness of the claimed legal status for the product. Where the advisory committee considers that a change is required from GSL to another status, then the applicant has the right to appeal against that advice.

17.7.6 Changing legal status

It is possible for a product licence holder or for other intertested parties — for example, professional bodies, consumer groups — to request that the legal status of a product be changed. Useful background information for anyone wishing to do so may be found in Medicines Act Information Letters 37 and 46. (These are available from the Medicines Control Agency.)

It is possible to end the product licence-imposed five-year POM restriction on a new active ingredient-containing product at any time by using a Section 59(2) Order under the Medicines Act. To do this, full supporting data (which will be discussed later) must be submitted, assessed, and found suitable. One mechanism for this is to submit a product licence application specifically to change the legal status. However, the legal status aspect of a full product licence application is not the subject of appeal rights to the advisory committees. The Licensing Authority will normally take advice on at least the legal status aspects of such applications from the appropriate section 4 committee, probably the Medicines Commission and possibly a panel of experts in the appropriate field. If the advice is in favour of the change and the Licensing Authority is minded to accept that advice, then a formal consultative process has to be followed involving all potentially interested parties. Assuming that this consultative procedure raises no new objections of substance, the Licensing Authority then prepares an amendment to the POM list, and, once this has been approved by Parliament, published, and brought into effect, the legal status of the product is changed.

If it is wished to add a product to the general sales list it is possible to obtain a temporary change in legal status by means of a change to an existing product licence or by means of a specific application for a product licence to achieve this end. In neither case is there an automatic right of appeal to an advisory committee. Supporting data are required to justify the inclusion of a new product in the GSL. This needs to address a number of points and to provide convincing evidence that the product contains 'safe' substances. In assessing the submission due account is taken of any need for the product to be taken only under professional supervision. Another factor that is taken into account is the need for a pharmacist's advice on the method of use of the product. A third factor to be considered is the suitability of the claimed indication(s) for advertising to the public.

The appropriate advisory committees and panel is usually consulted by the Licensing Authority, and, if this is successful and the Licensing Authority is minded to change the legal status of the product permanently, a formal consultative process follows. If this is also successful, then a Medicines (General Sales List) Amendment Order is placed before Parliament and, if approved, the legal status of the product is changed once the order has ben published and brought into effect.

Several types of supporting data might be included in an application to change legal status. Epidemiological data showing the safety of the product or ingredient are useful. Toxicological data may be required, including teratology and carcinogenicity studies where necessary (for example, where data have not previously been submitted or where the studies previously reported are not in accordance with current expectations). Pharmacokinetic studies showing the rate and extent of systemic absorption may be needed — for example, with a topically-applied product.

Comparisons with other formulated products may be useful. If the same drug has been marketed abroad for some time, then a summary of experience may be provided. Any candidate product for a lesser level of control than exists at the moment should be accompanied by data relating to considerable numbers of patients gained over a reasonable period.

Where the indications claimed for a product are changed it might be necessary to provide additional data to demonstrate the efficacy of the product in those indications. Where appropriate, particular attention should be drawn by the company to indications, warnings, pack sizes, labelling, and marketing plans relevant to the requested legal status. The company should also give particular thought to safety warnings appropriate to the intended use of the product.

17.7.7 Examples of special cases
17.7.7.1 Radiopharmaceuticals

The legal status of radiopharmaceuticals is determined by the ingredient, rather than by any inherent radioactivity. This has little practical effect since the supply and use of radioactive materials for the clinic is controlled separately.

The Medicines (Radioactive Substances) Order 1978 (Statutory Instrument [SI] 1978 No. 1004, or 1978 No. 1006) defines a radioactive substance for medicinal purposes as a substance containing one or more radionuclides of which the activity or the concentration cannot be disregarded as far as radiation protection is concerned. The Order, made under section 104 of the Medicines Act, extended the provisions of that Act to interstitial and intracavity appliances (other than nuclear powered cardiac pacemakers) intended to contain a radioactive substance sealed or bonded within the material and intended to be inserted into the human body or human cavities; and to surface applicators containing a sealed or bonded material intended to be brought into contact with the human body; to any apparatus capable of administering neutrons in order to generate a radioactive substance in the person to whom they are administered for the purpose of diagnosis or research; and to other substances or articles (not instruments, apparatus, or appliances) which consist of or contain or generate a radioactive substance which is administered in order to utilise the emitted radiation.

A separate Order controls the administration of radioactive substances. This is the Medicines (Administration of Radioactive Substances) Regulations 1978 (SI 1978 No. 1006). These regulations cover the use of radioactive materials for diagnosis, treatment, or research.

Radioactive medicinal products may be administered only by doctors or dentists specifically authorised (by means of the grant of a certificate) to do so, or persons acting in accordance with the directions of such a doctor or dentist. The authority to administer radioactive substances may specify particular descriptions or classes of radioactive medicinal product that may be used by a particular practitioner. In some cases the purposes for which radioactive materials may be administered may also be stated.

The provision of the certificates involves an advisory committee known as the Administration of Radioactive Substances Advisory Committee (ARSAC). The majority of the members of this Committee are required to be doctors, but membership is also extended to others with relevant and wide recent experience in the field of the administration of radioactive medicinal products and related scientific and radiological safety matters. It is possible for certificates to be suspended, revoked or varied, with an appeal mechanism to allow for hearings or written representations. ARSAC is set up under powers derived from EURATOM Directives.

17.7.7.2 Breathing gases
Under the terms of the Medicines (Breathing Gases) Order 1977 (SI 1977 No. 1488) oxygen, air, or any mixture of both or of either with any inert gases or nitrogen (whether compressed or not) which are administered to human beings other than for treatment or diagnosis of any disease caused or aggravated by conditions such as abnormal atmospheric pressure, lack or contamination of air, etc., are specifically exempted from the Medicines Act.

17.7.7.3 Surgical materials
The Medicines (Surgical Materials) Order 1971 (SI 1971 No. 1267) brought under the Medicines Act three classes of materials by means of a section 104 Order. The types of material included are: surgical ligatures and sutures made from the gut or other tissues of an animal for use in surgical operations on the human body; any other surgical ligature or suture for use in operations on the human body which is capable of being absorbed by the body tissues; and any absorbent or protective material used in surgical operations on the human body capable of being absorbed by the body tissues. The relevant part of Part III of the Medicines Act concerned with legal status was not activated in the Order. These products therefore have no legal status.

17.7.7.4 Contact lenses and contact lens care products
The Medicines (Specified Articles and Substances) Order 1976 (SI 1976 Number 968) enabled three classes of product to be controlled under the Medicines Act by means of an order made under section 104. These were contact lenses and blanks from which contact lenses could be prepared; products used in the care of contact lenses or lens blanks; and instruments, apparatus, or appliances inserted in the human uterus or cervix for the purpose of contraception (including intrauterine contraceptive devices).

The Order has been activated for intrauterine contraceptive devices and for contact lens care products. At the time of writing the Order has not been activated in connection with contact lenses or blanks.

The types of contact lens care products covered by the Order are those used for cleaning, disinfecting, irrigating, lubricating, wetting, or storing contact lenses or blanks, as well as any fluid in which the lens or blank is soaked or rinsed or used as a barrier between the lens and the eyeball, or any other substance used in connection with a lens or blank. The full provisions of Part III of the Medicines Act relating to legal status are not activated in the Order: these products do not have a legal status. (It is, however, the advice of the Committee on Dental and Surgical Materials that such products be supplied only through professional outlets.)

17.7.7.5 *Topical hydrocortisone creams and ointments*

Most hydrocortisone products are POMs. It is possible to have a pharmacy medicine ('P') status for hydrocortisone creams and ointments in certain circumstances.

To become a 'P' medicine, a hydrocortisone product should contain not more than one per cent of hydrocortisone or hydrocortisone acetate and be presented in a cream or ointment which does not contain any added ingredient which is likely to significantly increase the availability of the active ingredient. The container should hold 10 to 15 grams of the product. In the case of low-dose or novel formulations, data may be required to demonstrate efficacy.

Pharmacy sale-status hydrocortisone topical products should have limited clinical indications: irritant dermatitis, contact allergic dermatitis, and insect bite reactions. Eczema and rash should not be mentioned, nor 'dermatitis' unless suitably qualified. The product should be contra-indicated for use on the face or eyes, the anogenital region, and on broken or inflamed skin (including cold sores, acne, and athlete's foot).

The instructions for use should carry a direction that the product should be used sparingly over a small area once or twice daily for a maximum period of one week. It should be stated that if the condition does not improve, then a doctor should be consulted. Particular warnings should be included to the effect that the product should not be used on children under ten years of age without medical supervision; and a special warning concerning use during pregnancy should also be included.

To gain pharmacy sale-status it is necessary to submit a suitable abridged application. This should carefully take into account the guideline included in MAL 2 (guidelines for applications for product licences) for this type of application. Assuming the application to be successful, the status of the product becomes 'P' once a Medicines (Prescription Only Medicines) (Amendment) Order listing the name and product licence number comes into force.

17.7.8 An outline of the legal status position in the EC

There are restrictions on the sale and supply of medicinal products in all Member States of the EC. The nature of the controls varies from country to country and from product to product.

The supply of narcotics and drugs liable to abuse is controlled in all Member States of the EC. There are also restrictions in all Member States on products which may be supplied only by or on the prescription of an appropriate practitioner. There is reasonable consistency across the EC regarding the supply of certain products only through pharmacies, although differing levels of provision are allowed for dispensing by physicians, especially in rural areas.

The lists of controlled products are not identical between Member States. There may also be more than one set of controls that can be applied to products available only on prescriptions.

In some EC Member States there are restricted lists of non-prescription products that may be obtained other than through a pharmacy. For example, there are products that may be obtained from non-pharmacy outlets in Ireland and Germany (although some degree of specialist knowledge may be required of the suppliers of some products in the latter).

Mechanisms are available for the changes of legal status of a product from prescription only status to non-prescription status in some but not all Member States.

The original packs may not be opened for part of the contents to be supplied to patients in most countries. Exceptions may be made in the case of large containers in some countries. Pack leaflets are supplied to patients in many countries (although exceptions may be made for products supplied in hospitals). The UK is unique in the range of products it allows to be sold and supplied through non-professional outlets (GSL products).

The situation could be claimed to be a non-tarriff barrier to trade in the EC. In November 1989 the Commission of the European Communities (CEC) issued a draft directive on legal status for consultation. At the time of writing the consultation process had not resulted in a definitive proposal. It is therefore considered appropriate to restrict consideration to the original document.

With regard to products restricted to prescription it was envisaged that there would be more than one category, with differing restrictions on the provision of repeat prescriptions during the lifetime of the prescription. Some products might be supplied repeatedly within six months (unless otherwise restricted by the prescriber), while others might need the explicit approval of the prescriber before repeats could be supplied. In the case of narcotic substances and substances likely to result in psychological dependence there were likely to be special controls. Some products could be restricted to hospital or even specialist prescribing.

The criteria suggested for the inclusion of a substance in the prescription only categorisation are similar in many respects to those already in use in the UK: namely, the likelihood of the substance endangering human health under normal conditions of use (directly or indirectly) based on the findings of preclinical and clinical tests and trials as well as potentially serious adverse reactions found in normal use; whether the product could be potentially harmful in terms of dosage, pack size, or its potential for excessive extended use without professional supervision; whether there was the possibility for abuse, misuse, addiction, or possible criminal misuse; whether the indications for the use of the product require medical diagnosis or supervision; and the novelty of the active ingredient.

The proposals acknowledged that a second category of non-prescription status products would also be needed, and the products to be included could be substantially safe in use and indicated for easily identifiable conditions which did not require a professional consultation with a physician before the initiation of self-therapy. The nature of the non-prescription product outlets was not discussed in the proposals.

The CEC had suggested that each Member State should decide how products holding marketing authorisations would be classified in their own territories. It would be required that lists of the categorisation be published, however. The status of each product would also be the subject of review every five years (when the marketing authorisation came up for renewal).

APPENDIX 1
Statutory Instruments relating to the Medicines Act

Year	Number	Title
1968	1699	The Secretary of State for Social Services Order
1969	388	The Transfer of Functions (Wales) Order
1970	746	The Medicines Commission and Committee Regulations
	1256	The Medicines (British Pharmacopoeia Commission) Order
	1257	The Medicines (Committee on Safety of Medicines) Order
1971	972	The Medicines (Standard Provisions for Licences and Certificates) Regulations
	973	The Medicines (Applications for Product Licences and Clinical Trial and Animal Test Certificates) Regulations
	974	The Medicines (Applications for Manufacturer's and Wholesale Dealer's Licences) Regulations
	1153	The Medicines (First Appointed Day) Order
	1198	The Medicines (Exportation of Specified Products for Human Use) Order
	1200	The Medicines (Control of Substances for Manufacture) Order
	1267	The Medicines (Surgical Materials) Order
	1326	The Medicines (Importation of Medicinal Products for Re-exportation) Order
	1410	The Medicines (Exemption from Licences) (Foods and Cosmetics) Order
	1445	The Medicines (Retail Pharmacists — Exemptions from Licensing Requirements) Order
	1447	The Medicines (Applications for Product Licences of Right and Clinical Trial and Animal Test Certificates of Right) Regulations
	1448	The Medicines (Applications for Manufacturer's and Wholesale Dealer's Licences of Right) Regulations
	1450	The Medicines (Exemption from Licences) (Special and Transitional Cases) Order
1972	640	The Medicines (Exemption from Licences) (Wholesale Dealing) Order
	717	The Medicines (Closing Date for Applications for Licences of Right) Order
	788	The Medicines Act 1968 (Commencement No. 1) Order
	1198	The Medicines (Termination of Transitional Exemptions) (No 1) Order
	1199	The Medicines (Exemption from Licences) (Manufacturer and Assembly Temporary Provisions) Order

	1200	The Medicines (Exemption from Licences) (Special Cases and Miscellaneous Provisions) Order
	1226	The Medicines (Standard Provisions for Licences and Certificates) Amendment Regulations
	1255	The Medicines Act 1968 (Commencement No 2) Order
	2076	The Medicines (Data Sheet) Regulations
1973	367	The Medicines (Extention to Antimicrobial Substances) Order
	1529	The Medicines Act 1968 (Commencement No 3) Order
	1822	The Medicines (Pharmacist) (Applications for Registration and Fees) Regulations
	1849	The Medicines (Pharmacist) (Appointed Day) Order
	1851	The Medicines Act 1968 (Commencement No 4) Order
	2079	The Medicines (Exemption from Licences) (Foods and Cosmetics) Amendment Order
1974	316	The Medicines (Exemption from Licences) (Emergency Importation) Order
	498	The Medicines (Exemption From Licences) (Clinical Trials) Order
	832	The Medicines (Renewal Applications for Licences and Certificates) Regulations
	1149	The Medicines (Termination of Transitional Exemptions) (No 2) Order
	1150	The Medicines (Exemption from Licences) (Ingredients) Order
	1523	The Medicines (Standard Provisions for Licences and Certificates) Amendment Regulations
1975	298	The Medicines (Advertising of Medicinal Products) Regulations
	533	The Medicines (Dental Filling Substances) Order
	681	The Medicines (Application for Product Licences and Clinical Trial and Animal Test Certificates) Amendment Regulations
	761	The Medicines (Termination of Transitional Exemptions) (No 3) Order
	762	The Medicines (Exemption from Licences) (Wholesale Dealing in Confectionery) Order
	1006	The Medicines (Committee on the Review of Medicines) Order
	1169	The Medicines (Medicines Act 1968 Amendment) Regulations
	1326	The Medicines (Advertising of Medicinal Products) (No 2) Regulations
	1473	The Medicines (Committee on Dental and Surgical Materials) Order
	2000	The Medicines (Child Safety) Regulations

1976	74	The Medicines Act 1968 (Commencement No 5) Order
	968	The Medicines (Specified Articles and Substances) Order
	1643	The Medicines (Child Safety) Amendment Regulations
	1726	The Medicines (Labelling) Regulations
1977	189	The Medicines (Renewal Applications for Licences and Certificates) Amendment Regulations
	640	The Medicines (Importation of Medicinal Products for Re-exportation) Amendment Order
	670	The Medicines (Bal Jivan Chamcho Prohibition) (No 2) Order
	675	The Medicines (Standard Provisions for Licences and Certificates) Amendment Regulations
	996	The Medicines (Labelling) Amendment Regulations
	1038	The Medicines (Manufacturer's Undertakings for Imported Products) Regulations
	1039	The Medicines (Standard Provisions for Licences and Certificates) Amendment (No 2) Regulations
	1050	The Medicines (Medicines Act 1968 Amendments) Regulations
	1051	The Medicines (Applications for Product Licences and Clinical Trial and Animal Test Certificates) Amendment Regulations
	1052	The Medicines (Applications for Manufacturer's and Wholesale Dealer's Licences) Amendment Regulations
	1053	The Medicines (Standard Provisions for Licences and Certificates) Amendment (No 3) Regulations
	1054	The Medicines (Exemption from Licences) (Wholesale Dealing) Order
	1055	The Medicines (Leaflets) Regulations
	1068	The Medicines Act 1968 (Commencement No 6) Order
	1399	The Medicines (Certificates of Analysis) Regulations
	1488	The Medicines (Breathing Gases) Order
	2126	The Medicines (Pharmacy and General Sale) (Appointed Day) Order
	2128	The Medicines Act 1968 (Commencement No 7) Order
	2130	The Medicines (Retail Sale or Supply of Herbal Remedies) Order
	2131	The Medicines (Prohibition of Non-medicinal Antimicrobial Substances) Order
	2168	The Medicines (Labelling) Amendment (No 2) Regulations
1978	40	The Medicines (Fluted Bottles) Regulations
	41	The Medicines (Labelling and Advertising to the Public) Regulations
	1004	The Medicines (Radioactive Substances) Order

Ap. 1] Appendix 1 275

	1006	The Medicines (Administration of Radioactive Substances) Regulations
	1020	The Medicines (Advertising to Medical and Dental Practitioners) Regulations
	1138	The Medicines (Intra-Uterine Contraceptive Devices) (Appointed Day) Order
	1139	The Medicines (Intra-Uterine Contraceptive Devices) (Amendment to Exemptions from Licences) Order
	1140	The Medicines (Licensing of Intra-Uterine Contraceptive Devices) (Miscellaneous Amendments) Regulations
	1421	The Medicines (Collection and Delivery Arrangements Exemption) Order
1979	382	The Medicines (Chloroform Prohibition) Order
	1114	The Medicines (Exemption from Licences) (Assembly) Order
	1181	The Medicines (Phenacetin Prohibition) Order
	1535	The Medicines (Committee on Dental and Surgical Materials) Amendment Order
	1539	The Medicines (Contact Lens Fluid and Other Substances) (Appointed Day) Order
	1585	The Medicines (Contact Lens Fluids and Other Substances) (Exemption from Licences) Order
	1745	The Medicines (Contact Lens Fluids and Other Substances) (Exemption from Licences) Amendment Order
	1759	The Medicines (Contact Lens Fluids and Other Substances) (Labelling) Regulations
	1760	The Medicines (Contact Lens Fluids and Other Substances) (Advertising and Miscellaneous Amendment) Regulations
1980	263	The Medicines (Chloroform Prohibition) Amendment Order
	1467	The Medicines (Intra-Uterine Contraceptive Devices) (Termination of Transitional Exemptions) Order
	1806	The Medicines (Pharmacists) (Applications for Registration and Fees) Amendment Regulations
	1923	The Medicines (Sale or Supply) (Miscellaneous Provisions) Regulations
	1924	The Medicines (Pharmacy and General Sale — Exemption) Order
1981	164	The Medicines (Exemption from Licences) (Clinical Trials) Order
	1633	The Medicines (Data Sheet) Amendment Regulations
	1689	The Medicines (Contact Lens Fluids and Other Substances) (Labelling) Amendment Regulations

Year	SI No.	Title
	1690	The Medicines (Contact Lens Fluids and Other Substances) (Termination of Transitional Exemptions) Order
	1791	The Medicines (Labelling) Amendments Regulations
1982	27	The Medicines (Pharmacy and General Sale — Exemption) Amendment Order
	28	The Medicines (Sale or Supply) (Miscellaneous Provisions) Amendment Regulations
	1335	The Medicines (British Pharmacopoeia Commission) Amendment Order
	1789	The Medicines (Renewal Applications for Licences and Certificates) Amendment Regulations
1983	1212	The Medicines (Products Other Than Veterinary Drugs) (Prescription Only) Order
	1724	The Medicines (Medicines Act 1968 Amendment) Regulations
	1725	The Medicines (Applications for Manufacturer's and Wholesale Dealer's Licences) Amendment Regulations
	1726	The Medicines (Applications for Product Licences and Clinical Trial and Animal Test Certificates) Amendment Regulations
	1728	The Medicines (Exemption from Licences) (Wholesale Dealing) Amendment Order
	1729	The Medicines (Labelling) Amendment Regulations
	1730	The Medicines (Standard Provisions for Licences and Certificates) Amendment Regulations
1984	187	The Medicines (Cyanogenic Substances) Order
	673	The Medicines (Exemption from Licences) (Importation) Order
	756	The Medicines (Products Other Than Veterinary Drugs) (Prescription Only) Amendment Order
	769	The Medicines (Products Other Than Veterinary Drugs) (General Sale List) Order
	1261	The Medicines (Committee on Radiation from Radioactive Medicinal Products) (Revocation) Order
	1886	The Medicines (Pharmacies) (Application for Registration and Fees) Amendment Regulations
1985	1403	The Medicines (Control of Substances for Manufacture) Order
	1539	The Medicines (Control of Substances for Manufacture) (Appointed Day) Order
	1540	The Medicines (Products Other Than Veterinary Drugs) (General Sale List) Amendment Order
	1558	The Medicines (Labelling) Amendment Regulations
	1878	The Medicines (Pharmacies) (Applications for Registration and Fees) Amendment Regulations

1986	586	The Medicines (Products Other Than Veterinary Drugs) (Prescription Only) Amendment Order
	1761	The Medicines Act 1968 (Hearings by Persons Appointed) Rules
1987	674	The Medicines (Products Other Than Veterinary Drugs) (Prescription Only) Amendment Order
	877	The Medicines (Child Safety) Amendment Regulations
	910	The Medicines (Products Other Than Veterinary Drugs) (General Sale List) Amendment Order
	1250	The Medicines (Products Other Than Veterinary Drugs) (Prescription Only) Amendment (No 2) Order
	2099	The Medicines (Pharmacies) (Applications for Registration and Fees) Amendment Regulations
	2202	The Pharmaceutical Qualifications (EEC Recognition) Order
1988	2017	The Medicines (Products Other Than Veterinary Drugs) (Prescription Only) Amendment Order
	2113	The Medicines (Pharmacies) (Applications for Registration and Fees) Amendment Regulations
1989	192	The Medicines Act 1968 (Commencement No 8) Order
	418	The Medicines (Fees Relating to Medicinal Products for Human Use) Regulations
	684	The Medicines (Fixing of Fees Relating to Medicinal Products for Human Use) Order
	969	The Medicines (Products Other Than Veterinary Drugs (General Sales List) Amendment Order
	1183	The Medicines (Data and Labelling) Amendment Regulations
	1184	The Medicines (Exemption from Licences) (Special and Transitional Cases) Amendment Order

APPENDIX 2
Medicines act leaflets (MALs)

MAL 1	Guide to the licensing system (9.84)
MAL 2	Now published by HMSO as *Guidance notes on applications for product licences* (1989)
MAL 2(PI)	Note for applications for product licences (parallel importing)(medicines for human use) (4.87)
MAL 4	Now published by HMSO as *Guidance notes on applications for clinical trial certificates and clinical trial exemptions* (1985;1986)
MAL 5	Applications for manufacturer's ordinary licences (8.88)
MAL 6	Applications for wholesale dealer's licences (9.88)
MAL 7	Licensing fees (9.87)

MAL 8	A guide to the status of borderline preparations under the Act (7.82)
MAL 9	Licensing provisions affecting retail pharmacists (3.85)
MAL 10	Applications for product licences for veterinary medicinal products*
MAL 11	(temporarily withdrawn)
MAL 13	Licensing of products sold as chemists' own brands (1972)
MAL 14	Special dispensing services (1972)
MAL 18	Licensing requirements involved in the packing and labelling of medicinal products (9.80)
MAL 21	(temporarily withdrawn)
MAL 22	The licensing of ingredients (8.74)
MAL 23	The application of licensing to non-NHS hospitals (1972)
MAL 24	Supply in the course of giving advice as to treatment (10.83)
MAL 25	Notes on data sheets (5.84)
MAL 26	Guide to provisions on medicated animal feeding stuffs*
MAL 28	Guide to provisions on labelling of and supply of leaflets with medicated animal feeding stuffs*
MAL 29	Notes on export certificates (5.86)
MAL 30	A guide to the provisions affecting doctors and dentists (6.85)
MAL 32	Clinical trials using marketed products (11.81)
MAL 36	Notes for guidance on reproduction studies (1981)
MAL 37	The promotion of sales of medicinal products (1980)
MAL 38	Notes for guidance on veterinary reproduction studies*
MAL 39	Products containing herbal ingredients (11.85)
MAL 41	Additional notes for guidance — biological medicinal products (5.82)
MAL 42	Notes on the Medicines (Labelling) Regulations 1976 (10.83)
MAL 44	Implementation of the EEC Directives about the Marketing and Manufacture of Medicinal Products (1977)
MAL 45	EEC requirements about the 'Qualified Person' (2.82)
MAL 46	EEC requirements for the importation of proprietary medicinal products for human use (1.82)
MAL 47	Leaflets supplied with proprietary medicinal products (8.83)
MAL 49	Medicines (Labelling) (Amendment) Regulations 1977 (2.83)
MAL 52	Retail sale of certain veterinary medicines to commercial manufacturers of animal feeding stuffs*
MAL 53	(Now incorporated into MAL 2)
MAL 55	Labelling and advertising to the public (1978)
MAL 56	Guidance on the assessment of efficacy of growth promoters*
MAL 57	Advertising to medical and dental practitioners (8.83)
MAL 58	Notes on licensing procedure in connection with the review of product licences (medicines for human use) (6.87)
MAL 59	Hearings and representations under Part II of the Medicines Act 1968 (9.84).
MAL 60	Colouring matters permitted in medicinal products (1979)

MAL 61	Applications for product licences and clinical trial certificates for intrauterine contraceptive devices (1979)
MAL 62	(Now included in MAL 4)
MAL 63	Animal tests arranged by veterinary surgeons or veterinary practitioners in private practice*
MAL 64	Guidelines for the use of antibiotics in the manufacture of veterinary vaccine*
MAL 65	Guidelines on the production and control of mammalian live virus vaccine*
MAL 67	Use of substances of animal origin in the manufacture of veterinary vaccine*
MAL 68	Medicines Acts 1968 and 1971: Notes on European Community requirements for the importation of proprietary medicinal products and ready-made drugs for veterinary use*
MAL 69	Medicines Acts 1968 and 1971: Notes on European Community requirements about the 'Qualified Person' for veterinary medicinal products*
MAL 70	Guideline for the production and control of killed infectious bursal disease vaccines*
MAL 71	Guidelines for the production and control of killed avian vaccines*
MAL 72	Animal test exemption scheme*
MAL 99	The control of medicines in the United Kingdom of Great Britain and Northern Ireland (*under revision — out of print*)

Unless otherwise indicated, available from Medicines Control Agency, Department of Health or, for items marked * from the Ministry of Agriculture, Fisheries, and Food.

18

The other national authorities in the EC

18.1 INTRODUCTION

Chapter 17 has described the United Kingdom (UK) system for assessing and granting marketing authorisations and in particular its network of advisory committees and subcommittees. The present chapter illustrates some of the differences between the UK and other European Community (EC) Member States. Even after 1992 these differences will remain very important in relation to both national applications and applications made through the 'decentralised' procedure (see Chapter 21). The information in this chapter was made available to the author by friends and colleagues in the other EC Member States in the course of many discussions at the Committee for Proprietary Medicinal Products (CPMP) and elsewhere, and this assistance is gratefully acknowledged. Some of the information was made available as answers to a questionnaire. Some of the replies to the questionnaire were, however, incomplete; in other areas the information was regarded as confidential and not available for publication. Within these limits the author has tried to present as complete a picture as possible.

18.2 THE EC MEMBER STATES

All of the EC Member States are bound by the same framework of European legislation (Directives, Decision, Commission Communication, Council Recommendations, and CPMP guidelines). However, the national agencies differ substantially in their internal organisation and procedures.

As might be expected, the size of the national agencies roughly depends on the populations of the Member States and national resources (gross domestic product), as shown in Table 18.1.

The size of the national agencies are set out in Table 18.2. The total staff numbers are those actually in post (i.e. not staff complement) in December 1989 in whole-time

Table 18.1 — Member States — population and 1987 gross domestic product (GDP)

Country	Population (millions)	GDP ($ billions)†
Federal Republic of Germany	61.149	806
(Combined FRG and German Democratic Republic)	(77.910)	(—)
Italy	57.193	441
United Kingdom	55.776	553
France	55.600	634
Spain	38.815	204
Netherlands	14.669	181
Portugal	10.229	26
Greece	10.002	43
Belgium	9.858	99
Denmark	5.124	71
Ireland	3.543	21
Luxembourg	0.366	3.7

† USA billion = 10^9.

equivalents. Thus, the totals can be less than the sum of the numbers of professional staff, since some of them are employed part-time.

Table 18.2 — The staffing levels of some of the national agencies

Country staff	Numbers of staff			Total
	Clinicians	Pharmacists	Scientists	
Federal Republic of Germany	54	67	31	523
Italy	26	18	15	138
United Kingdom	19	47	43	331
Spain	12	43	1	101
Netherlands	11	25	7	25
Belgium	1	20	—	40
Denmark	3	9	2	19
Ireland	5	10	2	45
Portugal	2	33	—	124
France	†	†	†	150‡

† Information not available.
‡ About 60 involved with product evaluation.

The numbers of staff are only a crude measure of the size of the national agencies. It is necessary to consider their role and organisation in more detail.

In some countries, such as Germany, France, Italy, and the UK, substantial numbers of staff are employed in work on the national pharmacopoeia. In some countries, such as Ireland, the assessment staff is also concerned with the assessment of veterinary and feed additive products, whereas in other countries (such as the UK) there is a completely separate team of veterinary and pharmaceutical assessors who are responsible for these products.

The numbers of staff above include the medicines inspectors (responsible for inspection of pharmaceutical manufacturers, wholesalers, etc.), and the role of these inspectors can vary in the different countries. In Italy, the inspectors inspect active ingredient manufacturers. In the UK, the Inspectorate inspects all human and veterinary manufacture whether in the UK or overseas (except for those countries which are part of the Pharmaceutical Inspection Convention (PIC) where the national inspectors undertake inspections on their behalf, and in Canada where there is a bilateral inspection convention). In France, the Départment de la Pharmacie et du Médicament (DPhM) has responsibility for inspecting and regulating pharmacies and pharmacists as well as medicinal products.

The numbers of staff employed in the national control laboratories (also often involved inextricably in the assessment of marketing authorisation applications) is given separately in Table 18.9.

In some cases (Italy), the numbers of staff include those responsible for good laboratory practice (GLP) inspection and audit. In the UK there is a separate GLP compliance unit in the Department of Health.

18.3 THE ORGANISATION OF THE ASSESSMENT OF MARKETING AUTHORISATION APPLICATIONS (Table 18.3)

In some countries (e.g. the UK and Denmark) the assessment of new applications is wholly by internal assessors (i.e., using a dedicated staff of professional pharmacists/clinicians/scientists who assess the dossier). An internal assessor may be employed full-time or part-time. Part-time assessors are often employed partly by a research institute or in a hospital or in an academic institution.

In other countries (e.g. France), the assessment is done wholly by external assessors who are independent 'experts' employed by national institutes, hospitals, clinics, academic colleges and universities. In these cases the role of the professional staff employed in the government agency is to coordinate this assessment process and to present the report to the advisory committee. In France there is a pool of about 500 such external experts who are available to the authorities, although the number used regularly is much smaller.

In both internal assessment or external 'expert' assessment, advice may be sought from an advisory committee. In those countries where all assessment is done externally, the role of the advisory committee is to oversee the assessment of all applications. In others (such as the UK) the committee may only see only some applications and their role is quite different.

Table 18.3 — Organisation of marketing authorisation application assessment — internal vs external assessment

Country	Pharmaceutical assessment	Toxicological/ clinical assessment
Federal Republic of Germany	Internal†	Mostly Internal
Italy	Internal	Internal/External
United Kingdom	Internal	Internal
France	External	External
Spain	Internal	Internal
Netherlands	Internal	Internal‡
Belgium	Internal/External	Internal/External
Greece	Internal/External	Internal/External
Denmark	Internal	Internal
Ireland	Internal	Internal
Luxembourg	Internal/External	Internal/External
Portugal	Internal/External	External

† External for generic products and review licence applications.
‡ Employed by the national authority but spending about 50% of their time on research or clinical practice.

18.4 THE ROLE OF THE NATIONAL COMMITTEES OF INDEPENDENT EXPERTS

All countries except Spain (Table 18.4) have at least one national committee of independent experts (Spain has only a pharmacovigilance advisory committee). In the Netherlands, the Committee for the Evaluation of Medicines (College ter beoordeling van geneesmiddelen) is the licensing authority and makes binding decisions on the applications. In all of the other Member States the national committees have an advisory role, i.e. they advise the licensing authority (the responsible Minister and his senior officials), but their advice is not binding (although in practice it is almost invariably taken).

In those countries which have a national committee, it is usually a multipurpose one dealing with all types of product (and sometimes, as in Ireland and Denmark, with both veterinary and human products). In Germany and the UK, however, there is more than one advisory committee.

The terms of appointment of the chairman of the national committee can vary very considerably as shown in Table 18.5. It should be noted that although a period of appointment is quoted, the appointment of the chairman is usually renewable.

The members of the national committees are usually drawn from hospitals, universities, government research institutes, the Ministry of Health, and other government departments. In some countries (Belgium and the Netherlands) the national control laboratory is also represented on either the main committee or one or more of its subcommittees. The members of the national committees are usually

Table 18.4 — The national committees

Country	Committee name	Remit of committee
Federal Republic of Germany	Commission A	Human New Actives
	Commission D	Homoeopathics
	Commission E	Vegetable drugs
Italy	Commissione Consultiva Unica del Farmaco	All products
United Kingdom	Committee on Safety of Medicines (CSM)	All products except dental/surgical
	Committee on Dental & Surgical Materials (CDSM)	Dental/surgical products
	Committee on Review of Medicines (CRM)	Review of old medicines
France	Commission d'Autorisation de Mise sur le Marché	All products
Spain	None	—
Netherlands	College ter beoordeling van geneesmiddelen	All products
Belgium	Medicines Commission	All products
Greece	Registration Committee	All products†
Denmark	Registration Board	All products
Ireland	National Drugs Advisory Board (NDAB)	All products
Luxembourg	Comité d'Experts charger de donner son avis sur les demandes des autorisation de mise sur le marché	All products
Portugal	Comissao Tecnica dos Novos Medicamentos (CTNM)	All products

† The Greek Committee is composed of a core membership of the chairman and three members with other added experts according to the product or subject under consideration. There are a number of registration subcommittees which deal with specialist products, e.g. herbals, blood products, biological products.

appointed by the Ministry of Health. In the Federal Republic of Germany, however, the members of the commissions are nominated by professional and other bodies. In Germany and France there is either a member or observer from the pharmaceutical industry/trade association.

Table 18.5 — The chairmen of national committees

Country	Who appoints	Period of appointment
Federal Republic of Germany	Elected by fellow commissioners	3 years
Italy	Minister of Health	3 years
United Kingdom	Secretary of State	3 years
France	Minister of Health	3 years
Netherlands	The Queen	4 years
Belgium	Minister (of Health)	6 years
Greece	Minister of Health	—
Denmark	Ministry of Health	4 years
Ireland	Minister of Health	4 years
Luxembourg	Minister of Health	No fixed term
Portugal	Elected by Commissao	No fixed term

Not surprisingly, as shown in Table 18.6, the size of the national committees can also vary quite considerably.

Table 18.6 — Size of the national committees

Country	Committee	Number of members
Federal Republic of Germany	Commission A	23†
	Commission D	13‡
	Commission E	12§
Italy	Commissione Consultiva	33¶
Britain	CSM	21¶
	CDSM	19¶
France	Commission d'AMM	28¶
Netherlands	College ter beoordeling van geneesmiddelen	14
Belgium	Medicines Commission	16
Greece	Registration Committee	4¶
Denmark	Registration Board	10
Ireland	NDAB	16
Luxembourg	Comité d'Experts	6 (6 subs)
Portugal	CTNM	11

† 46 Deputy members, 5 external experts.
‡ 26 Deputy members.
§ 24 Deputy members.
¶ Regular or occasional experts invited according to the nature of the product/subject under discussion.

In many countries the national committees are served by advisory subcommittees.

In France there are nine Groupes de Travail (GT) associated with the Commission d'AMM:

GT Médicaments antiinfectieux
GT Biotechnologie
GT Pharmaceutique
GT Plantes
GT Radiopharmaceutiques
GT Médicaments et SIDA (AIDS products)
GT Toxico-pharmaco-clinique
GT Validation qualité pharmaceutique
GT Validation qualité therapeutique.

In Greece there are eight Registration subcommittees associated with the Registration Committee:

Radiopharmaceuticals
Biological products and medical devices
Herbal remedies
Blood derivatives
Veterinary medicinal products
Dental materials
Nutritional supplements
Cosmetic products.

In the UK there are four subcommittees who serve both CSM and CDSM:

Biologicals
Chemistry, pharmacy, and standards (CPS)
Efficacy and adverse reactions (SEAR)
Adverse reactions group of SEAR (ARGOS).

In Italy there are three sub-groups:

Pharmaceutical/analytical
Pharmaco-toxicological
Clinical

In Ireland there are three advisory subcommittees serving the National Drugs Advisory Board (NDAB):

Committee for drug evaluation and toxicity
Committee for drug usage and adverse reactions
Committee for clinical trials.

Denmark has a Board for Adverse Drug Reactions, a clinical trials subcommittee, and a subcommittee for the Summary of Product Characteristics.

The frequency of meetings of the national committees also varies as is shown in Table 18.7.

Table 18.7 — Frequency of meetings of the national committees

Country	Committee	Frequency
Federal Republic of Germany	Commission A	11/year
	Commission D	6/year
	Commission E	7/year
Italy	Commissione Consultiva	Monthly
United Kingdom	CSM	Monthly
	CDSM	2 monthly
France	Commission d'AMM	2 weekly
Spain	—	—
Netherlands	College	Monthly
Belgium	Medicines Commission	2 weekly
Greece	Registration Committee	Monthly
Ireland	NDAB	Monthly
Luxembourg	Comité d'Experts	10/year
Portugal	CTNM	Weekly

18.5 THE APPEALS PROCEDURES

While there may be no major differences in overall standards and technical criteria for assessment in the different EC Member States, there are, as we have already seen, considerable differences in procedures. This also applies to appeals procedures where there are substantive issues that must be resolved before issue of an authorisation in the Member State.

In the UK and a number of the other EC Member States where internal professional assessment is available, many of the simpler marketing authorisation applications involving well-known active ingredients will be assessed without requiring the advice of the advisory committee or of external experts. In the vast majority of such cases, problems are dealt with directly between the applicant company and the professional assessors in the Member State concerned (in the UK this is known as 'the Licensing Authority route'). However, where there are major problems they will be referred to the advisory committee.

Major new active substance (either chemical or biological) products are almost invariably referred to the national committees. Many of these will be the subject of formal appeals as detailed questions about them are raised. In the UK, for example (see Chapter 17 for a more detailed analysis), over 50% are the subject of a formal letter from the CSM under Section 21(1) of the 1968 Medicines Act — which precipitates a formal first appeal back to the CSM either as a written representation or as a written representation with an oral hearing.

In France, if a product is not approved, there are two possibilities:

- the 'mesure d'instruction' (product held to be approved but more data/clarification to be provided to the Commission d'AMM within 12 months)
- the 'projet de rejet' (where the perceived risk/benefit is poor and the Commission asks for further clinical data).

In France a formal appeal to the Commission d'AMM is a comparative rarity and can proceed only with the permission of the Director of the Department de Pharmacie et du Médicament (DPHM).

The appeals stages and bodies are set out in Table 18.8.

18.6 THE NATIONAL CONTROL LABORATORIES AND THEIR INVOLVEMENT IN THE PREMARKETING TESTING OF SAMPLES OF ACTIVE INGREDIENTS, INTERMEDIATES, AND FINISHED PRODUCTS

In many cases a representative of the national control laboratory is a member of the national committee involved in considering marketing authorisation applications. Belgium, Spain, Greece, Ireland, Italy, Luxembourg, the Netherlands, and Portugal require samples of the finished product to test. Greece, Ireland, Luxembourg, the Netherlands, and Portugal require samples of all active ingredients to test. Belgium, Spain, the Netherlands, and Portugal require samples of excipients for testing where the applicant has introduced a new monograph. Belgium and Spain require samples of active ingredients for test where the applicant has introduced his own monograph. The other Member States may also request samples of active ingredients or finished product.

In many of the Member States there are specialist requirements for biological products (immunologicals, blood products, etc.), and samples of these may be tested in a special laboratory (e.g. the National Institute for Biological Standards and Control in the UK, the Institut Pasteur in France, or the Paul Ehrlich Institut in the Federal Republic of Germany). Samples may be tested before authorisation. There may also be requirements to provide samples for test after grant of the authorisation before an individual batch is released onto the market (batch release).

The names and approximate sizes of the national control laboratories concerned with testing of 'chemical' active ingredients (i.e. excluding the biological products) are given in Table 18.9.

Table 18.8 — Appeals and appeal bodies

Country	Appeal stages† and bodies
Federal Republic of Germany	5 Appeal stages — new data to the BGA, formal appeal to the BGA, Administrative Court, Administrative High Court, Federal Administrative Court
Italy	3 Appeal stages — to Consultative Committee, to Health Council, to Administrative Court
United Kingdom	2 Appeal stages — to CSM/CDSM/CRM and then to a separate body the Medicines Commission
France	See text
Spain	2 Appeal stages — to the Subdireccion General de Evaluacion de Medicamentos
Netherlands	2 Appeal stages — to the College and then after the final College decision to the Crown
Belgium	1 Appeal stage (if the applicant does not respond to an unfavourable decision within 2 months a refusal is issued)
Denmark	2 stages of appeal — in writing to the Registration Board and then to the Ministry of Health
Ireland	2–3 stages of appeal — to standing committees/Board, to special committee or to the Minister of Health
Luxembourg	Written appeal only to the Comité d'Experts. Further appeals possible to Court of Justice and the State Council
Greece	Appeals to the Scientific Council
Portugal	— (Information not available)

† Legal appeals are possible in most Member States on matters of law or procedure.

Table 18.9 — The national control laboratories

Country	Name of laboratory	Total staff
Federal Republic of Germany	None. But there are 10 laboratories in the Länder concerned with post-marketing assessment	—
Italy	Health Institute, Rome	67
United Kingdom	Medicines Testing Laboratory, Royal Pharmaceutical Society of Great Britain, Edinburgh	32
France	— (information not available)	—
Spain	Centro Nacional de Farmaco-biologia, Majadahonda	187
Netherlands	Rijksinstituut voor geneesmiddelenonderzoek, Leiden	39
Belgium	Instituut voor Hygiene en Epidemiologie, Brussels (laboratory responsible for both chemical drugs and vaccines)	18
Denmark	Medicines Control Office	19
Ireland	Galway Regional Laboratory	5
Luxembourg	Laboratoire de Santé	†
Greece	— (information not available)	
Portugal		14

† Information confidential.

18.7 THE NAMES AND ADDRESSES OF NATIONAL AUTHORITIES IN THE EC MEMBER STATES

BELGIUM:
Ministère de la Santé publique,
Inspection générale de la Pharmacie,
Cité Administrative,
Quartier Vésale,
B-1010 Bruxelles.
Tel: (32)(2) 210.49.01
Telefax (Telecopie): (32)(2) 210.48.80

DENMARK:
Sundhedsstyrelsen,
Laegemiddelafdelingen,
Frederikssundsvej 378,
DK-2700 Bronshoj.
Tel: (45)(42) 94.36.67
Telefax: (45)(42) 84.70.77

Names and addresses of the national authorities

GERMANY:
Institüt für Arzneimittel des Bundesgesundheitsamtes,
Seestrasse 10,
D-1000 Berlin 65.
Tel: (49)(30)1 450.24.49
Telefax: (49)(30)1 450.212.07

For immunological products (vaccines, sera, allergens etc.):

Paul-Ehrlich-institut,
Bundesamt für Sera und Impstoffe,
Paul-Ehrlich-Strasse 42–44,
Postfach 700810,
D-6000 Frankfurt am Main 70.
Tel: (49)(69) 63.60.16
Telefax: (49)(69) 63.44.02

SPAIN:
Ministereo de Sanidad y Consumo,
Direccion General de Farmacia y Productos Sanitarios,
Paseo del Prado, 18–20
E-28014 Madrid
Tel: (34)(1) 420.20.68
Telefax: (34)(1) 420.10.42

FRANCE:
Ministére de la Solidarité, de la Santé et de la Protection sociale,
Direction de la Pharmacie et du Médicament,
1 place de Fontenoy,
F-75700 Paris
Tel: (33)(1) 40.56.60.00
Telecopie: (33)(1) 405.65.355

GREECE:
E.O.F. (National Drug Oraganisation)
Voulis Str. 4,
Athens 10562
Tel: (30)(1) 323.09.11
Telefax: (30)(1) 323.86.81

IRELAND:
National Drugs Advisory Board,
63– 64 Adelaide Road,
Dublin 2
Tel: (353)(1) 76.49.71
Telefax: (353)(1) 76.78.36

ITALY:
Ministero della Sanita,
Servizio Farmaceutico,
Viale della Civilta Romana 7,
I-00144 Roma, EUR
Tel: (39)(6) 592.58.63
Telefax: (39)(6) 592.58.24

LUXEMBOURG:
Direction de la Santé,
Division de la Pharmacie et des Médicaments,
10, rue C. M. Spoo,
L-2546 Luxembourg
Tel: (352) 4.08.01
Telefax: (352) 48.49.03

NETHERLANDS:
College ter beoordeling van geneesmiddelen,
S. W. Churchilllaan 362,
PO Box 5811,
2280 HV Rijswijk (ZH).
Tel: (31)(70) 340.79.11
Telefax: (31)(70) 340.51.55

PORTUGAL:
Ministerio da Saude,
Direçao Geral dos Assuntos Farmaceuticos,
Av. Estados Unidos de America 37,
P-1700 Lisboa
Tel: (351)(1) 80.41.31
Telefax: (351)(1) 84.80.331

UNITED KINGDOM:
Medicines Control Agency,
Department of Health,
Market Towers,
1 Nine Elms Lane,
Vauxhall,
London SW8 5NQ
Tel: (44)(71) 7202188
Telefax: (44)(71) 7205647

CPMP Secretariat,
Directorate General III/C-2,
Commission of the European Communities,
200 rue de la Loi,
B-1049,
Bruxelles
Tel: (32)(2) 235.69.35
Telecopie: (32)(2) 236.15.20

REFERENCE

Bacou, J-P, (1990). Analyse des Obstacles Institutionnels et Economiques à l'Harmonisation Européenne en matière d'Enregistrement des Médicaments. Thèse pour le Doctorat en Medicine. Université Paris VII.

19

EEC guidelines — quality, safety, efficacy, and biotechnology

19.1 INTRODUCTION

The Committee for Proprietary Medicinal Products (CPMP) has always attached a great deal of importance to the preparation of guidelines on the quality, safety, and efficacy of medicinal products. The first sets of CPMP guidelines were published as recommendations from the Council of Ministers to the Member States. Two such sets of guidelines were adopted — Council Recommendation 83/571/EEC of 26 October 1983, and Council Recommendation 87/176/EEC of 9 February 1987.

The first Council Recommendation comprised five guidelines, the second a further fourteen.

The production of guidelines as Council Recommendations is a complex process — involving the CPMP, the Pharmaceutical Committee, the European Parliament, and the Council of Ministers. In July 1987, the Council of Ministers delegated to the Commission of the European Communities (CEC) (in Directive 87/19/EEC, adopted on 22 December 1986) the power to amend the 'norms and protocols' Directive (75/318/EEC) which contains all of the detailed technical requirements in terms of quality, safety, and efficacy for a marketing authorisation application. This permits the drafting of a so-called 'Commission Directive'. This is designed to be a rapid procedure.

In the light of this change, it no longer made sense to issue non-binding guidelines by a more cumbersome and bureaucratic process than that used to amend the legal requirements in 75/318/EEC. Thus, recent guidelines have merely been adopted by the CPMP and issued to the industry immediately after their adoption.

The guidelines issued up until March 1989 are all included in Volume III of *The rules governing medicinal products in the European Community* entitled 'Guidelines on the quality, safety, and efficacy of medicinal products for human use'. This text includes the previous Council Recommendations as well as a further thirteen guidelines on biotechnology (three guidelines), quality (four guidelines), safety and efficacy (six guidelines). Further guidelines have since been issued by the CPMP, and when sufficient have been collected together, they will be issued in additional volumes (the first in December 1990) as Appendices to Volume III.

19.2 THE PURPOSE OF GUIDELINES

Guidelines are intended for applicants for marketing authorisations for medicinal products. Their purpose is to avoid national differences in the interpretation of the detailed technical requirements for safety, quality, and efficacy in Directive 75/318/EEC by giving additional explanation; and to facilitate the preparation of applications for marketing authorisation which will be accepted by all of the EEC Member States.

Guidelines set out the main points to be dealt with in the dossiers and Expert Reports; the minimum requirements (such as the number of batches of a medicinal product in its intended pack which will need to be subjected to a stability test), and the methods in general terms (but taking care to maintain flexibility, so as not to restrict the freedom to use legitimate alternative test methods).

19.3 STATUS OF GUIDELINES

As pointed out by Cartwright (1990), guidelines are complementary to the Directive 75/318/EEC legal requirements; in accord with the current consensus of scientific regulatory opinion; approved by the national authorities in the Member States who all agree to see that they are observed and to follow them when assessing applications for marketing authorisations; and represent a published statement of the views of the EC authorities on the subject, which will help to promote international standardisation of test methods and their interpretation, and which may make it unnecessary for third (non-EC) countries to ask for other tests to be done.

Guidelines are by definition non-mandatory, but if an applicant company wishes to use procedures etc. which are radically different from those in the CPMP guideline, the relevant Expert will need to explain or justify this in the Expert Report.

19.4 WORKING PARTIES AND THEIR MEMBERSHIP

The CPMP and Commission working parties have been described in Chapter 13. Since 1989 they now include one representative from the group of Nordic countries (Sweden, Norway, Finland), and (since 1990) one from the European Free Trade Area countries (Switzerland, Austria, etc.) in addition to the delegates from the EC Member States. Thus, all those countries which have close economic and political links with the EC, and which have accepted the need for pan-European technical cooperation and agreement, are involved in the work of drawing up new technical guidelines or amending the existing ones.

19.5 PROCEDURE FOR DRAWING UP GUIDELINES

The procedure is as follows. The topics to be considered are selected and approved by the CPMP. The guideline is then drawn up by the relevant working party or parties (some may need input from more than one working party). The first draft(s) are drawn up by a rapporteur from one of the Member States with a particular interest in the subject.

There may be some preliminary discussion with experts from the pharmaceutical industry — usually drawn from the European Federation of Pharmaceutical Industry Associations (EFPIA) and Association Européenne des Societés Grand Publique (AESGP) member companies. The discussion may be either before the draft is written, or before it is formalised.

The draft text is approved for consultation and is then submitted to the national authorities in the EC Member States, the European pharmaceutical industry associations, the Japanese Ministry of Health and Welfare, and the Food and Drug Administration of the USA. Normally, a six-month period is allowed for submission of comments and their consideration.

On the basis of the written comments received, supplemented usually with a meeting with experts from the European industry groups to clarify their views, the working party draws up a final document. The final text is then submitted to the CPMP for adoption. After any final amendment by the CPMP, the text is adopted. The adoption of the new guideline is announced in the press release of that meeting from the CPMP.

The adopted text is sent to the European pharmaceutical industry associations, for them to circulate to their national associations in the different countries. The national pharmaceutical industry trade associations then circulate to their member companies. The adopted text is included in a published volume of CPMP guidelines. Each new guideline includes a date of coming into force. It is recognised that guidelines may sometimes represent fundamental changes in the way in which information is generated, and the industry will need a 'lead-in' period to adapt to this change.

19.6 REVISION OF EXISTING GUIDELINE TEXTS

As science and technology alter, so the existing guidelines need amendment and updating. It is part of the task of the CPMP working parties to keep the requirements under continuous review. A revised guideline goes through the same process of consultation before its adoption as set out in section 19.5.

REFERENCE

Cartwright, A. C. Introduction to CPMP quality guidelines. *BIRA Journal* **9**(3), 1–2, 1990.

20

The new general Directive, immunologicals etc. Directives

20.1 INTRODUCTION

In May and June 1989, the Council of Ministers adopted four new Directives extending the scope of the existing pharmaceutical Directives to include products previously excluded from their scope under Article 34 of Directive 75/319/EEC. These products were previously exempted because it was felt that the existing provisions of 75/318/EEC (the 'norms and protocols' Directive) and 75/319/EEC (the administrative and general provisions Directive) would need adaptation to their special requirements. The new Directives adopted in 1989 are collectively called the 'extension Directives'.

Three Directives were adopted on 3 May 1989 — 89/341/EEC a new general Directive amending 65/65/EEC, 75/318/EEC and 75/319/EEC; 89/342/EEC a Directive on vaccines, serums, and toxins; and 89/343/EEC a Directive on radiopharmaceutical products.

A new Directive on blood products (89/381/EEC) was adopted by the Council of Ministers on 14 June 1989.

This chapter will deal mainly with 89/341/EEC — the new general Directive. Chapter 8 deals with the special requirements for radiopharmaceutical products.

20.2 DIRECTIVE 89/341/EEC. THE NEW GENERAL DIRECTIVE

20.2.1 Implementation date

The Directive has a latest implementation date in the EC Member States of 1 January 1992.

20.2.2 Objectives of the Directive
The main objectives of the Directive are stated to be to improve the information given to consumers of medicines by requiring more systematic provision of patient leaflets; to improve the guarantee of quality of medicinal products by requiring compliance with the principles of good manufacturing practice (GMP); to provide for a system for rapidly amending the requirements of the Directives as far as GMP is concerned (to create Commission Directives) using a regulatory committee procedure; to improve the information provided with exports to Third World countries; and to extend the scope of the existing Directives to cover other industrially produced medicinal products hitherto excluded.

20.2.3 Change of terminology
Article 1 of the Directive replaces the previous terminology in Directive 65/65/EEC of 'proprietary medicinal product' by 'medicinal product'. Previously, some Member States had felt that it was not clear whether the Directives were supposed to include generic products or not. Although the Commission of the European Communities (CEC) had always felt that the previous definition did include generics, the change makes it unambiguous.

20.2.4 New categories of exemptions from the Directives
A number of exemptions from the Directive requirements are created (in line with the existing practice in the UK with the Medicines Act 1968 exemptions, and in most other EC Member States). These categories of product are exempted from the need to hold a marketing authorisation, the labelling requirements, the suspension and revocation requirements, and the general provisions. The new exempt categories are:

(1) medicinal products prepared on the basis of a 'magistral' formula or official formula;
(2) medicinal products for research and development trials (i.e. clinical trials);
(3) intermediate products intended for further processing by an authorised manufacturer; and
(4) products supplied in response to a *bona fide* unsolicited order, formulated in accord with the specifications of an authorised health care professional, and for use on his individual patients on his direct responsibility.

'Magistral' products are defined as products 'prepared in a pharmacy for individual patients in accord with a prescription'. 'Official' products are defined as products prepared according to a prescriptions of a pharmacopoeia in a pharmacy, and intended to be supplied directly to the patients served by the pharmacy in question.

20.2.5 Amendment to the Summary of product characteristics (SPC) requirements
Article 1 adds a new requirement to Part 6 of the SPC (the pharmaceutical particulars):

> 6.6. special precautions for disposal of unused product waste or waste materials derived from such products, if appropriate.

20.2.6 Amendment to the labelling requirements

Article 1 amends Article 13 of Directive 65/65/EEC to add a requirement about information on precautions about waste disposal (see 20.2.5 above).

20.2.7 Labelling of ampoules: batch number added

Because of their small size, ampoules were exempted from most of the labelling requirements except for product name, quantity of active ingredient, route of administration, and expiry date. The new Directive adds the requirement for batch number.

20.2.8 Replacement of the term 'proprietary medicinal product' by 'medicinal product' in Directive 75/318/EEC

Article 2 of the Directive amends Directive 75/318/EEC. Thus, all of the technical and scientific requirements for a marketing authorisation application will apply to all medicinal products which are industrially produced.

20.2.9 Testing of samples

Article 3 amends Directive 75/319/EEC to allow the national control laboratories in the Member States to ask for samples of starting materials and intermediates (as well as finished product as previously allowed) for evaluation of the suitability of test methods, specification limits, etc.

20.2.10 Mandatory package leaflet

Article 3 amends Directive 75/319/EEC to make a package leaflet obligatory except where all information can be included on the outer container or the immediate container. The objective, as the preamble to the Directive states, is to ensure that information to consumers of medicines (the patients) is improved. The effect of this change will be that even where a generic medicine is prescribed, it will have to include a patient leaflet. The only class of medicine likely to be able to claim the exemption, because all information is included on the outer pack or immediate container, is likely to be some of the over-the-counter (OTC) medicines packed in relatively large pack sizes. In the UK this change is likely to be particularly noticeable because relatively few of the prescription or pharmacy sale products currently contain a leaflet. In other countries (such as Belgium, Italy, Federal Republic of Germany) leaflets are the norm.

20.2.11 A manufacturing authorisation required even for export only products

Article 3 introduces the new requirement for a manufacturing authorisation even where the product is intended only for export, and not for sale on the 'home' market. This will guarantee that all products are manufactured under GMP, and the premises, equipment, etc. are subject to regular inspection. This will help to give a further guarantee of quality for products intended for export (and perhaps particularly those intended for the Third World).

20.2.12 Inspections and good manufacturing practice

Article 3 now introduces an obligation on the manufacturer of a medicinal product to 'comply with the principles and guidelines of good manufacturing practice . . .'. Even before this Directive comes into force, the EC has issued its GMP guide (Volume IV of *The rules governing medicinal products in the European Community* entitled 'Guide for good manufacturing practice for medicinal products').

Article 3 introduces a provision which will enable a GMP directive to be promulgated or revised by using the regulatory committee procedure (Article 2c of Directive 75/318/EEC — the Committee on the Adaptation to Technical Progress . . . . — see Chapter 13 for details). This Directive was adopted in early 1991.

The authorities in the Member States are now required to ensure by means of 'repeated inspections' that the legal requirements governing manufacture and testing of medicinal products are complied with. After each inspection, the inspectors are required to report as to whether the manufacturer complies with GMP. A copy of the report is to be sent to the manufacturer. Hartley (1990) has commented on the new GMP requirements.

20.2.13 Exports and export certificates

Article 3 now introduces certain additional checks on the quality of exported products. As stated previously, these checks are mainly intended to protect the interests of Third World importing countries, but do in fact apply to all countries outside the EC. The new requirements are that the exporter, the manufacturer, or the authorities in the importing country can request a certification that the manufacturer is authorised; that the certificates comply with the current World Health Organization requirements; that for products which are also approved for marketing in the exporting country, a copy of the summary of product characteristics should be supplied; and that if the product is not authorised in the exporting EC Member State an explanation should be provided.

20.2.14 Communicating the results of GMP inspections between the authorities

Article 3 adds a new requirement for results of inspections of manufacturers to be communicated between authorities on receipt of a 'reasoned request'. If the authority receiving the report feels that it cannot accept the conclusions of the report, it can ask for further information. If, at the end of the day, there are still serious differences existing, the CEC becomes concerned with the matter.

The implementation of the new GMP requirements will mean that inspections in the Member States will be carried out by the authorities of that Member State working to an agreed common standard of GMP.

20.2.15 Notification of suspensions and revocations

Article 3 places a new obligation on the holder of the marketing authorisation to notify the Member States concerned (i.e. those where the product is marketed) of any action he takes to suspend or withdraw the marketing on grounds of safety or efficacy. The Member States then have an obligation to notify the CPMP and the World Health Organization.

The CEC is required to publish an annual list of medicinal products which are prohibited in the EC.

20.3 DIRECTIVES 89/342/EEC (IMMUNOLOGICALS), 89/343/EEC (RADIOPHARMACEUTICALS), AND 89/381/EEC (BLOOD PRODUCTS)

These Directives have the following features — definitions of these specialist products (e.g. allergen); definition of quantitative particulars in relation to these products (e.g. mass of active, International Units); requirements for special handling precautions to be included in the SPC; provision for detailed technical requirements to be laid down, using the regulatory committee procedure (Article 2c of Directive 75/318/EEC — see Chapter 13 for details); and a requirement for all of the existing authorisations to be reviewed between the date of adoption of the Directive and 31 December 1992.

In most Member States this last requirement means a review of all existing licences between 1 January 1992 and 31 December 1992. Before that, a Commission Directive amending Directive 75/318/EEC will be issued with the special technical requirements for a marketing authorisation application for these categories of product. In addition, new sections of the 'Notice to Applicants...' will be drafted and detailed technical guidelines issued.

REFERENCE

Hartley, B. (1990). Manufacturing harmonisation — EC export/import. *BIRA Journal* **9** (2), 12–15.

21

The Single Market after 1992: new directions

21.1 INTRODUCTION

In its 1985 White Paper on the completion of the Internal Market, the Commission of the European Communities (CEC) announced that it would bring forward proposals on a future system for the authorisation of medicinal products — whether human or veterinary.

21.2 THE CONSULTATION PROCESS

On 22 March 1988 the services (staff) of Directorate-General III brought forward one of its regular reports on the work of the Committee for Proprietary Medicinal Products (CPMP). This included a review of the use of the existing multistate and concertation procedures.

DGIII then began a series of consultations with the delegates from the CPMP, the national authorities (through the Pharmaceutical Committee), the European pharmaceutical industry, the health professions, and consumer groups. The objective was to elicit views on possible future institutions and procedures which would achieve the Single Market in pharmaceutical products.

In April 1989, the DGIII staff issued another document entitled 'Memorandum on the future system for the authorisation of medicinal products in the European Community'.

After considering the results of these further discussions another document entitled 'Future system for the authorisation of medicinal products within the European Community' was issued in December 1989.

During the first six months of 1990, the Commission reviewed the comments and proposals it had received in response to these ideas. It then formulated an Explanatory Memorandum to the Council of Ministers, with proposals for a Council Regulation and three Council Directives. These were put to the Council of Ministers in September 1990 as the first formal proposals for the legislative framework for the Future System to be introduced from 1 January 1993.

21.3 REVIEW AND ADOPTION OF THE FUTURE SYSTEM LEGISLATIVE PROPOSALS

During the remainder of 1990 and much of 1991 there will be further detailed discussions in a Council of Ministers Expert Working Party and the Committee of Permanent Representatives (COREPER), as well as in the European Parliament, the Economic and Social Committee, etc. This process was described in chapter 2. It is only at the end of this process with their final adoption by the Council of Ministers, that the final shape of the new Community institutions and procedures will become clear. A detailed analysis of the working of the post-1992 future system as finally adopted will therefore need to await a future edition of this book. For this edition, it is only possible to summarise factually the September 1990 proposals, without any attempt being made to forecast how they might be amended.

In the lead-up to 1993, the working methods of the existing CPMP will also need to be modified and the practical details of the new procedures elaborated and stated in a new (third) edition of the 'Notice to Applicants'. It is also certain that this period will see some experiments in processing of marketing authorisation applications to try out some ideas in preparation for the future system — using the Working Parties of the CPMP, *ad hoc* groups of Experts, etc.

21.4 THE PROPOSALS FOR PROCEDURES AFTER 1992

The Commission Explanatory Memorandum envisages the use of three procedures as being available to the industry after 1992:

- a 'decentralised procedure',
- a 'centralised procedure', and
- national procedures.

The function of the decentralised procedure is envisaged as enabling smaller companies to progressively penetrate the pharmaceutical Euro-market. It would probably be the most frequently used Community procedure, and any company which had obtained an authorisation in any one Member State would then be able to apply for acceptance of the authorisation in one or more of the other European Community (EC) Member States. If the Member State(s) concerned considered that they could not accept the authorisation, even after bilateral discussion and negotiation with the first country, the matter would then be referred to the CPMP for binding arbitration at Community level.

The function of the centralised procedure would be to provide major innovative products with direct access to the whole Euro-market. It is envisaged as being compulsory for biotechnology products, but optionally available to companies for new active substance products and (if the CPMP agrees in the cases concerned) also for certain high technology products.

National procedures are seen as eventually only necessary for registering purely local products in one country. Where products are traditionally marketed in several countries together — such as the United Kingdom (UK) and Ireland, or the Benelux countries (Belgium, the Netherlands, and Luxembourg), it would automatically involve the decentralised procedure.

21.5 PHASING AND TRANSITIONAL ARRANGEMENTS FOR THE NEW PROCEDURES

21.5.1 National applications

Proposed transitional arrangements for national applications are envisaged as follows:

1993–1996: Parallel applications in two or more Member States allowed, but if one or more Member State(s) wishes to suspend its evaluation and wait for the other Member State to complete its assessment it can do so.

1996 onwards: Parallel applications not permitted after one Member State has authorised. After the first authorisation, all subsequent applications would be handled via the decentralised procedure.

21.5.2 Centralised applications

Transitional arrangements for a new active substance (NAS) marketing authorisation application are envisaged as follows:

1993–1999: Applications to be made either centrally or using the national/decentralised route at the choice of the company.

1999 onwards: The categories of product where applications would have to be made compulsorily via the centralised procedure would be reviewed. It seems likely, if the new European Medicines Agency is working well by this time, that the procedure would be extended to NAS applications.

21.6 PRODUCTS AUTHORISED NATIONALLY BEFORE 1993

In the case of products authorised nationally before 1993, the Member States would still be responsible for the management of the authorisations — dealing with variations, renewals, suspensions, revocations, etc. However, reference may be made to the CPMP in cases where:

- Community interests are involved (Article 12 of Directive 75/319/EEC), or
- where divergent decisions have been made (Article 11 of 75/319/EEC).

There will also need to be Community consideration of the pre-1993 products in relation to pharmacovigilance, defect reports, and proposals to revoke or suspend authorisations which exist in more than one Member State.

21.7 THE OBJECTIVES OF THE NEW INSTITUTIONS AND PROCEDURES

The future system must meet certain agreed criteria from the points of view of public health, industrial policy, and the CEC. These were discussed in the CPMP and Pharmaceutical Committee and are now set out in the CEC's 1990 Explanatory Memorandum. Some of the main points are detailed below.

21.7.1 Public health

A new future system should provide a scientific evaluation of the marketing authorisation application by the best possible Community experts; and it should have clearly defined harmonised criteria for quality, safety, and efficacy; it should define clear legal responsibilities for each authority concerned with marketing authorisations as far as grant/refusal/suspensions etc. It should have the ability to restrict or withdraw a product on the basis of pharmacovigilance reports or product surveillance information (counterfeits or defects); provide identical product information throughout the Community (i.e. a single summary of product characteristics, identical product labelling and patient information leaflet texts in the national languages); and give an equivalent legal status in all EC Member States. Finally, it should provide encouragement to carry out preclinical and clinical research in Europe.

21.7.2 Industrial policy

The new future system should provide clear uniform requirements for format and content of marketing authorisation applications, an assessment based on a single dossier sent to one authority, and consider using simple administrative procedures, rights to appeal against adverse decisions, and reasonable fees related to the level of work caused to the authorities.

21.7.3 EC interests

The new future system should provide the ability for innovatory companies to consult the authorities during the development and testing of a new product — thus encouraging the development of the European industry. It should give access to the whole European market for innovatory new products. It should make allowance for local and regional marketing of products. It should provide for the implementation of a complete system for inspection, enforcement, and validation of the data in the application dossier (good clinical practice, good laboratory practice, and good manufacturing practice). The new institutions should encourage the continuation of the international harmonisation of test requirements, format for applications, etc., to minimise unnecessary (and scientifically unjustified) extra work needed to register the same product in different world markets.

21.8 THE EUROPEAN MEDICINES EVALUATION AGENCY (EMEA)

The draft Regulation proposes the establishment of a new European Medicines Evaluation Agency, which would be responsible for both veterinary and human pharmaceutical products.

The main tasks of the agency would be the coordination of the scientific and technical assessment of the quality, safety, and efficacy of medicinal products subject to EC procedures; and the presentation of assessment reports, summaries of product characteristics (SPCs), labels, and patients and healthcare professional information leaflets. It would be involved in the continued supervision of products authorised at a Community level, and in the coordination of manufacturing and testing requirements, enforcement, and inspection (GCP, GLP, GMP). It would promote co-operation with the European Pharmacopoeia Commission. It would co-ordinate national pharmacovigilance reporting arrangements.

The European Medicines Evaluation Agency would, it is proposed, be composed of the following elements:

(a) managerial and administrative support — an executive director and the Agency secretariat;
(b) an administrative management board consisting of two representatives from each Member State (one for human products and one for veterinary products), and two representatives from the CEC;
(c) the scientific and technical support for the EMEA which will consist of the rapporteurs from the Member States, and the experts drawn from the Member States;
(d) the scientific and technical committees — the Committee for Proprietary Medicinal Products (CPMP), the Committee for Veterinary Medicinal Products (CVMP), the working parties of the above, and *ad hoc* Expert groups of the above;
(e) the Scientific Council of five to nine persons of outstanding and internationally recognised ability with particular knowledge of the ethical and scientific issues in the development and testing of veterinary and human pharmaceutical products.

21.8.1 Managerial and administrative support

It is proposed that the executive Director would be nominated by the Council of Ministers acting on a proposal from the CEC.

The administrative support for the Agency would service the technical and scientific committees; be concerned with the management of the dossiers; keep a databank on the products; provide personnel, legal, translation, and accounting services.

It should be noted that the funding of the Agency would be based partly on fees paid by companies for the assessment of their applications, and partly by funds from the Community budget.

21.8.2 Administrative board

The function of the administrative board would be to ensure the efficient functioning of the Agency. Each year it would consider the annual report, the programme of work for the next year, the draft annual accounts for the past year, and the estimates of income and expenditure for the next year.

The general report of the activities of the Agency would be forwarded each year to the Member States, the CEC, the Council of Ministers, the European Parliament, and the Scientific Council. The financial report would be submitted by 31 March each year to the EC's Court of Auditors.

21.8.3 Scientific and technical support for the EMEA

This will consist of the rapporteurs and experts drawn from the national agencies, national advisory committees, etc. in the Member States. It is these experts who will be asked by the CPMP (or the CVMP for veterinary products) to do the preliminary assessment work on a centralised application, or to provide a separate assessment if the arbitration process is invoked through the decentralised procedure.

It is proposed that the rapporteurs and Experts would be commissioned to deliver their report and be remunerated on a fixed scale of fees.

The scientific assessment of applications by these rapporteurs and Experts for the Agency will mean a continued role for the national agencies in providing these experts. In some senses the Agency could be envisaged as consisting of a core with an administrative support team surrounded by a group of experts to be drawn on as needed. The experts will be drawn from the full-time employees of national agencies, part-time employees of the national agencies and the outside advisory experts used in many of the national agencies (see Chapter 19).

21.8.4 The scientific and technical committees

These consist of the CPMP, the CVMP, and their working parties and expert groups.

The CPMP and CVMP will each consist (it is proposed) of scientific advisors nominated by each Member State for a renewable term of five years. The Member States are required to consult so that the composition of the committee reflects the various scientific and medical disciplines necessary for the evaluation of medicinal products.

The members of the CPMP and CVMP act as a link to coordinate with the work of the national advisory committees (see Chapter 18).

It is not yet clear what standing ('institutional') working parties will be needed to assist the CPMP and CVMP. At present, as explained in Chapter 13, there are quality, safety, efficacy, biotechnology/pharmacy, pharmacovigilance, and operational working parties.

It is likely that expert groups will be convened as needed to consider particular problems or applications for a particular product or group of associated products.

21.8.5 The Scientific Council

It is proposed that the Scientific Council will consist of five to nine persons of outstanding and internationally recognised ability, with particular knowledge of the scientific and ethical issues relating to development and testing of medicinal products. Issues would be referred to them by the CPMP and CVMP. They would also see the draft Agency annual report and be able to comment on it.

21.9 THE CENTRALISED PROCEDURE

This procedure is intended to give innovative products easier access to the whole Euro-market.

21.9.1 Products eligible for the procedure

The procedure would be obligatory for those biotechnology products in List A to the Regulation (which are the same as those in Directive 87/22/EEC) and in addition for the veterinary growth promoters.

The procedure would be optional (i.e. it would be a matter of choice for the applicant) for new active substance products. These are defined as being products which on 1 January 1993 had not been authorised in any of the EC Member States. It is likely that an explanation of this definition will be given in the next edition of the 'Notice to Applicants....', and new chemical active substance products will, for example, almost certainly include products containing the separate desired enantiomers (the eutomers) of active ingredients previously marketed as racemic mixtures/racemates.

The procedure would be optional for new medicinal products derived from human blood or human plasma.

The procedure would again be optional for certain defined categories of high technology products. However, in the case of these products the Agency is envisaged as having a 'gatekeeper' role, in that the company would apply for them to be included, but would have to produce arguments in their Expert Report as to the innovative nature etc. of the product, which the Agency would then consider and decide whether to admit the product to the procedure. The categories of high technology product for which this applies would include the following:

- medicinal products developed by other biotechnological processes (i.e. other than those in List A of the Regulation) which, in the opinion of the Agency, constitute a significant innovation;
- medicinal products administered by mean of new delivery systems which, in the opinion of the Agency, constitute a significant innovation;
- medicinal products for an entirely new indication which, in the opinion of the Agency, is of significant therapeutic interest;
- medicinal products based on radioisotopes which, in the opinion of the Agency, are of significant therapeutic interest; and
- medicinal products the manufacture of which employs processes which, in the opinion of the Agency, demonstrate a significant technical advance such as two-dimensional electrophoresis under microgravity.

As stated earlier, the categories of product for which a compulsory procedure is applicable, and those for which it is optional, will be subject to review in 1999. It seems likely that there will then be an extension of the procedure to ensure that all the major innovative products intended for sale in most countries of the Euro-market would be considered by the compulsory centralised Community procedure.

21.9.2 The working of the centralised procedure

Much of the detail of the procedure remains to be worked out. Discussions on these details are likely to take place in the period 1990 to 1992, in order to produce a new (third) edition of the 'Notice to Applicants'. This will lay down, for example, the number of copies of the dossier needed for a centralised application, the fee payable, the languages needed for the various parts of the dossier, etc.

After validation of the application, it would be referred to the CPMP for assessment. The assessment would be coordinated by a rapporteur appointed by the CPMP, using experts nominated by the CPMP to consider individual parts of the dossier — probably one for quality aspects, one for preclinical safety aspects and one for clinical aspects.

The job of the rapporteur is to produce the assessment report for the product, a draft SPC, and draft labelling and package inserts for the product. These would then be referred to the CPMP and its working parties and panels.

It is likely that for nearly all applications there will be a need to ask the applicant for clarification and comment. The overall time allowed for consideration of the application would be 210 days, but this would be the net time, and the clock would be stopped while the applicant provided further information and comment as necessary.

After allowing the applicant to present this further information, the draft assessment report would be presented to the CPMP with the draft SPC/label/leaflet texts. The CPMP would then issue a scientific Opinion, which would become binding under the new 'regulatory mechanism'.

21.9.3 Appeals in the centralised procedure

The draft Regulation envisages three stages of appeal.

The first is during the assessment by the CPMP, when the applicant is allowed to make oral or written explanations. The second is after the issue of a wholly or partly negative scientific opinion (e.g. proposed refusal, need to amend the applicant's proposed SPC, authorisation subject to special conditions), where the applicant has 15 days to notify in writing his wish to appeal, and the CPMP has 60 days in which to consider the appeal. The third is after the issue of a draft Decision, when the applicant would be able to submit written observations on the draft Decision for consideration by the CEC.

The existing concertation procedure could be used as a model for the likely working of the first appeal stage in the new centralised procedure. Thus, informal appeals (in writing and orally) have generally been to the biotechnology/pharmacy working party on quality aspects, and as formal appeals (again in writing and orally) to the CPMP itself on any issues of quality that remained after the informal hearing, on the preclinical safety and human clinical risk/benefit. In the CPMP, the hearings have concentrated on the issues that remained after consideration of the written data, and the rapporteur has briefed the applicant company on these issues. A hearing has usually lasted between 40 minutes and 1 hour, with about 20 minutes of presentation in answer to the remaining issues and the remainder for question and answer between the company's representatives and the CPMP delegates. The company usually has a team of four to six Experts who attend the hearing.

The details of the second and third appeal stages will no doubt be published in the next edition of the 'Notice to Applicants...'.

21.10 THE DECENTRALISED PROCEDURE

Just as the centralised procedure is a development of the concertation procedure, the decentralised procedure is based on the present multistate procedure. It is envisaged as a means whereby medium or small companies can gain progressive access to the pharmaceutical Euro-market.

The proposals for the decentralised procedure are laid down in one of the new draft Directives.

21.10.1 Products eligible for the decentralised procedure

Products eligible for the procedure are all those except the biotechnology List A products defined in the draft Regulation. They could include new active substance products, blood products, and 'abridged' or 'second applicant' products containing existing active ingredients.

21.10.2 The working of the decentralised procedure

To use the procedure, the applicant company first obtains a national authorisation by applying in one or more of the EC Member States. The authorities in the Member State would then consider the application in the usual way. They would systematically issue a detailed assessment report, text of the approved SPC, and the label and leaflet texts.

As with the current multistate procedure, the applicant company would then apply for recognition of the first authorisation to other countries of the EC (but with the proposed threshold now lowered to one or more, instead of two or more as with the current procedure). The applicant would apply, using the same application dossier as approved in the first country with the same SPC, label text, leaflet text, etc. In addition, the first country would furnish its assessment report — so that all of the issues it considered in its evaluation were clear to the other countries.

The expectation is that there might then need to be bilateral or multilateral discussion and negotiation on the contents of the dossier, between the rapporteurs and co-rapporteurs in the countries involved. If they could reach agreement, then authorisations would be issued in the other countries.

If the countries concerned with the decentralised application cannot reach an agreement, and important substantive (probably clinical) issues remain, the decentralised procedure then envisages that a compulsory arbitration scheme would be brought into play. Thus, the rapporteur and co-rapporteurs would present an agreed statement of the problem for the CPMP to consider, together with their assessment reports, draft SPC texts, etc.

The arbitration procedure uses an independent rapporteur and set of experts appointed by the CPMP who would then review the information supplied by the other countries — the assessment reports, draft SPC texts, etc. The conclusions of these experts would be submitted via working parties and panels (as appropriate) to the CPMP. The CPMP would then issue an Opinion. The Opinion would become a binding decision (for the concerned countries only) using the regulatory mechanism.

As mentioned in section 21.5.1, it is planned for there to be transitional arrangements for national applications between 1993 and 1996.

It is also intended that Member States can informally work-share the assessment. Thus, if a Member State becomes aware that another EC country has received the same application, it can defer its national consideration until it has received the assessment report of the first country. However, it then has only 90 days to decide whether to recognise the first decision or not. If it does not, the matter would be referred to the CPMP for arbitration.

Thus, the decentralised procedure can be seen as really comprising two separate modes:

- sequential applications (first obtaining one authorisation, then using that authorisation to gain access to other countries), and
- concurrent national applications (but where a final decision is likely to await the result of the first assessment).

It remains to be seen whether a major innovative (say a new active substance) product would be put into simultaneous national applications, if there was the probability that there would then be a sequential application process, and a risk of subsequent reference to the CPMP for arbitration. It might be seen as being simpler and quicker to use the centralised procedure in the first place. However, this question will probably remain an open one — at least until actual experience with the various procedures is gained after 1 January 1993.

As with the centralised procedure, the timescale for a decision in the decentralised procedure is 210 days, with the facility for stopping the clock for further information or comment. However, in the sequential procedure, each subsequent national stage can take up to 90 days, with additional time (another 90 days) if the CPMP is used for arbitration.

21.10.3 Appeals in the decentralised procedure

The following appeal stages (or at least stages when the applicant's views can be heard) can be identified in the Directive proposals for the decentralised procedure:

(a) national appeals during the first national processing of the application (the number of appeal stages depends on national laws — see Chapters 17 and 18 for details);
(b) facility for oral or written comment during the bilateral/multilateral negotiation when the application is being considered by the other Member States;
(c) facility for oral or written explanation during the CPMP arbitration process before the Opinion is issued;
(d) facility for the applicant to ask to comment within 15 days, and then to provide that comment on a wholly or partly negative opinion (e.g. proposed refusal, proposed amendment to the applicant's summary of product characteristics,

grant subject to conditions, or requirement to suspend, withdraw, or amend an existing authorisation);
(e) facility for the applicant to comment to the Commission on the draft Decision.

21.11 THE 'REGULATORY MECHANISM' — TURNING OPINIONS INTO DECISIONS

In both the centralised and decentralised procedures, the same so-called 'regulatory mechanism' is proposed. This mechanism consists of the following stages:

(a) The opinion is sent to the CEC, with the following documents:
- the draft SPC,
- draft text of the label and package leaflet,
- details of any conditions that may be imposed on the sale or supply of the product (such as legal status).
(b) Within 30 days, the CEC prepares a draft Decision. If it is a decision in favour of grant of an authorisation, the draft SPC, label, and leaflet are attached to it.
(c) The draft Decision is circulated to the Member States and the applicant company.
(d) Member States have 30 days to object to the draft Decision by commenting to the CEC and the other Member States.
(e) The applicant has the same 30 days to comment to the CEC on the draft Decision.
(f) The CEC reviews any request received under (d) or (e) above with the Agency.
(g) If the request received raises technical or scientific questions, these may be sent back to the Agency for a second CPMP opinion within a 60 day time limit.
(h) If the request raises other than technical or scientific questions, the matter is then referred to a regulatory committee of the Member States, where a decision is presumably taken by a qualified majority vote (see Chapter 14).

21.12 THE SUPERVISORY AUTHORITY

In the proposals for the Future System, much of the responsibility for the supervision of manufacturers and any necessary inspection and enforcement measures will still lie with the national authorities of the Member States. The draft Regulation establishing the Future System embodies the concept of the national supervisory authority performing delegated functions for the whole EC. The supervisory authority would be responsible for inspection and control of manufacturers and wholesalers in their own national territories, and for ensuring that test and controls on importation are carried out for products from third (non-EC) countries.

In relation to inspections outside the EC, use will obviously be made of the reciprocal arrangements of the Pharmaceutical Inspection Convention (PIC) where appropriate. However, where non-PIC members are concerned, the proposals allow for coordinated inspections using national inspectors or inspectors employed by the European Medicines Evaluation Agency.

The new legal framework envisaged for after 1992 still includes the possibility of suspension or withdrawal of a European marketing authorisation on a temporary basis where it is a matter of urgency. However, the matter would obviously need to be referred to the Agency for the application of Community procedures as soon as possible.

Certain types of illegal conduct in relation to European authorisations (e.g. sale or supply to outlets other than those permitted in the authorisation, promotion for indications other than those approved) would also necessitate national enforcement measures. The penalties would be the same as for such misconduct involving purely national authorisations.

The whole Future Systems proposals are in fact a delicate balance between the powers given to the new European Agency and powers delegated to the existing national authorities (for assessment on behalf of the Community, for GMP inspections, for enforcement, for pharmacovigilance etc.). It will be essential, if the proposals for the Future System are to become fully effective, for the balance to be maintained in such a way that it enables both the new Agency and the existing national agencies to work efficiently and harmoniously together.

REFERENCE

Future system for the free movement of medicinal products in the European Community. COM(90) 283 final — SYN 309 to 312. Brussels, 14 November 1990. Commission of the European Communities.

Appendix
Abbreviations and acronyms

More than one hundred abbreviations or acronyms used in this book. Although each is defined at its first appearance, the following glossary may be helpful.

ABPI	Association of the British Pharmaceutical Industry
ADR	adverse drug reaction
AE	adverse event
AESG	Association Européennes des Societés Grands Publiques
AFNOR	French Standardisation Committee
AIDS	acquired immune deficiency syndrome
AIII	Association of International Industrial Irradiation
AIM	active ingredient manufacturer
ANDA	abbreviated new drug application
ARSAC	Administration of Radioactive Substances Advisory Committee
BAN	British Approved Name
BGA	Bundesgesundheitsamt
BP	*British Pharmacopoeia*
BPC	British Pharmacopoeia Commission
CANDA	computer assisted new drug application
CAPLA	computer assisted product licence application
CDSM	Committee on Dental and Surgical Materials
CEC	Commission of the European Communities
CEE	Commaunité Européen Economique (=EEC)
CEN	European Standardisation Committee
CENELEC	European Electrotechnical Standardisation Committee
CJEC	Court of Justice of the European Communities
COCIR	Coordination Committee of Radiological and Electrotechnical Equipment

Abbreviations and acronyms

COREPEPER	Committee of Representatives of the EC Ammbassadors
COWS of WASP	Commission on World Standards of the World Association of Societies of Pathology
CPMP	Committee for Proprietary Medicinal Products
CPS	Chemistry, Pharmacy, and Standards Subcommittee
CRM	Committee on the Review of Medicines
CSD	Committee on Safety of Drugs
CSM	Committee on Safety of Medicines
CSP	Comité de Specialités Pharmaceutiques
CTC	clinical trial certificate
CTX	critical trial certificate exemption
CVMP	Committee for Veterinary Medicinal Products
DAB	*Deutsches Arzneibuch*
DDX	doctors' and dentists' exemption
DHAEMAE	Disposable Hypodermic and Allied Equipment Manufactuers' Association of Europe
DMF	drug master file
DPLM	Direction de la Pharmacie et du Médicament
EASSI	European Association of Surgical Sutures Industry
EC	European Community(ies)
ECJ	European Court of Justice
EDMA	European Diagnostic Manufacturers Association
EEC	European Economic Community (ies)
EFPIA	European Federation of Pharmaceutical Industries Associations
EFTA	European Free Trade Association
EMEA (EMA?)	European Medicines Evaluation Agency
EN	European Standard
EUCOMED	European Confederation of Medical Suppliers Association
EURATOM	European Atomic Energy Community
EuroDMF	European drug master file
Euromcontact	European Federation of National Associations of Contact Lens Manufacturers
Eurom VI	European Federation of Precision Mechanical and Optical Industries
FDA	Food and Drug Administration
FIDE	Federation of European Dental Industry
GCP	good clinical practice
GDP	gross domestic product
GMP	good manufacturing practice
GP	gas permeable (contact lenses)
GSL	general sales list

HD	harmonisation document
IAPM	International Association of Medical Prosthetics Manufacturers
IASBM	International Association of Surgical Blade Manufacturers
ICDRA	International Conference of Drug Regulatory Authorities
ICSH	International Committee for Standardisation in Haematology
IEC	International Electrotechnical Commission
IFCC	International Federation of Clinical Chemistry
IFPMA	International Federation of Pharmaceutical Manufacturers Associations
IND	investigatory new drug application
INN	International Nonproprietary Name
ISC	Iron and Steel Community
ISO	International Standards Organization
IUCD	intrauterine contraceptive device
IUPAC	International Union of Pure and Applied Chemistry
MA	market authorisation
MAIL	Medicines Act information letter
MAL	medicines advice leaflet (or Medicines Act leaflet)
MC	Medicines Commission
MCA	Medicines Control Agency
MDD	Medical Devices Directorate
MEP	Member of the European Parliament
MI	Medicines Inspectorate (UK)
MHW	Japanese Ministry of Health and Welfare
MIMS (UK)	*Monthly Index of Medical Specialities*
MLA	medicines licence application
NAS	new active substance
NBAS	new biological active substance
NCAS	new chemical active substance
NCE	new chemical entity
NDAB	National Drugs Advisory Board
NSAID	non-steroidal steroid anti-inflammatory drug
OTC	over-the-counter
P	pharmacy sale medicine
PER	product evaluation report
Ph. Eur.	*European Pharmacopoeia*
PIC	Pharmaceutical Inspection Convention
PL	product licence
PL(PI)	parallel import product licence
PLR	product licence of right
PMS	postmarketing surveillance
POM	prescription only medicine

Abbreviations and acronyms

RAPS	Regulatory Affairs Professionals Society
SEAR	Safety Efficiency, and Adverse Reactions
SKF	Smith Kline and French Laboratories
SI	Statutory Instrument
SM	Single Market
SOP	standard operating procedures
SPC	summary of product characteristics
UK	United Kingdom of Great Britain and Northern Ireland
US/USA	United States of America
USAN	United States Adopted Name
USP	*United States Pharmacopeia*
VPC	Veterinary Products Committee

Index

35 days, 262
120 days, 227, 255
1992
   procedures after, 303–4, 305–6
     transitional arrangements, 304

abbreviations, 314–7
abridged applications, 40, 93–105, 170, 174, 175, 190, 198–208, 222, 223, 227, 256, 309
   before July 1987, 93–4
   data requirements, 100–105
   medically targeted, 243
   piggy-back, 243
   simple, 243
absorption, 79
Acanthamoeba spp., 164
accreditation and certification, 138
accuracy, 61
acquired immune deficiency syndrome, 217
acronyms, 314–7
active implantable medical devices, 130, 138–49, 156
   Directive, 138–49, 161
active ingredient, 58, 59, 70, 99, 106, 182, 236, 262
   amount, 58
   combinations, 78
   drug master file procedure, European, 110–12
   manufacturer, 58
   specification, 66–7
active medical device, 130, 131
administrative information, 57–8, 96
adverse drug reaction, 22, 52, 170, 187, 195, 196, 197, 217, 223
adverse event, 87, 88, 125, 141, 154, 165
advertising and promotion, 44
advertising material, 59
advisory body, 256–60
advisory committee (UK), 256, 257, 261, 263, 264, 267
   advice, 257
     grant, 257
     grant on condition, 257
     refuse, 257, 258
     recommendation, 258

     grant, 258, 260
     grant on condition, 258, 260
     refuse, 258, 260
allergen product, 52
allopurinol, 108
amoxycillin trihydrate, 108
ampicillin trihydrate, 108
analysis
   of application
     CPMP procedure, 222
     defects in, 190–212
     multistate, 223
   pooled, 90
analytical
   aspect, 182
   development, 69, 101
   method, 61, 110
   validation, 61, 66, 69, 101, 110, 173, 184, 203, 204, 215
anticancer product, 26
antimicrobial preservative, 182
   absence of, 120
   efficacy, 72, 101, 164, 254
     inocula, low level, 164
     preservative inactivation, 164
     recovery experiment, 164
     validation, 164
appeal, 170, 180, 190, 205, 206, 228, 229, 258, 259, 262, 263, 267, 287–9, 305, 309, 311
   concertation procedure, 239–40
   data, 170
   delay due to, 207
   national, 229
   outcome, 205–8
applicant's signature, 58
application
   cross-referral, 188
   date of, 58
   defects in, 190–212
   deficiencies, 254
   drug, 52
   forms (UK), 251, 253, 261, 263
   incomplete, 190–1
   number granted, 191
   number of copies, 58, 252

Index 319

number received, 191
  Part I, 56–60
  Part II, 60–72
  Part III, 73–84
  Part IV, 89–92
  Part V, 72–73
  referred to CPMP
    deficiencies, 205–8
    processing (UK), 261
  referred to CSM
    deficiencies, 205–8
  rejection rate, 196–7
approved name, 109
arbitration, 37
  binding, 303, 310
Article 4(8)(a), 95, 110, 175, 253
  (i), 95, 225
  (ii), 95, 100, 102, 174, 175, 185, 225
  (iii), 95, 99, 175, 225
Article 4(8)(b), 96, 175
assay
  active ingredient, 68, 101, 123, 203
  biological activity, 69
  excipient, 68, 123, 203
  limits, 69
assembly, 64
assent procedure, 49
assessment report, 168, 169, 170, 222, 227, 229, 230, 240, 247, 258, 306, 308, 310
  contents, 230
assessors (UK), 255, 256, 262, 263
assurance of production quality, 147–8, 156
atenolol, 108
Australia, 172, 247
Austria, 22, 52, 135, 247
authenticity, statement of, 104
authorization and marketing, 96–7
  10-year rule, evidence of, 96–7
  first authorization, 253
authors and editors, 24

batch analysis, 67, 69, 87, 109, 111, 184, 200, 201, 204
batch control, 39
batch size, 63
Belgium, 34, 46, 48, 58, 73, 114, 132, 135, 163, 221, 230, 233, 234, 280–93
bibliography, 94
bioavailability, 36, 52, 59, 88, 99, 103–4, 109, 143, 144, 154, 158, 178, 186, 201, 202, 254, 256
  study design, 103
  verification, 104
bioburden, 166, 203
biocompatibility, 143
biodistribution, 119, 120, 122, 123, 124
bioequivalence, 88, 90, 103–4, 110, 201, 203, 254
  decision rule, 104
  study design, 103
  verification, 104
biological product, 255, 262
biological standardization, 31
biological testing, 31

biopharmaceutics, 173
biostudy, analytical validation, 204
biotechnology, 214, 235
  procedure, 41, 236–7
  processes, 237, 238
    new (*see also* List A), 237
    other (*see also* List B), 237
blood products, 37, 43, 187, 218, 223, 224, 236, 255, 297, 301, 309
borderline products, 130, 187
breathing gases, 269
bridging summary (*see also* within summary), 175, 193, 195
British Approved Name, 64, 199
British Pharmacopoeia, *see under* Pharmacopoeia, British
British Pharmacopoeia Commission, 33, 257
Bundesgesundheitsamt, 34, 185
Bureau of Chemistry, 31

CE work, 138, 139, 141, 142, 149, 153, 156, 156, 156, 160
  wrongly applied, 152
CEC, *see* Commission of the European Communities
CPMP, *see* Committee for Proprietary Medicinal Products
Canada, 172, 247
carconogenicity, studies, 83–4, 125, 167, 185, 212
carrier, 116, 122
case report forms, 88
centralized procedure, 41, 215, 303–4, 308–10
centrapharm, 38
certificate
  clinical trial, *see under* clinical trial
  design examination, 145
  of batch conformity, 147
  type-examination, 147
certification, 160
chairman, 213, 215–7
changes (*see also* variations), 170, 226, 249, 263
characteristics and performance, 142, 152, 154
chemical active ingredient
  deficiencies in applications, 199–205
Chemie Grunethal, 32
chemistry and pharmacy data requirements, 54–75, 100–102, 109–10, 111–2, 118–20, 122–4, 164–5, 166, 226, 253, 259
child-resistant containers, 62
chirality (*see also* stereochemistry, eutomer), 34
chromatographic methods, 66, 110
cimetidine, 97
classification (medical devices), 151–2, 157–9
clinical
  data, 226
  database, 192, 194
  data requirement, 85–92, 120–1, 125, 165, 167
  documentation, 90
  dossier, 192–198
  evaluation, 148–9, 159
  experience, 90
  Expert, *see under* expert, clinical

indication, 59, 90, 110
investigation, 141, 148, 153, 156, 161
interaction, 59
patient safety, 142, 154
pharmacology, 89–90, 186, 195
trials
  application, 87, 188
  certificate, 107, 131, 188, 250–61, 263
  exemption, 131, 161, 188, 250, 251, 262–3
  final report, 87
  individual reports, 196–8
  investigator, 86, 88
  monitor, 86, 87–8
  sponsor, 86–7
clock, 238, 261, 309
college ter Beoordeling van geneesmiddeln, 33
co-rapporteur, 229–30
colour, 37–8
combination products, 78, 96, 246
commission
  communication, 38, 49, 51
  decisions, 51
  directives, 40, 50
  of the European Communities, 23, 47
committee, 170
  Administration of Radioactive Substances, Advisory, 120, 268
  applications, consideration of, 205–8
  Economic and Social, 47, 49, 136–7
  ethics, 86, 87, 153
  for Proprietary Medicinal Products, 24, 29, 37, 47, 51, 52, 54, 58, 76, 99, 110, 168, 175, 180, 190, 204, 213–7, 236, 238, 250, 255, 256, 261, 280, 294, 302, 306
    procedure, 37, 220, 221–2
  for the Adaptation to Technical progress, 40, 50, 218–9
  for the Evaluation of Medicines, 33
  for Veterinary Medicinal Products, 33, 257, 306
  Membership, 257
  of Permanent Representatives (COREPER), 47, 137
  on Dental and Surgical Materials, 33, 131, 164, 190, 205, 257, 266, 269
  on Radiation from Radioactive Medicinal Product, 257
  on Safety of Drugs, 33
  on Safety of Medicines, 33, 117, 170, 190, 194, 199, 227, 257
  on the Review of Medicines, 257, 266
  Pharmaceutical, 37, 47, 217–8, 294, 302
  standing, 138, 140, 153
  veterinary products, 257
compatibility, 62, 63, 143, 154, 201
  study, 164
compliance certificate, 145
component, 166
composition, 62, 70, 99, 100, 182, 226
computer-assisted application, 196
concerned Member State, 220, 227
concertation procedure, 29, 41, 117, 169, 171, 214, 216, 235–41, 243, 244, 302

confidentialityy, 142, 153
conformity assessment, 141, 152, 156
connector, 154, 155
consolidated list, 239
constituent, unusual, 63
consultative process, 136
contact lens, 129, 162–6, 269
  care product, 129, 162–6, 223, 256, 262, 269
container, 59, 107, 118, 165
contamination, risk of, 154
contergan, 32
contraceptive, 256
contraindication, 59, 144, 174, 187, 217, 224, 226, 246
control test (*see also* specification)
  active ingredient, 66–7, 100, 101, 110, 111, 183
  biodistribution, 123
  finished product, 68–9, 101, 119, 123, 166, 184
  impurity, 106, 183
  intermediate, 64, 68, 101, 109, 166, 184, 199, 202
  radiochemical purity, 123
  starting material, 64–8, 101, 123, 199
cooperation procedure, 49, 51
Coordination Committee of Radiological and Electromedical Equipment, 130
copies, number of, 58, 252
copy products, 40, 94, 175
Council
  common position, 130, 137
  Decisions, 51, 134, 137
  of Europe, 41
  of Ministers, 44, 47, 130, 137
  Recommendation, 39, 51, 78, 79, 80, 82, 83, 211, 212, 294
  Working Group, 47, 137
Court of Justice of the European Communities *see* European Court of Justice
critical
  analysis, 171, 173, 180, 193, 194
  overview, 176
  review, 171
cross-referral applications, 188
custom-made device, 138-9, 148, 156
cytokine, 26, 215

Dalli-Werke, Maürer and Wirtz, 32
data recording, 86
data sheets, 26, 59, 194
date
  authorization, 225
  of guideline application, 26
decentralized procedure, 173, 215, 221, 243, 280, 303, 310–2
decision, 47, 51, 229
declaration of conformity, 144–5, 147–8, 156
Declaration of Helsinki, 86
decomposition product, 70
defects in applications, 190–212
definitions, 137
degradation
  pathway, 101

product, 178, 185, 203
Denmark, 34, 41, 46, 58, 73, 95, 107, 114, 132, 135, 163, 179, 221, 225, 230, 233, 234
dental product, 253, 256
description, 64
design, 143, 154
 and construction, 143, 154
 dossier, 145
 examination certificate, 145
Dictionnaire Vidal, 224
De Peijper, 38, 49, 51
Deutsches Arzneibuch, 42, 100
development
 chemistry, 65–8, 69
 pharmaceutics, 36, 62, 100, 173, 182, 201, 202
Directives
 65/65/EEC, 22, 35, 55, 73, 93, 108, 114, 116, 121, 126, 136, 139, 143, 151, 154, 158, 159, 160, 174, 175, 185, 213, 218, 220, 225, 236, 250, 253, 297
 75/318/EEC, 36, 41, 55, 60, 77, 78, 79, 80, 81, 83, 85, 85, 89, 90, 100, 102, 108, 114, 121, 143, 154, 169, 174, 203, 216, 218, 294, 297
 76/319/EEC, 36, 55, 108, 127, 168, 169, 175, 213, 217, 220, 223, 236, 239, 297
 76/579/EURATOM, 117
 78/25/EEC, 37
 80/386/EURATOM, 117
 83/189/EC, 134, 140
 83/570/EEC, 36, 55, 81, 94, 168, 216, 220, 221
 84/359/EEC, 131
 84/467/EURATOM, 117
 86/609/EEC, 77
 87/18/EEC, 76
 87/19/EEC, 40, 55, 218, 294
 87/21/EEC, 40, 55, 94, 95
 87/22/EEC, 41, 55, 95, 159, 187, 214, 224, 235, 236, 240, 245
 88/182/EEC, 134
 88/320/EEC, 77
 89/105/EEC, 43
 89/336/EEC, 139
 89/341/EEC, 43, 44, 55, 297–301
 89/342/EEC, 43, 55, 223, 297
 89/343/EEC, 43, 45, 114–28, 223, 297
 89/381/EEC, 43, 55, 223, 297
 90/336/EEC, 138–49
 EC, 34, 47, 50, 110, 117, 250
 EURATOM, 117, 121, 143, 155, 269
 exemptions from, 298
 medical device, 129–61
 proposal for new, 218
Directorates-General
 III, 23, 24, 47, 227, 302
 VI, 47
 list of, 48
disinfection, 63
disintegration, 203
dissolution, 63, 101, 184, 201, 203, 204
Distillers (biochemicals) Ltd, 32
distomer, 34
distribution, 79, 124

distributor, 58, 111
doctor and dentist exemption, 250
documents and particulars, 36, 93, 168, 169
dosage form, 72, 77
dose, 59, 90, 123, 125, 174, 195, 262
dosimetry, 119, 125
dossier, 23, 55, 172, 244
drafting groups, 216
drive, ability to, 59
drug
 information
 Law, 34
 master file, 60, 98, 106–13, 198, 218, 253
 substance, 175, 199–201
duration of therapy, 110, 262

EC, *see* European Communities(y)
eastern Europe, 23, 46
economic importance, 22
economic value, 22
Economic and Social Committee, *see* Committee, Economic and Social
editors and authors, 24
effective date, 142
efficacy, *see* safety, quality and efficacy
elimination, 124
emission energy, 123
emission type, 123
enforcement, 313
enzyme induction/inhibition, 79
erythromycin, 108
essential requirements, 134, 138, 139, 142–4, 153, 154–6, 160, 161
essential similarity, 40, 41, 97–9, 110, 175, 236, 253
ethics committee, *see* committee, ethics
ethylene oxide sterilization, 166
European Confederation of Medical Suppliers Associations, 130
European Community(ies), 21, 29, 46–8
 institutions, 46, 47
 Member States, 48
 procedures, 29
 regulation, 46
 structure, 46
European Court of Justice, 38, 49
European Diagnostic Manufacturers Association, 131
European drug master file procedure, 26, 110–12, 218
European Economic space, 52
European Electrotechnical Standardization Committee, 135
European Federation of Pharmaceutical Industries Associations, 215
European Free Trade Area (Association), 22, 52, 171, 247, 248
European Medicines Evaluation Agency, 21, 23, 306–8
European Parliament, 47, 49, 137, 161, 294
European Patent, 235
European Pharmacopoeia, *see* Pharmacopoeia,

322 Index

European
European Pharmacopoeia Commission, 113
European Pharmacopoeia Convention, 41, 136
European Standardization Committee, 135–6
European Standards, 135
European summary of product characteristics, 232–3, 240
eutomer, 34, 308
evaluation report, 52
excipient, 59, 63, 69, 100, 106, 118, 123, 203, 262
expert, 23, 37, 168–89, 231, 236, 238, 244, 245, 246, 310
  clinical, 91, 102, 104, 169, 172, 173, 174–5, 178, 185, 192, 198, 224
  consultant, 176
  duties of, 178–80
  foreign, 176–7
  links between, 177–8
  multiple, 175–6
  national, 176–7
  pharmaceutical, 59–60, 70, 72, 98, 104, 110, 169, 172, 173, 174, 178, 194, 198, 238
  pharmacotoxicological, 70, 72, 77, 82, 83, 98, 102, 110, 169, 172, 173–4, 178, 183, 185, 194, 198
  qualifications, 59–60, 172–3
  report, 52, 56, 59–60, 109, 110, 111, 117, 163, 168–9, 216, 223, 226, 243, 244, 245, 246, 252, 254, 308
    chemical, pharmaceutical and biological, 59
    clinical, 59, 186–7, 193–4, 223, 224, 226, 254
    combined, 174
    pharmaceutical, 66, 69, 182–4, 198
    pharmacotoxicological, 59, 66, 185, 223
    product profile and, 177
excretion, 79
exports, 299, 300
exposure in man, 195
extended release, 26

Farmacopoeia Ufficiale della Repubblica Italiana, see Pharmacopoeia, Italian
fast track, 243, 247
favourable regulatory environment, 235
Federal Health Office (Germany), 34
final report, clinical trial, 87
finished product, 68–9, 96, 201–4
Finland, 22, 52, 135, 247
flowchart, synthetic, 65
foetal toxicity, 80–1
format, applications, 55, 57, 194, 231, 232, 305
formats, Expert Report, 60, 180, 185
formula, 62
formulated product, 62
formulation, 178
Food and Drug Administration (US), 31, 104, 107–8, 113, 174, 216, 253
Food Drug and Cosmetic Act (US), 31, 33
Food Drug and Insecticide Administration (US), 31
framework Directives, 50
France, 34, 46, 58, 73, 107, 114, 132, 135, 163, 170, 221, 231, 233, 234, 236, 243
frusemide, 108
function, ingredient, 62, 100
future system, 21, 23, 37, 43, 214–5, 217, 243, 302, 303, 308–13
  centralized procedure, 308–10
  decentralized procedure, 310–12
  regulatory mechanism, 312
  supervisory authority, 312–3

general sales list, *see under* legal status
generator, *see* radiopharmaceutical generator
generic, 236, 254, 298
Germany, 34, 41, 46, 48, 56, 58, 73, 107, 114, 131, 135, 163, 221, 226, 231, 233, 234, 243, 247
global analysis, 186, 187, 226
global application, 172
good clinical practice, 26, 86–9, 214, 305, 306
good laboratory practice, 174, 305, 306
good manufacturing practice, 22, 39, 43, 87, 117, 121, 131, 298, 299, 305, 306
Greece, 34, 48, 58, 73, 94, 107, 114, 135, 163, 225, 230, 231, 234
Grippex, 32
grounds for rejection, 197–8
growth promoter, veterinary, 308
guidance note, *see* guideline
guideline
  ABPI, 193
  development of, 295–6
guidelines
  EC, 39, 54, 60, 108, 111, 117, 215, 246, 250, 255, 294–6
    analytical validation, 55
    anticancer products, 88
    application date of, 26
    bioavailability, 89
    carcinogenic potential, 39, 76
    chemistry of active ingredient, 55
    development pharmaceutics, 55
    European drug master file, 55
    fixed combination, 39
    good clinical practice, 86–9
    good manufacturing practice, 121
      radiopharmaceutical supplement, 121, 126
    herbal remedies, 55
    hypnotic agents, 89
    investigations
      in children, 89
      in the elderly, 89
    local tolerance testing, 55
    long-term use, 89
    metabolic studies, 39, 76
    mutagenic potential, 76
    non-clinical testing strategies, 76
    pharmacodynamics, 76
    pharmacokinetics, 39, 76
      in man, 89
    preclinical safety, 76
    processor validation, 55
    radiopharmaceuticals, 55

based on monoclonal antibodies, 121
repeated dose toxicity, 39, 76, 79, 80
reproduction studies, 39, 76
single-dose toxicity, 76, 79
stability, tests, 55, 70, 72, 203
statistical, 88, 89
stereoisomerism, 76
therapeutic class, 89
national, 214, 250, 255
UK, 117, 121, 163, 166, 203, 250, 255, 262, 270
list of, 56
purpose, 295
revision, 296
status, 295
Guild of Pepperers, 30

harmonization, 22, 43, 44, 94, 96, 129, 214
Document, 135
harmonized standard, 138, 140, 152, 161
heparin sodium, 108
herbal product, 181, 262
high technology, 235
procedure, 41, 59, 117, 237–8
products, 41, 59, 117, 179, 236, 237–8, 245–6, 253, 308
status, 179
High Court (UK), 261
history, 29–45
hearings, 205, 228, 231–2, 239–40, 245, 246, 258, 259, 261
Horner, Frank W., 32
homeopathic, 37, 223
homogeneity, 63, 101
human blood product, 308
human monoclonal antibodies, 26
human plasma product, 308
Hungary, 247
hybridoma, 247
hydrocortisone, 270

ibuprofen, 108
Iceland, 22, 52, 135
identity, 64
test, 68, 101, 110, 123, 166, 203
immunological product, 37, 43, 218, 223, 256, 301
implantation, 167
import test, 202
importer, 58, 111
impurity, 65, 106, 110, 112, 113, 123, 174, 184, 199, 201, 203
analytical method validation, 204
named, 201
profile, 76, 77, 98, 123, 170, 178, 183, 199, 201, 211
specification limit, 183
toxicology, 110, 112, 174, 183
in vitro diagnostic, 131
independent consultant, 176
index, application, 89, 193
information
device, 143–4, 155–6

drug, 52
informed consent, 86, 88
ingredient, 62, 119
innovation
protection of, 40, 94, 235–6
significance of, 238
innovator product, 103
in-process control, *see* control test, intermediate
inspection, 31, 37, 300
contract test laboratory, 37
ingredient manufacturer, 108
manufacturer, 31, 37, 108, 112
institution, *see* European Community institution
instruction leaflet
device, 144, 152, 155–6
radiopharmaceutical, 127–8
intended performance, 142
intended use, 112, 120, 164
interaction, 125, 187, 195, 197, 200
internal audit, 86
intermediate (*see also* control test, intermediate), 65, 199
international application, 24, 221
International Association of Medical Prosthetics Manufacturers, 130
International Atomic Energy Agency, 126
international dossier, 23, 221
International Electrotechnical Commission, 135
International Nonproprietary Name, 57, 59, 109
International Standard, 135
International Standards Organization, 135
intracervical contraceptive, 129, 162, 166–7, 262, 269
intrauterine contraceptive, 129, 162, 166–7, 262, 269
introduction, 29
dossier, 193
invasive device, 157
investigational radiation, 143
ionizing radiation, 143
Ireland, Republic of, 34, 41, 46, 48, 58, 73, 95, 107, 114, 135, 163, 178, 221, 230, 231, 233, 234
isomer, 65, 67, 200
isomerism, 77
potential, 65, 109
isotropic abundance, 123
Italy, 34, 46, 48, 58., 73, 114, 131, 135, 163, 173, 230, 233, 236, 247

Japan, 23, 26, 131, 216

Kefauver–Harris Drug Amendments, 33
Kevadon, 32
kit, radiopharmaceutical, *see* radiopharmaceutical kit

label
devices, 143–4, 152
inaccuracies, 152
pharmaceutical, 32, 35, 52, 70, 72, 73–5, 87, 126–7, 140, 165, 202, 230, 264, 299, 310

Index

lactation, 59, 174, 185
language, 56, 230
leaching, 154
legal instrument, 50
legal status
  EC, 270–1, 305
  UK, 44, 163, 202, 260, 264–71
letter
  access, 111, 253
  authorization, 108
  section 21, 109
  section 21(1), 194, 205, 258, 259
  section 21(3), 260
  section 44, 109
licensable product, 246
Licensing Authority, UK, 257, 258, 260, 264
limit of detection, 61, 66
limit of quantification, 61, 66
limulus amoebocyte lysate test, 124, 203, 204
linearity, 61, 62
list
  A product, 41, 95, 117, 187, 224, 236, 308
  B product, 41, 95, 117, 179, 187, 224, 237, 245
  published references, 94
long-term (device), 157
Luxembourg, 34, 41, 46, 48, 58, 73, 95, 114, 135, 163, 178, 221, 230, 231, 234

machinery, operation of, 59
manipulation of radiopharmaceuticals, 119, 120, 122
manufacture, 70, 143, 166
  active ingredient, 65, 111
  dosage form, 63–4
  nuclear reaction, 122
  radionuclide, 119, 122
  separation, 122
manufacturer
  active ingredient, 58, 106–13
  drug master file, 109
  facilities, 131
  inspection, 37, 108, 112, 131, 132
  licences, 249
  medical device, 131
  product, 70, 183
  registration scheme, 131
  surveillance, 148
manufacturing
  authorization, 37, 73, 117, 249, 260
  for export, 299
  method, 63, 65, 101, 111, 122, 166, 201, 202, 206, 226, 236
    nonstandard, 64
    novel, 201
    validation, 63, 64, 101, 122, 201
  site, 65, 183, 254
market exclusively, 94
marketing, 58
  10 years, 97
  authorization, 21, 35, 37, 58, 73, 106, 107, 213, 223, 249
  applications, 24, 39, 58, 93–105, 172

    abridged, 93–105
    deficiencies, 190–212
    reviewed, 170, 223
    unreviewed, 223
    current, 97
material balance, 72, 184
mass balance, 72, 184
Massengill Company, Samuel, 31
media
  diluting, 119
  reconstituting, 119
medical device, 129–61
  classification, 151–2, 157–8
  definitions, 138–9, 149–50
medical Directives, 129–61
medical Directorate (UK), 131
medicated device, 129–61
medicinal product, 35, 43, 87, 116, 298, 299
  character of, 30
  name of, 59
medicines
  act (Netherlands), 33
  act (UK), 33, 115, 117, 131, 205, 249–79, 264
  orders under, 115, 162, 260, 268–9
  section
    2, 257
    4, 257
    21, 258, 260
    44, 256
    59, 267
    104, 268, 269
  act information (UK), 251, 252, 267
  advisory leaflet (UK), 250, 253, 262, 277–9
  Commission (UK), 33, 131, 257, 260, 267
  Control Agency (UK), 22, 24, 33, 106, 110, 117, 161, 190, 250, 251, 252, 253, 255, 257, 261
    Businesses, 253, 255, 263
  Inspectorate (UK), 203, 254, 263
Member State, 22, 48
  concerned, 220
Merrell Co., William S., 32
metabolism, 79, 186, 195, 200
metabolite, active, 195
method of sale (see also legal status), 264–5
methyldopa, 108
microbiological contamination, 154
microbiological controls, 68
microbiological studies, 164
Ministry of Health and Welfare (Japan), 216
modified release, 103, 253
monoclonal antibody, 41, 117, 236
  human, 26
multistate procedure, 29, 37, 58, 59, 91, 117, 169, 171, 173, 179, 214, 216, 220–34, 243, 246, 247, 302
application
  analysis of, 233–4
  format of, 231–2
  language, 231
assessment report, 230
authorizations for, 222–7

Index

changes and, 226
hearing, 231
label, 230
leaflet, 230
rapporteur, 229–30
rules, 222
samples, 230-1
second applicant product and, 225–6
summary of product characteristics, 232
timing, 227–9
Münich Convention on Patent, 235
mutagenic potential, 125
mutagenicity, 36, 185, 211
   studies, 81–2, 120, 125, 165, 211
mutsahib, 29

name
   active ingredient, 57, 62
   excipient, 62
   product, 57
national agencies (EC), 290–3
   addresses, 280–3
   organization, 282–3
national authorities (EC), 280–93
national appeal, 229
national application, 243, 246, 247, 280, 304, 310
   transitional arrangements, 304
national committees (EC), 283–5
national control laboratories (EC), 288–90
national decision, 229
national guidelines, 214
national language, 56, 140, 153
national standards, 135
   organizations, 136
national subcommittees, 286
negative vetting, 250
Netherlands, 33, 34, 46, 48, 58, 73, 107, 114, 135, 162, 170, 221, 230, 231, 233, 234, 247
new active substance, 168, 170, 177, 190, 194, 220, 223, 237, 238, 242, 243, 247, 253, 254, 256, 304, 308, 310
new approach Directive, 129, 130, 134–8
new biological active substance, 168, 236, 255
new biotechnology process, 237
new chemical active substance, 54–92, 168, 198–208, 255
   data requirement
      clinical, 85–84
      preclinical, 76–84
      quality, 54–75
new clinical indication, 237
new compound dispensatory, 30
new delivery system, 237, 238, 253
new ester, 54, 253
new molecular compound, 54
new salt, 54, 253
nifedipine, 108
no-carrier added, 124
non-active medical device, 130, 131
non-animal test system, 165
nomenclature, 64, 109
norms and protocols, 36, 39, 40, 169

Nordic Council, 52, 53
   guidelines, 52
Norway, 22, 52, 135, 247
note for guidance, *see under* guidelines
Notice to Applicants, 52, 54, 55, 60, 102, 108, 111, 117, 121, 168, 169, 173, 174, 175, 180, 181, 182, 185, 186, 192, 193, 194, 195, 216, 226, 227, 250, 254, 255, 308
notified body, 141, 149, 159
   decisions, period of validity, 152
novel excipient, 54, 63
number of copies, 58

observer status, 136
ocular irritation, 165
old approach Directive, 131, 134–8
ophthalmic product, 255
opinion, 47, 51, 213, 214, 228, 229, 244, 246, 311
   binding, 309, 311
organoleptic properties, 68, 70
orphan drug, 36
other ingredient, 67
overage, 63, 165
overdose, 59

package inset, 44, 72, 299
packaging, 72, 87, 143, 166, 182, 184
page numbering, 193, 252
pagination, 193, 252
parallel import, 38, 218, 256
parallel Directive, 38
parametric release, 69, 124, 166, 184, 203
patent
   law, 94
   term, 94
patient information (*see also* product information), 43, 44, 298
person appointed procedure, 258, 260
pharmaceutical data requirements, *see* chemistry and pharmacy data requirements
pharmaceutical development, 36, 62, 100
pharmaceutical Directives, 34, 47, 54, 110, 111, 117, 250, 255, 264
pharmaceutical excipient, 54, 63
   novel, 54
   Expert, *see* Expert, Pharmaceutical
pharmaceutical Expert Report, *see* Expert report, pharmaceutical
pharmaceutical form, 57, 59, 99
pharmaceutical incompatibility, 59
Pharmaceutical Inspection Convention, 177, 312
pharmaceutical tests, 68, 203
pharmacological data requirements, *see under* toxicological data requirements
pharmacological properties, 59, 174
pharmacology, 175, 254
   primary, 196
   profile, 77
   relevant to therapeutic use, 78, 210
   secondary, 78, 210
Pharmacopée Française, 42
Pharmacopeia, United States, 30, 54, 100

Pharmacopeial Forum, 30
Pharmacopoeia, 30, 52, 106, 119, 183, 184, 189, 254
  British, 30, 42, 164
  Edinburgh, 30
  European, 41, 42, 62, 64, 67, 68, 100, 107, 109, 111, 113, 114, 116, 119, 123, 126, 131, 136, 152, 161, 184, 203
  Italian, 42
  London, 30
  Japanese, 100
pharmacopoeia, national, 42, 100, 107, 109, 111, 119, 123, 131
pharmacodynamics, 77–8, 125, 167, 185
pharmacokinetics, 78–9, 125, 167, 185, 200, 202, 210
pharmacotoxicological Expert, *see* Expert, pharmacotoxicological
pharmacotoxicological tests, 36, 40
pharmacovigilance, 22, 170, 305, 313
pharmacy medicine, 264
Pharmeuropa, 30
photoprinting quality, 252
physical characteristics, 62, 109, 110, 166, 199
physical properties, 70, 101
physicochemical biological and microbiological tests, 36
physicochemical properties, 66
piggy-back, 243
plasma protein binding, 79
Portugal, 34, 46, 48, 58, 73, 94, 107, 135, 163, 223, 230, 231
posology, *see* dose
post-marketing
  experience, 187
  surveillance, 22, 144, 147, 170, 226
pre-assessment period, 239
precautions, 59, 187
precision, 61
preclinical data requirements, 76–84, 102, 120, 165, 166
preclinical dossier deficiencies, 208–12
precursor radiopharmaceutical, 116, 122
preface, 21–7
pregnancy, 59, 174, 185
prescription only medicine, 264, 265
pricing, 43, 44
  transparency, 43
problem statement, 186
process validation, 36, 173, 183, 184, 203
Procurement Directive, 131
product
  development, 166
  Evaluation Report, 171, 247–8
    scheme, 171, 247–8
  information, 77, 81, 305, 306, 309, 310
  licence, 250, 261, 263
    application, 249
      defects in, 190–212
  profile, 60, 69, 177
  quality assurance, 156
product–container interaction, 72, 164

professional assessment, 255–6
prolonged action, 26
promotion and advertising, 44
proposed clinical use, 76
propranolol hydrochloride, 108
proprietary medicinal product, 35, 93, 94, 298, 299
protection of innovation, 40, 94, 235–6
protocol, 86
public domain application, 99
Pure Food and Drugs Act (US), 31
purity, 123
  profile, 59
  requirements (radiolabelling), 122
  tests, 101
pyrogens test, 124, 203

qualified majority voting, 40, 219
Qualified Person, 37, 120
qualitative and quantitative particulars, 59
quality, *see* safety, quality and efficacy
quality (assurance) system, 69, 123, 131, 144, 147, 166
quality control, 121
Quality Working Party, 42
quinine sulphate, 30

racemate, 65, 308
radiation sterilization, 166
radioactivity, amount of, 122
radiochemical purity, 116, 118, 119, 122, 123, 124
radiolabelled compound, 67, 199, 237
radiolabelling, 119, 122, 123
radionuclide, 122
radionuclidic purity, 116, 119, 123
radiopharmaceutical, 37, 43, 52, 114–28, 181, 187, 218, 223, 236, 268, 297, 301
  generator, 116, 118, 119, 121, 122, 123
  kit, 116, 118, 122, 123, 124
rapporteur, 169, 179, 227, 228, 229, 230, 231, 236, 239, 240, 244, 245, 246, 306, 309, 310
reasoned objection, 227, 229
recipient countries, 222, 234
reclassification (devices), 132
recombinant DNA technology, 41, 236
Recommendation, 39, 47, 51, 78, 79, 80, 82, 83, 211, 212, 294
reconstituting media, 119
reference material, 66, 109, 204
reference number (UK), 252
reference product, 103
refused or restricted marketing (device), 142, 153
registration scheme, manufacturers, 131
regulations, 43, 47, 50, 249
  and orders (UK), 249
regulatory environment, 235
regulatory mechanism, 312
regulatory strategy, 171, 221, 242–8
rejection, grounds for, 197–8
related substance, 199, 203
removal from the market, 138, 140
renewal, 249, 263

Index

repeat dose toxicity study, 80
Repertorio, 224
reproductive function, 80–1, 125, 167
reproductive toxicity, 80–1, 125, 167
  information (product literature), 211
results, 66, 70, 72
retest interval, 70
review of old products, 37, 224
reviewed marketing authorization, 170, 223
reviewed product licence, 170, 254, 266
revocation, 305
  notification of, 300
rheological properties, 101
risk/benefit assessment, 82, 187, 198, 231
risks, minimize (devices), 143, 154–5
robustness, 61
role of CPMP, 214
Role List, 224
route of administration, 58, 59, 96, 106, 253, 262
Rules governing medicinal products (EC), 22, 24, 35, 42, 214, 215
  Volume I (*see also* Directives), 25, 35, 42, 43, 85
  Volume II (*see also* Notice to applicants), 25, 42, 85
  Volume III (*see also* guidelines), 25, 42, 85, 100, 173, 182, 216, 294
  Addendum, 25, 187
  Volume IV, 25, 42, 121, 217, 300
  Volume V, 25, 43

safety data, 195
safety, quality and efficacy, 22, 29, 34, 69, 125, 131, 205, 214, 256, 257, 294, 306
safety, quality and usefulness, 154, 160
Salvarsan, 31
samples, 73, 230–1, 299
Samuel Massengill Company, 31
scale of licensing activities (UK), 190
Secretary of State for Health (UK), 257
second applicant
  product, 96, 99–100, 223, 225–6, 310
  protection, 95, 235–6
sensitization, 165
sensitivity, 61, 62
serums, 187, 223, 236, 297
shelf life, 59, 70, 184
short term, 157
side effect, 174
significant innovation, 180, 308
significant technical advance, 180, 308
significant therapeutic interest, 237, 238, 308
similarity, essential, 40, 44, 97–9, 110, 175, 236, 253
single dose toxicity study, 79–80
single European Act, 29, 49, 51
single isomer, 65
single Market, 23, 29, 43, 44, 51, 134, 221, 242, 302–13
Smith, Kline and French Laboratories, 97
  judicial review (UK), 97
source countries, 221, 223

Spain, 36, 46, 48, 58, 73, 94, 107, 114, 135, 163, 225, 230, 231, 234
special particulars, 72–3
specific (radio) activity, 116, 122, 123
specification
  active ingredient, 66–7, 100, 101, 110, 111, 183, 201, 202, 236
  excipient, 100, 110
  finished product, 68–9, 101, 119, 202, 203, 226, 236
  impurity, 106
  intermediate, 68, 101, 109
  method validation, 204
  release, 68, 119
  shelf life, 69, 119, 185
  starting material, 64–8, 101, 109, 226
specificity, 61
spectra, 65, 109, 110
stability, 69–72, 77, 100, 102, 110, 120, 124, 166, 173, 182, 184, 200, 226, 254
  accelerated studies, 70
  active ingredient, 69, 102, 173, 178, 182, 184, 200
  chemical, 72
  finished product, 69, 102, 173, 184
  in vivo (radiolabel), 125
  method validation, 204
  radionuclide, 120, 124
  study, 70
standard operating procedure, 86
standards
  European, 135
  ingredient, 62
starting material, 64–9, 199
state laboratories, 31
statistical analysis, 88
Statutory Instrument (UK), 250, 260, 272–7
stereochemical properties, 65, 109
stereochemistry, 190, 200
stereoisomer, 34, 195
stereoselectivity, 200
sterilization, 63, 123, 154, 165, 203, 253
sterility test, 124, 166, 203
storage conditions, 70
storage precautions, 59, 184
structure, proof of, 65, 109, 199, 200
subcommittees (UK), 257
'subject to', 245, 246
substance, 117, 159
sulfanilamide elixir, 31
summary
  basis of approval, 174, 175
  information, 180
  product characteristics, 39, 58–9, 174, 186, 193, 194, 197, 214, 221, 232–3, 240, 298, 306, 309, 310
Supreme Court (UK), 261
surgical dressing, 131
surgical product, 253, 256
surgical suture, 131
surgically invasive (device), 157
suspension

authorization, 305
  notification of, 305
  redispersability, 101
Sweden, 22, 41, 52, 135, 221, 247
Switzerland, 22, 41, 52, 135, 221, 247
synthesis, 65
  alternate, 65, 109
synthetic route, 65, 106, 109, 110, 178, 199, 200, 201, 253
  alternate, 65, 106, 109

tabulated information, 171
tagamet tablets, 97
Talimol, 32
tamoxifen citrate, 108
tamper evident container, 62, 165
timetable, concertation, 238–9
technical Directives (Commission Directives), 40, 50
teratogenic potential, 77
  and product information, 77
thalidomide, 29, 32, 34
Therapeutic Substances Act (UK), 31
therapeutic use, 96
therapeutically important, 223
Third World, 298, 299
time limit, 35, 227
toxicity, 110, 124, 143, 154, 174, 178, 185, 197
  studies, 183, 201, 210
    exposure to drug, 210
    local toxicity, 165
    pathological change, 210–1
    repeat dose, 80, 120, 125, 210
    single dose, 79–80, 120, 125, 210
toxicology, 79, 175, 178, 210, 226, 254
  data requirements (*see also* preclinical data requirements), 76–84, 124–5, 165, 166
toxins, 187, 297
transfer of authorization, 188
toothpaste, medicated, 256
trade mark, 203, 255, 236
trade name, 202, 203
transient, 157
Treaty of Rome, 46, 49, 51
type examination
  procedure, 145–6, 156
  certificate, 146, 147

undesirable effects, 174
uniformity of content, 68
United States Adopted Name, 64, 109
United States of America, 26, 31, 107, 112, 131, 160, 174, 196, 216, 221, 253
United Kingdom, 34, 41, 46, 48, 54, 58, 73, 106, 114, 135, 162, 173, 181, 188, 190, 196, 199, 205, 221, 225, 227, 231, 233, 234, 243, 247, 248, 249–79, 280
  system, 249–79
unusual constituent, 63

vaccines, 187, 223, 236, 297
validation
  analytical, 61, 66, 69, 101, 110, 173, 184, 203, 204, 215
  application (UK), 253–5
  clinical trial data, 88
  manufacturing process, 63, 64, 101, 122, 201
variations, 170, 226, 243
verapamil hydrochloride, 108
verification procedure, 146–7, 156, 160
vertical standard, 161
volunteer study, 250

warnings, 59, 187, 217
wholesale dealer, 249
withdrawal from market, 141
written evidence, 258
written representation, 205, 228, 239, 258
written response, quality of, 245
written summary, 90, 171, 180, 185, 193, 195
working parity (CPMP) (*see also* drafting group) 215–7, 295, 306
  ad hoc, expert reports, 216
  ad hoc pharmacovigilance, ???
  efficacy, 215
  operational, 217
  plant origin, products of, 215
  quality, 215
  safety, 215
working party (Commission) (*see also* drafting group), 217
  biotechnology/pharmacy, 215, 217, 236
  inspection, 217